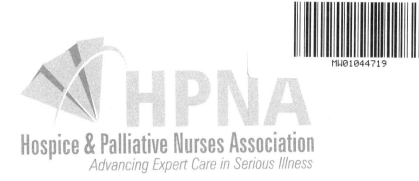

Hospice & Palliative Nurses Association
Advancing Expert Care in Serious Illness

MW01044719

CORE CURRICULUM FOR THE HOSPICE AND PALLIATIVE REGISTERED NURSE

Fourth Edition

Coordinating Editors:

Holli Martinez, FNP-BC, ACHPN®, FPCN®
Program Director
Palliative Care Service, University of Utah Health Care
Salt Lake City, UT

Patricia Berry, PhD, RN, ACHPN®, FPCN®, FAAN
Professor
Director, Hartford Center of Gerontological Nursing Excellence at OHSU
School of Nursing
Oregon Health and Science University
Portland, OR

Hospice and Palliative Nurses Association
One Penn Center West, Suite 425
Pittsburgh, PA 15276-0109
www.AdvancingExpertCare.org

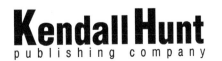

Kendall Hunt
publishing company

> **HPNA Mission Statement:**
>
> Advancing Expert Care in Serious Illness

Cover image: art_of_sun/Shutterstock.com

Kendall Hunt
publishing company

www.kendallhunt.com
Send all inquiries to:
4050 Westmark Drive
Dubuque, IA 52004-1840

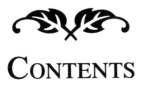

CONTENTS

CHAPTER I: AN OVERVIEW OF HOSPICE AND PALLIATIVE CARE
CHERYL BROHARD AND CORRINE ANDERSON

CHAPTER II: INTERDISCIPLINARY COLLABORATIVE PRACTICE IN HOSPICE AND PALLIATIVE SETTINGS
PAULA LARSEN AND SANDRA JENSE

CHAPTER III: PATTERNS OF DISEASE PROGRESSION
NIKI KOESEL AND MARLENE A. S. FOREMAN

CHAPTER IV: PAIN MANAGEMENT
JUDITH A. PAICE

CHAPTER V: SYMPTOM MANAGEMENT
AMY Z. McDEVITT, MARGARET DONEGAN, AND SANDRA MUCHKA

CHAPTER VI: PSYCHIATRIC/PSYCHOLOGICAL SYMPTOMS AND DIAGNOSES
NAN GROTTANELLI AND PAMELA SHOCKEY STEPHENSON

CHAPTER VII: CARE OF THE FAMILY
KATHERINE P. SUPIANO, JUDITH C. LENTZ, AND BRIDGET SUMSER

CHAPTER VIII: PALLIATIVE CARE ACROSS CARE SETTINGS
SHERRA STEWART-REGO AND DENA JEAN SUTERMASTER

CHAPTER IX: ADVANCE CARE PLANNING AND GOALS OF CARE
BEVERLY J. DOUGLAS AND CATHERINE PARSONS EMMETT

CHAPTER X: CARE OF THE PATIENT AND FAMILY IN THE FINAL DAYS
KAREN A. KEHL AND PATRICIA BERRY

CHAPTER XI: ETHICAL ISSUES IN END-OF-LIFE CARE
KAREN WAHLE AND SUSAN LYSAGHT HURLEY

CHAPTER XII: POLICY AND ECONOMIC ISSUES IN PALLIATIVE CARE
JOY BUCK

CHAPTER XIII: NATIONAL GUIDELINES AND RN PRACTICE
CONSTANCE DAHLIN AND JUDITH C. LENTZ

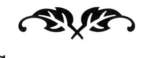

CONTRIBUTORS

Corrine Anderson, MSN, RN
Retired
Grapevine, TX

Patricia Berry, PhD, RN, ACHPN®, FPCN®, FAAN
Professor
Director, Hartford Center of Gerontological
    Nursing Excellence at OHSU
School of Nursing
Oregon Health and Science University
Portland, OR

Cheryl Brohard, PhD, RN, AOCN®, CHPCA®
Director of Education
Houston Hospice
Houston, TX

Joy Buck, PhD, RN
Professor
West Virginia University
Martinsburg, WV

Constance Dahlin, ANP-BC, ACHPN®, FPCN®,
    FAAN
Director of Professional Practice
Hospice and Palliative Nurses Association
Pittsburgh, PA

Margaret Donegan, MSN, APRN, NP-BC,
    ACHPN®
Nurse Practitioner, Palliative Care Team
Medical College of Wisconsin
Milwaukee, WI

Beverly J. Douglas, MSN, GNP-BC, ACHPN®,
    ARNP
Nurse Practitioner
Life Path Hospice, Division of Chapters Health
    Services
Tampa, FL

Catherine Parsons Emmett, PhD, ARNP, ACHPN®
Professional Development Facilitator, Advance
    Clinical Practice
Suncoast Hospice
Clearwater, FL

Marlene A. S. Foreman, RN, BSN, ACNS-BC,
    ACHPN®
Clinical Nurse Specialist/Education Coordinator/
    Veteran Coordinator
Hospice of Acadiana, Inc.
Lafayette, LA

Nan Grottanelli, ARNP, AGPCNP-BC, CHPN®
Nurse Practitioner
Caremore
Richmond, VA

Susan Lysaght Hurley, PhD, GNP-BC, ACHPN®
Nurse Practitioner
North Shore Medical Center
Salem, MA

Sandra Jense, DNP, ACNP-BC
Nurse Practitioner
University of Utah
Salt Lake City, UT

Karen A. Kehl, PhD, RN, ACHPN®, FPCN®
Assistant Professor
University of Wisconsin-Madison, School of
    Nursing
Madison, WI

Niki Koesel, ANP, ACHPN®, FPCN®
Director of Palliative Care, Levine Cancer Institute
Carolinas Healthcare System
Charlotte, NC

Paula Larsen, LCSW, ACHP-SW
Palliative Care Social Worker
University of Utah Hospital and Clinics, Social
    Work Office
Salt Lake City, UT

Judith C. Lentz, RN, MSN, FPCN®
Retired
Moon Township, PA

Amy Z. McDevitt, MSN, ANP, ACHPN®
Nurse Practitioner
Roper St. Francis Healthcare
Charleston, SC

Sandra Muchka, MSN, RN, APNP, ACNS-BC,
    ACHPN®, FPCN®
Clinical Nurse Specialist
Froedert Hospital
Milwaukee, WI

Judith A. Paice, PhD, RN
Director, Cancer Pain Program
Northwestern University, Feinberg School of
    Medicine
Chicago, IL

Pamela Shockey Stephenson, PhD, RN, AOCNS,
    PMHCNS-BC
Assistant Professor
Kent State University
Kent, OH

Sherra Stewart-Rego, RN, BSN, MPH, CHPN®
Hospice Director
VNS of Connecticut Hospice at Home
Trumbull, CT

Bridget Sumser, LMSW
Director of Palliative Social Work
Winthrop University Hospital
Mineola, NY

Katherine P. Supiano, PhD, LCSW, FT, F-GSA
Associate Professor
Director, Caring Connections: A Hope & Conflict
    in Grief Program
University of Utah College of Nursing
Salt Lake City, UT

Dena Jean Sutermaster, RN, MSN, CHPN®
Education Specialist
Hospice and Palliative Nurses Association
Pittsburgh, PA

Karen Wahle, RN, MSN, JD, CHPN®
Hospice RN
Capital Caring
Falls Church, VA

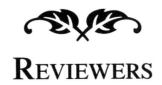

REVIEWERS

Kathleen Beaver, RN, BSN, CHPN®
Palliative Care Nurse Program Manager
Fort Belvoir Community Hospital
Fort Belvoir, VA

Kathryn M. Beck, BSN, RN, CHPN®
QAPI Coordinator/Staff Educator
Saint Mary's Hospice of Northern Nevada
Reno, NV

Colleen Fleming-Damon, PhDc, APRN,
    ACHPN®, CT
Director of Education and Training
MJHS Hospice and Palliative Care
New York, NY

Annette M. Feierman, RN, MSN, CPHQ, CHPN®
Hospice Staff Educator
MJHS Hospice and Palliative Care
New York, NY

Kim Goff, RN, BSN, MBA, CHPN®, CHPCA®
Clinical Director
Grace Hospice
Kansas City, MO

Deborah Imbach, RN, MS, CHPN®
Director of Clinical Operations
Seasons Hospice & Palliative Care of Maryland
Glen Burnie, MD

Elizabeth B. McGrath, MSN, APRN, AGACNP-
    BC, AOCNP, ACHPN®
Nurse Practitioner
Norris Cotton Cancer Center Dartmouth Hitchcock
    Medical Center
Lebanon, NH

Kay Mueggenburg, PhD, MSN, RN, CHPN®
Associate Professor and Palliative Care
    Coordinator
McKendree University, Division of Nursing
Lebanon, IL

Deborah L. Nicholson, RN, BS, CCM, CHPN®
Inpatient Oncology Case Manager Palliative Care
    RN Coordinator
St. Joseph Regional Health Network
Reading, PA

Deanne Sayles, RN, MN, CHPN®
Director of Quality, Education & Clinical Practice
Hinds Hospice
Fresno, CA

Debbie Stoughton, RN, BSN, PHN, CHPN®
Director of Patient Care Services
Sea Crest Hospice
Costa Mesa, CA

Dena Jean Sutermaster, RN, MSN, CHPN®
Education Specialist
Hospice and Palliative Nurses Association
Pittsburgh, PA

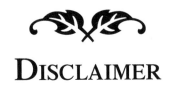

DISCLAIMER

The Hospice and Palliative Nurses Association,
its officers and directors and the authors and reviewers of this Core Curriculum
make no claims that buying or studying this publication will guarantee a passing score
on the CHPN® Certification examination.

The Hospice and Palliative Nurses Association will not be held liable
or responsible for individual treatments, specific plans of care,
or patient and family outcomes. This core curriculum is intended for
professional education purposes only.

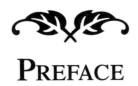

PREFACE

The practice of hospice and palliative care nursing is evolving and growing, enabling this specialty to be fully integrated into the spectrum of all practice settings. This has propelled nurses into thinking about the continuum of care in creative ways and enhanced the bedside delivery of hospice and palliative care. It is an exciting time to be in this amazing field and our resources must reflect this growth.

In preparing nurses for this expanding role, it is vital to include up to date evidence to guide practice in this new edition. Compared to previous editions, you will find the authors have included the latest evidence while retaining some of the classic literature, which provides important context and background. We are hopeful this evidence-packed edition will serve as a preparatory guide for the board certification exam and a practice guide for the hospice and palliative care nurse.

We extend our sincere thanks to the chapter authors and reviewers—a talented group of hospice and palliative professionals who volunteered their time and expertise to create this edition. Sincere thanks also to Dane Semonian, who kept all of this organized, in its proper format, and copyedited. And to Dena Jean Sutermaster—your continued patience, kindness, persistence, and organization made this all possible. Many thanks.

Holli Martinez, Salt Lake City, Utah
Patricia Berry, Portland, Oregon

CHAPTER I

AN OVERVIEW OF HOSPICE AND PALLIATIVE CARE

Cheryl Brohard, PhD, RN, AOCN, CHPCA®
Corrine Anderson, MSN, RN

I. Hospice

A. Origins of Hospice

1. Concept antedates 475 AD

2. The term *hospes*, a Latin word, from which the term hospice is derived, means to be both host and guest and implies an interaction and mutual caring between patient, family, and hospice staff

3. Self-sustained communities evolved after 335 AD where ill, weary, homeless, and dying persons received care

4. During the early middle ages, the words *hospice*, *hospital*, and *hostel* were used interchangeably

5. Also during the middle ages, hospitia or travelers' rests at monasteries and convents provided food, shelter, as well as care for those sick or dying

6. The care and support of the whole person (the body, soul, mind, and spirit) evolved in these early hospices

7. In the 1800s, hospice evolved to care for the sick and incurables

8. The word *hospice* became synonymous with care of the terminally ill late in the 1800s with the founding of Our Lady's Hospice in Dublin by Sister Mary Aikenhead of the Irish Sisters of Charity, who was a colleague of Florence Nightingale

9. St. Joseph's Hospice was established in 1900 in London, England

10. Dame Cicely Saunders, MD, began refining the ideas and protocols that formed the cornerstone of modern hospice care in the 1950s and 1960s

11. By the 1960s, Dame Cicely Saunders opened St. Christopher's Hospice in suburban London, marking the beginning of the modern hospice movement

12. Dame Cicely Saunders visited the United States in 1963 and spoke to medical and nursing students and interested others at Yale University

13. Florence Wald, Dean of Yale School of Nursing, resigned to plan and found the Connecticut Hospice[1]

14. The palliative care service at the Royal Victoria Hospital, Montreal, Canada, was started by Balfour Mount, MD, and opened in 1975; first use of the term *palliative care* to refer to a program of care for terminally ill persons and their families; this became the first hospice palliative care program in North America

15. The first hospice in the United States was the Connecticut Hospice, incorporated in 1971. They began seeing home care patients in 1974, and opened a 44-bed inpatient facility in 1979

16. In 1983, the Tax Equity Fiscal Responsibility Act created the Medicare Hospice Benefit and defined hospice care in the United States as legitimate medical care but with a 1986 sunset provision

B. **Notable Influences on Hospice Development and Acceptance**

1. Development of current concepts of palliative care are, in large part, through the work of Dame Cicely Saunders at St. Christopher's Hospice in London, including the use of scheduled oral opioids for pain management

2. Elizabeth Kübler-Ross's work in the 1960s demystified death and dying and opened the debate on care of the dying for healthcare professionals and the lay public; *On Death and Dying* was published in 1969, which lead to increased knowledge and research regarding grief, loss, and bereavement

3. In 1996, major grant-makers began to fund research, program initiatives, public forums, and conferences to transform the culture of dying and improve care at the end of life

4. General dissatisfaction (among the public and some factions of the healthcare system) about how dying persons and their families are treated in the U.S. healthcare system, which generally emphasizes technological intervention and overtreatment to prevent death[2]

5. Development of a more holistic nursing practice model

6. Increased attention to cost of care

7. Physician-assisted suicide movement and the 1995 results of the Study to Understand Prognosis and Preferences for Outcomes and Risks of Treatment (SUPPORT) study, showing high incidence of uncontrolled pain (from 74% to 95%) in very ill and dying adults in spite of planned interventions from nurses, encouraged physicians to attend to pain control[2]

8. In 1986, the Medicare Hospice Benefit is made permanent by Congress and hospices are given a 10% increase in reimbursement rates. States are given the option of including hospice in their Medicaid programs. Hospice care is now available to terminally ill nursing home residents

9. In 1993, hospice is included as a nationally guaranteed benefit under President Clinton's healthcare reform proposal. Hospice is now an accepted part of the healthcare continuum

10. The *natural death* consumer movement similar to the natural childbirth movement, with increasing attention to care at home

11. In 1997, the Institute of Medicine (IOM) published the report *Approaching Death: Improving Care at the End of Life,* citing inadequacies in end-of-life care, and goals to improve that care

12. In 1997, the National Hospice Organization (NHO) published *A Pathway for Patients and Families Facing Terminal Illness*

13. In 2000, the now National Hospice and Palliative Care Organization's (NHPCO) developed *Hospice Standards of Practice for Hospice Programs*[3]

C. Definitions of Hospice

1. Centers for Medicare & Medicaid Services (CMS)—"a holistic approach to treatment that recognizes that the impending death of an individual warrants a change from curative to palliative care. Palliative care means 'patient- and family-centered care that optimizes quality of life by anticipating, preventing, and treating suffering. Palliative care throughout the continuum of illness involves addressing physical, intellectual, emotional, social, and spiritual needs and to facilitate patient autonomy, access to information, and choice'"[4]

2. The National Hospice and Palliative Care Organization (NHPCO)—hospice is considered to be the model for quality, compassionate care for people facing a life-limiting illness or injury. Hospice care involves a team-oriented approach to expert medical care, pain management, and emotional and spiritual support expressly tailored to the patient's needs and wishes. Support is provided to the patient's loved ones as well. At the center of hospice and palliative care is the belief that each of us has the right to die pain-free and with dignity, and that our families will receive the necessary support to allow us to do so. Hospice focuses on caring, not curing, and in most cases care is provided in the patient's home. Hospice care also is provided in freestanding hospice centers, hospitals, and nursing homes and other long-term care facilities. Hospice services are available to patients of any age, religion, race, or illness. Hospice care is covered under Medicare, Medicaid, most private insurance plans, health maintenance organizations (HMOs), and other managed care organizations[5]

3. Hospice and Palliative Nurses Association (HPNA)—hospice nursing as the provision of palliative nursing care for the terminally ill and their families with the emphasis on their physical, psychosocial, emotional, and spiritual needs. This care is accomplished in collaboration with an interdisciplinary team through a service that is available 24 hours a day, 7 days a week. The service comprises pain and symptom management, bereavement, and volunteer components. Hospice nursing, then, is holistic practice conducted within an affiliative matrix. The hospice nurse, in developing and maintaining collaborative relationships with other members of the interdisciplinary team, must be flexible in dealing with the inevitable role blending that takes place. In functioning as a case manager, coordinating the implementation of the interdisciplinary team developed plan of care, the hospice nurse also shares an advocacy role for patients and their families with other members of the team[6]

D. Key Concepts in Hospice Philosophy

1. The patient and family (as defined by the patient) are considered the unit of care

2. Hospice uses a core interdisciplinary team to address the physical, social, emotional, and spiritual needs of the patient and family

3. Hospice provides for the medical treatment of pain and other distressing symptoms associated with serious or life-threatening, progressive illness, but does not provide interventions to cure the disease or prolong life

4. The interdisciplinary team develops the overall plan of care, in accordance with the wishes of the patient and family, in order to provide coordinated care that emphasizes supportive services such as home care, symptom management, and limited inpatient services

5.   Hospice care actively engages the community by utilizing volunteer support in delivering hospice services. To meet Medicare's Conditions of Participation (CoPs), volunteers must provide day-to-day administrative and/or direct patient care services in an amount that, at a minimum, equals 5% of the total patient care hours of all paid hospice employees and contract staff[7]

6.   The patient's home or place of primary residence, no matter where that may be (e.g., skilled nursing or residential care facility, prison, shelter, daycare center for the elderly), is the primary site of hospice care

7.   The philosophy of hospice emphasizes comfort, dignity, and quality of life, with the focus on spiritual and existential issues throughout dying, death, and bereavement

8.   Patients and families are empowered to achieve as much control over their lives as possible

9.   Bereavement services are provided a minimum of 1 year after the patient's death to an average of 2 family members. Over 90% of hospices offer community support services[8]

E.   Issues that Affect Hospice Utilization

1.   Life expectancy of 6 months or less (should the disease run its usual course) is often difficult to determine in non-cancer diagnoses, and thus, some physicians may be reluctant to refer to hospice

2.   Physicians may be reluctant to discuss end-of-life matters such as do not resuscitate (DNR) orders, feeling that the patient and family may not be ready to accept this (Note: DNR orders are not required for hospice admission)

3.   Referrals often occur when death is imminent, thus rushing hospice to quickly bond with family and initiate symptom management in crisis mode. Between 2010 and 2013, the median length of hospice stays has steadily decreased from 19.7 to 18.5 days exhibiting the need for earlier referrals to hospice[8]

4.   Significant barriers to the management of pain and other symptoms continue to exist, although progress can be seen in this area

5.   Close scrutiny of patient medical records for documentation of the appropriateness for hospice is needed, including more frequent audits of medical records. In 2013, fiscal intermediaries provided detailed hospice eligibility criteria that included the International Classification of Functioning

F.   The first set of performance measures for hospice care is in the data collection and/or data submission phase. Refer to Chapter 13 for an in-depth discussion

G.   Hospice Care in the United States[8]

1.   Programs

   a)   In 2012, there were approximately 5800 operational hospice programs in all 50 states, District of Columbia, Puerto Rico, Guam, and U.S. Virgin Islands (see Chart 1-1)

      i.   Tax status[8]

         (a)   30% were nonprofit (charitable organization subject to 501(c)3 tax provisions)

Chart 1-1. Types of Hospices in the United States[8]

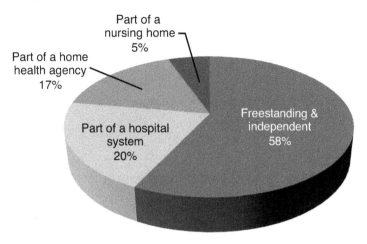

Part of a
nursing home
5%

Part of a home
health agency
17%

Part of a hospital
system
20%

Freestanding &
independent
58%

      (b)   66% were for-profit (privately-owned or publically-held entities), reflecting a steady increase

      (c)   5% were government-run

   ii.   CMS certification[8]

      (a)   92.7% were Medicare certified

      (b)   Most states have hospice licensure laws that define specific requirements for operating as a hospice program

2.   Patient demographics[8]

   a)   In 2013, an estimated 1.5 to 1.6 million patients received services from a hospice program, reflecting a steady increase over the past several years

     i.   1.13 million patients died while receiving hospice care

     ii.   54.7% were female; 45.3% male

     iii.   0.4% were younger than 24 years

     iv.   0.4% were between the ages of 25 and 34 years

     v.   15.3% were between the ages of 35 and 64 years

     vi.   16.6% were between the ages of 65 and 74 years

     vii.   26.1% were between the ages of 74 and 84 years

     viii.   41.2% were 85 years and older

     ix.   Patients of minority (non-Caucasian race) accounted for nearly 1 in every 5 hospice patients in 2013, unchanged since 2008

        (a)   80.9% were Caucasian

        (b)   8.4% were Black/African-American (slight increase since 2008)

        (c)   6.8% were Hispanic or Latino

        (d)   2.9% were Asian or Hawaiian/Pacific Islander

        (e)   7.5% were multiracial or "another race"

3.   Reimbursement

    a)   Medicare—in 2000, Medicare spent $2.9 billion on hospice, which rose to $15.1 billion in 2012, and this continues to rise as more people utilize hospice services[9]

    b)   Medicaid—hospice is covered under Medicaid in the District of Columbia and all states except Oklahoma

    c)   Private insurance—most private insurance plans include a hospice benefit though reimbursement can vary greatly

4.   Patient information[8]

    a)   Percentage of hospice admission by primary diagnosis in 2013

       i.   36.5% cancer

       ii.   Non-cancer diagnoses accounted for the remaining 63.5%

          (a)   Dementia—15.2%

          (b)   Heart disease—13.4%

          (c)   Lung disease—9.9%

          (d)   Unspecified debility—5.4%

          (e)   Stroke or coma—5.2%

          (f)   Kidney disease (end-stage renal disease [ESRD])—3.0%

          (g)   Liver disease—2.1%

          (h)   Non-amyotrophic lateral sclerosis (ALS) motor neuron—2.0%

          (i)   Amyotrophic lateral sclerosis—0.4%

          (j)   Human immunodeficiency virus/acquired immunodeficiency syndrome (HIV/AIDS)—0.2%

          (k)   Other—6.9%

    b)   Average length of service in 2013 was 72.6 days, reflecting a gradual increase; median length of service was 18.5 days, reflecting a decrease each year since 2008

       i.   34.5% of patients served by hospice either died or were discharged in 7 days or less

       ii.   48.8% of patients either died or were discharged within 14 days of their hospice admission

       iii.   11.5% died or were discharged in 180 days or more

    c)   Place of death for patients served by a hospice program

       i.   66.6% died at the patient's place of residence

          (a)   Private residence—41.7%

          (b)   Nursing home—17.9%

          (c)   Residential facility—7.0%

        ii.   Hospice inpatient facility—26.4%

        iii.   Acute care hospital—7.0%

    d)   Total number of patient admissions within a hospice agency

        i.   16.1% of agencies had 1–49 patients

        ii.   29.5% of agencies had 50–150 patients

        iii. 33.1% of agencies had 151–500 patients

        iv. 16.4% of agencies had 501–1500 patients

        v.   4.9% of agencies had > 1500 patients

    e)   Level of hospice care for patients

        i.   94.1% receive routine home care

        ii.   5.6% receive general inpatient care or continuous (crisis) care

        iii. 0.3% receive respite care

    f)   Payer sources for hospice

        i.   Medicare—91.2% of all hospice patient days are paid by Medicare

        ii.   Private insurance—4.0%

        iii. Medicaid—3.1%

        iv. Uncompensated or charity care—0.6%

        v.   Self-pay or other payer sources—0.6%

  5.   Cost savings—a recent study demonstrated that hospice services save money for Medicare, on average $2,309 per hospice patient. In addition, the research also found that Medicare costs could be further reduced with longer lengths of stays in a hospice program[10]

II. Leading the Way—Development of HPNA and Related Organizations

  A. **Hospice Nurses Association (HNA) is a national organization that was founded in 1986 to establish a network for nurses in this specialty[11]**

  B. **Incorporated in California as a "non-profit public benefit organization"[12]**

  C. **Purpose—promote education, study, research, and advocacy in standards of care for hospice patients and families[13]**

  D. **Established a National Office in Pittsburgh, Pennsylvania. Findings from a 1991 survey of hospice nurses desiring specialty certification led to the appointment of a 7-member geographically representative group to form the National Board for the Certification of Hospice Nurses (NBCHN®) in 1992[14]**

E.   **Changed its name to Hospice and Palliative Nurses Association (HPNA) in 1998**

F.   **2013 mission statement—"To advance expert care in serious illness"[11]**

G.   **Four Pillars of Excellence and their related goals are[6,11,15]**

   1.   Education—to be the primary resource for cutting-edge knowledge pertaining to the care and culture of serious illness

   2.   Advocacy—to be the leading voice for the transformation of the care and culture of serious illness

   3.   Leadership—to empower members to transform the care and culture of serious illness

   4.   Research—to translate evidence about the care and culture of serious illness into action

H.   **The Hospice and Palliative Nursing Foundation (HPNF) incorporated in 1998, with a stated purpose to enhance nursing excellence in hospice and palliative care with grants, scholarships, and awards to generate nursing education, research, and leadership[16]**

I.   **National Consensus Project—through a Robert Wood Johnson Foundation grant, a coalition of U.S. palliative care leaders met to determine standardization and quality of care throughout hospice and palliative care. This group became a task force in 2003, adopting the name of the Coalition of Hospice and Palliative Care and designated HPNA as the administrative home for their ongoing efforts. The third edition of the *Clinical Practice Guidelines for Quality Palliative Care* was released in March of 2013[17]**

III. **Specialty Certification Development**

A.   **1991—a survey of nurses to determine interest and desire for specialty recognition was conducted by Hospice Nurses Association (HNA) and the National Hospice Organization (NHO). The results supported interest in certification; the National Board for Certification of Hospice Nurses (NBCHN) was founded[18]**

   1.   1993—first meeting of NBCHN[18]

   2.   1994—first examination offered to registered nurses (RNs) with the credential of Certified Registered Nurse Hospice (CRNH)[18]

B.   **1997—role delineation/practice analysis conducted by NBCHN to compare the RNs practicing in hospice and palliative care to determine if a single certification exam was appropriate; the results indicated enough similarity that the exam included palliative care[14]**

   1.   1998—name changed for Certification Board to National Board for Certification of Hospice and Palliative Nurses (NBCHPN®)[6]

   2.   1999—palliative nurses included in exam and new credential of Certified Hospice and Palliative Nurse (CHPN®) in use[18]

      a)   2002—CHPN® examination achieved accreditation by the American Board of Nursing Specialties (ABNS)[6]

   3.   2014—named changed to Hospice and Palliative Credentialing Center (HPCC)

C.   **Other HPCC Certification Exams—HPCC is the only specialty organization that offers certification to all members of the nursing team**

   1.   2002—Certified Hospice and Palliative Nursing Assistant (CHPNA®) exam began[18]

   2.   National certification for advanced practice nurses initiated by the American Nurses Credentialing Center (ANCC) in 2001 and in 2003 became a joint project with NBCHPN®, credential was Board Certified, Palliative Care Management (BC-PCM)

       a)   NBCHPN® acquired full ownership of the advanced practice nurse exam in 2004. The credential was renamed Advanced Certified Hospice and Palliative Nurse (ACHPN®)[6]

       b)   In 2007, the ACHPN® received accreditation from the American Board of Nursing Specialties (ABNS)[6]

   3.   2003—NBCHPN® developed the certification examination for the hospice and palliative licensed practical/vocational nurse (LP/VN). Credential is Certified Hospice and Palliative Licensed Nurse, or CHPLN®[6]

   4.   2008—Certification for the hospice and palliative administrator was developed. Credential is Certified Hospice and Palliative Care Administrator (CHPCA®)[6]

   5.   2011—Certification for RNs working in pediatric hospice and palliative care was initiated. Credential is Certified Hospice and Palliative Pediatric Nurse (CHPPN®)[6]

   6.   2013—NBCHPN® initiated its first interdisciplinary (RNs, physicians, psychologists, counselors, child life specialists, social workers, and chaplains) certification examination for perinatal loss (pregnancy loss or infant death) care professionals. Credential is Certified in Perinatal Loss Care (CPLC®)[6]

IV. **Palliative Care**

   A.   **Origins of Palliative Care**

       1.   Attends to the whole person, including the family and/or close others

       2.   Is not limited to those who have progressive predictable disease

       3.   Contrasting views exist about the evolution of palliative care

           a)   Hospice and palliative care are often seen as synonymous (e.g., in England and Canada, hospice is also referred to as palliative care)

           b)   Hospice is a subset of palliative care

           c)   Many believe palliative care found its roots in hospice

           d)   Hospice includes the elements of palliative care, but not all palliative care includes all the elements of hospice care

   B.   **Development of the Palliative Care Movement**

       1.   Major factors have influenced the recent development of palliative care programs in the United States

           a)   Consumer demand

               i.   Advances in medical technology and treatment to prolong life

               ii. Aging of the population

      iii.   Prevalence of chronic, critically ill

      iv.   Growing public interest in assisted suicide and euthanasia

      v.   Congressional debates over requiring advance care planning discussions with primary care physicians and its reimbursement

      vi.   Growing gap between what people with serious or life-threatening illness desire and what they experience from healthcare systems and providers

      vii.   Supreme Court's ruling on the right to die and its affirmation of right to care at the end of life in 1976 with the ruling on the Nancy Cruzan case

b) Acknowledgment by the healthcare community that care of dying was in need of attention and improvement

      i.   Position papers from major palliative care organizations on withdrawing or withholding medical interventions, artificial nutrition and hydration, palliative sedation, and nursing care of the patients with DNR order

      ii.   Standardization of palliative care programs across the United States by a formal accrediting body

      iii.   World Health Organization (WHO) *Guidelines on Cancer Pain Relief and Palliative Care* (1990)

      iv.   SUPPORT study results (1995)[2]

      v.   Development of WHO *Standards for Cancer Pain Relief* (1996)

      vi.   Institute of Medicine's report on end-of-life care (1997)

      vii.   AHCPR Cancer Pain Guidelines (now Agency for Healthcare Research and Quality [AHRQ]); revised by the American Pain Society[19]

      viii.   Grassroots development of State Cancer Pain Initiatives in the late 1980s and early 1990s (most recently the American Alliance of Cancer Pain Initiatives, now inactive)

      ix.   Efforts of Project on Death in America (1994),[20] LAST ACTS Initiative (1995),[21] and the Rand Center to Improve the Care of the Dying (1990s)

      x.   Americans for Better Care of the Dying (ABCD, 1990s)

      xi.   Center to Advance Palliative Care (CAPC, 1999)[22]

      xii.   In 2001, The Joint Commission (formerly known as JCAHO) included pain assessment and management as part of the accreditation process for hospitals, home health, long-term care, long-term care pharmacies, ambulatory care, behavioral health, managed behavioral health, and healthcare networks

      xiii.   National Consensus Project for Quality Palliative Care[23]

          (a)   Made up of 6 consortium organizations

              (i)   American Academy of Hospice and Palliative Medicine

              (ii)   Center to Advance Palliative Care

              (iii)   Hospice and Palliative Nurses Association

              (iv)   National Hospice and Palliative Care Organization

              (v)   National Association of Social Workers

              (vi)   National Palliative Care Research Center

(b) Released the first edition of the Clinical Practice Guidelines for Quality Palliative Care in 2004; the second edition in 2009; the third edition was released in 2013

(c) In 2006, the National Quality Forum (NQF) adopted the Clinical Practice Guidelines for Quality Palliative Care within the document A National Framework for Palliative and Hospice Care Quality Measurement and Reporting

C. In 2011, The Joint Commission's Advanced Certification Program for Palliative Care was initiated. It "recognizes hospital inpatient programs that demonstrate exceptional patient- and family-centered care and optimize the quality of life for patients (both adult and pediatric) with serious illness"[24]

D. Philosophy of Palliative Care

1. Definitions of palliative care

a) The National Consensus Project for Quality Palliative Care reaffirms its definition of palliative care in its revision: "Palliative care means patient and family-centered care that optimizes quality of life by anticipating, preventing, and treating suffering. Palliative care throughout the continuum of illness involves addressing physical, intellectual, emotional, social, and spiritual needs and to facilitate patient autonomy, access to information, and choice."[23, p. 9] Common features of a palliative care program are care provided by an interdisciplinary team; collaboration is key among the patient, family, palliative care, and nonpalliative care health providers; services are provided concurrently or independent of the goals of care (i.e., curative, control); and the hope of life with peace and dignity are supported by the interdisciplinary team across the continuum of illness[23]

b) The National Hospice and Palliative Care Organization defines palliative care as: "Treatment that enhances comfort and improves the quality of an individual's life during the last phase of life. No specific therapy is excluded from consideration. The test of palliative treatment lies in the agreement between the individual, physician(s), primary caregiver(s), and the hospice team that the expected outcome is relief from distressing symptoms, the easing of pain, and/or enhancing the quality of life"[25]

c) The WHO defines palliative care as: "Palliative is an approach that improves the quality of life of patients and their families facing the problem associated with life-threatening illness, through the prevention and relief of suffering by means of early identification and impeccable assessment and treatment of pain and other problems, physical, psychosocial and spiritual"[26]

i. "Palliative care

(a) Provides relief from pain and other distressing symptoms;

(b) Affirms life and regards dying as a normal process;

(c) Intends neither to hasten or postpone death;

(d) Integrates the psychological and spiritual aspects of patient care;

(e) Offers a support system to help patients live as actively as possible until death;

(f) Offers a support system to help the family cope during the patient's illness and in their own bereavement;

(g)   Uses a team approach to address the needs of patients and their families, including bereavement counseling, if indicated;

(h)   Will enhance quality of life, and may also positively influence the course of illness;

(i)   Is applicable early in the course of illness, in conjunction with other therapies that are intended to prolong life, such as chemotherapy or radiation therapy, and includes those investigations needed to better understand and manage distressing clinical complications"[26]

ii.   The WHO recognizes the need and inclusion of palliative care for pediatric patients[26]

2.   Eight domains of palliative care are defined by the National Consensus Project for Quality Palliative Care. Excellence in specialist-level palliative care requires expertise in the following domains in order to provide consistent and high quality care. The eight domains are[23]

a)   Domain 1: Structure and Processes of Care

b)   Domain 2: Physical Aspects of Care

c)   Domain 3: Psychological and Psychiatric Aspects of Care

d)   Domain 4: Social Aspects of Care

e)   Domain 5: Spiritual, Religious, and Existential Aspects of Care

f)   Domain 6: Cultural Aspects of Care

g)   Domain 7: Care of the Patient at the End of Life

h)   Domain 8: Ethical and Legal Aspects of Care

3.   Issues that affect palliative care utilization include

a)   Patients, families, and staff may have difficulty transitioning from curative to palliative care

b)   Most programs are located in hospital-based, hierarchical medical institutions

c)   Some programs may not provide continuity and communication with primary care physicians and community-based programs

d)   Some programs may not provide supportive services such as social work, spiritual, volunteer, or bereavement follow-up, as compared to hospice care

4.   Palliative care in the United States[27]

a)   Policy initiatives for palliative care include

i.   Access and quality

ii.   Workforce

iii.   Research

b)   Palliative care programs

i.   First formal program was St. Luke's in New York City started in the 1970s, relied on philanthropic support

        (a)   Comprehensive interdisciplinary team saw patients in the emergency department and on nursing units

        (b)   Closed in mid-1980s due to lack of support

    ii.   *Get Palliative Care* is a searchable website, maintained by the Center to Advance Palliative Care, for the public to locate hospitals offering this service today[28]

c)   Access and quality

    i.   It is estimated that over 66% of hospitals (meaning over 1600) have palliative care programs in the United States[29]

    ii.   Ninety million people in the United States have serious disease or illness that has or will constrain the quality of life for those people. That number is expected to double with the aging baby boomer generation[27]

    iii. Cost savings/avoidance well-documented

    iv. Access to a palliative care program is limited due to geographical location and the size of the hospital

    v.   Common issues for the underserved people are

        (a)   Uncontrolled symptoms

        (b)   Poor communication between providers

        (c)   Fragmented care leading to inadequate follow-up care

        (d)   Family caregivers strain and inadequate knowledge

d)   Workforce

    i.   An increasing role for advanced practice nurses with palliative care experience

    ii.   1:1200 ratio for board-certified hospice and palliative care physicians to patient populations

    iii. CAPC reported the overall palliative care report card grade moved from a C in 2008 to a B in 2011[27]

e)   Research

    i.   Endorsement for research funding by National Institutes of Health and Institute of Medicine

    ii.   Revenue/cost savings projected/reported; CAPC has a formula to assist hospitals in projecting cost savings and increased revenue from instituting a palliative care program

    iii. Funding sources for research and clinical programs

        (a)   Federal grants

        (b)   Private and public foundations

        (c)   Industry grants

        (d)   Endowments and other philanthropic efforts

        (e)   In-kind support

E. Accreditation

1. There is currently no mandatory nationwide certification or accreditation for palliative care programs

2. In 2011, The Joint Commission offered an Advanced Certification for Palliative Care Programs for hospital-based inpatient programs that provide gold standard adult and pediatric palliative care. To achieve this designation, a palliative care program must demonstrate high quality standards for patient- and family-centered care, quality of life for patients, and care for patients' physical, emotional, social, and spiritual needs while maintaining the patient's autonomy and decision-making[24]

3. In 2012, the American Academy of Hospice and Palliative Medicine (AAHPM) endorsed, funded, and appointed an organizing board of directors for the purpose of creating a hospice medical director certification[30]

4. Being recognized as a subspecialty by 11 different medical residency programs in 2006 was paramount in making hospice and palliative care a legitimate medical specialization.[30] Hospice and palliative care medical fellowships are an outgrowth of this specialization

5. Certification for nursing and related disciplines (see earlier section in this chapter)

F. Examples of patients who may be appropriate for palliative care rather than hospice care include

1. Those on experimental protocols and/or who are receiving palliative chemotherapy, immunotherapy, and/or radiation therapy

2. Those individuals who are terminally ill and need assistance clarifying goals of care

3. Those patients who are still receiving active treatment for their incurable illness but who can also benefit from support services and symptom management

4. Children with severe congenital anomalies who will die quickly and often will remain in the hospital or those with a serious or life-threatening illness, but are considered to be far from the terminal stage

5. Persons who have sustained an injury or a complication from treatment where recovery is unlikely

G. Cost Savings and Revenue

1. Goal of palliative care is to improve quality of life

2. Potential savings for healthcare organizations, third party payers, and for patients/families

   a) Palliative care frees up beds for other patients, for example, intensive care beds

   b) Shortened hospital stays

   c) Reduced ancillary costs

   d) Reduces unnecessary tests and procedures

3. Cost savings are well-documented

4. Research continues on the impact of palliative care programs and units on cost, quality, patient outcomes, and family satisfaction

CITED REFERENCES

1. Lentz J. A conversation with Florence Wald. *J Hosp Palliat Nurs.* 2004;6(1):9-10.

2. The SUPPORT Principle Investigators. A controlled trial to improve care for seriously ill hospitalized patients: the Study to Understand Prognosis and Preferences for Outcomes and Risks of Treatments (SUPPORT). *JAMA.* 1995;274(20):1591-1598.

3. National Hospice and Palliative Care Organization (NHPCO). *Preamble and Philosophy.* 2014. www.nhpco.org/ethical-and-position-statements/preamble-and-philosophy. Accessed July 11, 2014.

4. Centers for Medicare & Medicaid Services (CMS), HHS. Medicare Program; FY 2014 hospice wage index and payment rate update; hospice quality reporting requirements; and updates on payment reform. *Fed Regist.* 2013;78(152):48233-48281.

5. National Hospice and Palliative Care Organization (NHPCO). *Hospice Care.* 2014. www.nhpco.org/about/hospice-care. Accessed July 9, 2014.

6. Dahlin CM, Sutermaster DJ, eds; Hospice and Palliative Nurses Association, American Nurses Association. *Palliative Nursing: Scope and Standards of Practice—An Essential Resource for Palliative and Hospice Nurses.* Silver Spring, MD: nursesbooks.org; 2014.

7. Centers for Medicare & Medicaid Services (CMS). *Electronic Code of Federal Regulations. Title 42; Chapter IV, Subchapter B, Part 418; Subpart D. Hospice Conditions of Participation.* U.S. Government Printing Office. 2014. www.ecfr.gov/cgi-bin/text-idx?c=ecfr&sid=818258235647b14d29 61ad30fa3e68e6&rgn=div5&view=text&node=42:3.0.1.1.5&idno=42#42:3.0.1.1.5.3.4.12. Accessed September 25, 2014.

8. National Hospice and Palliative Care Organization (NHPCO). *NHPCO's Facts and Figures: Hospice Care in America.* 2014. www.nhpco.org/sites/default/files/public/Statistics_Research/2014_Facts_ Figures.pdf. Accessed December 10, 2014.

9. Medicare Payment Advisory Commission. *A Data Book: Heath Care Spending and the Medicare Program.* 2014. medpac.gov/documents/publications/jun14databookentirereport.pdf. Accessed October 6, 2014.

10. Taylor DH Jr, Ostermann J, Van Houtven CH, Tulsky JA, Steinhauser K. What length of hospice use maximizes reduction in medical expenditures near death in the US Medicare program? *Soc Sci Med.* 2007;65(7):1466-1478.

11. Hospice and Palliative Nurses Association (HPNA). *Shared Mission, Vision & Pillars.* 2014. advancingexpertcare.org/about/shared-mission-vision-pillars/. Accessed October 20, 2014.

12. Amenta MO. History of the Hospice Nurses Association 1986–1996. *J Hosp Palliat Nurs.* 2001;3(4):128-136.

13. Hospice Nurses Association. *Articles of Incorporation.* San Diego: HNA; 1987. kepler.sos.ca.gov/. Accessed September 25, 2014.

14. Head B. Hospice and palliative nurse certification: evolution of a nursing specialty. *J Hosp Palliat Nurs.* 2001;3(4):137-139.

15. Welsh S. Association news. *J Hosp Palliat Nurs.* 2014;16(7):384-385. doi: 10.1097/NJH. 0000000000000097.

16. Hospice and Palliative Nurses Foundation (HPNF). *The Foundation's Purpose.* 2014. hpnf.advancingexpertcare.org/about/the-foundations-purpose/. Accessed October 20, 2014.

17. National Consensus Project (NCP) for Quality Palliative Care. *About Us.* www.nationalconsensusproject.org/DisplayPage.aspx?Title=About%20Us. Accessed October 8, 2014.

18. Hospice and Palliative Credentialing Center. *History of HPCC.* 2014. hpcc.advancingexpertcare.org/about/history-of-hpcc/. Accessed October 8, 2014.

19. Miaskowski C, Cleary J, Burney R, et al. Guidelines for the management of cancer pain in adults and children. *APS Clinical Practice Guidelines Series #3.* Glenview, IL: American Pain Society; 2005. apps.americanpainsociety.org/Default.aspx?TabID=251&ProductId=472. Accessed September 26, 2014.

20. Aulino F, Foley K. The Project on Death in America. *J R Soc Med.* 2001;94(9):492-495.

21. De Milto L. *Assessment of Last Acts Program Provides Recommendations for Future Direction.* Princeton, NJ: Robert Wood Johnson Foundation; 2002. www.rwjf.org/en/research-publications/find-rwjf-research/2002/10/assessment-of-last-acts-r--program-provides-recommendations-for-.html. Accessed August 14, 2014.

22. Nakashian M. *Center to Advance Palliative Care.* Princeton, NY: Robert Wood Johnson Foundation; 2012. www.rwjf.org/en/research-publications/find-rwjf-research/2012/05/center-to-advance-palliative-care0.html. August 14, 2014.

23. National Consensus Project for Quality Palliative Care. *Clinical Practice Guidelines for Quality Palliative Care.* 3rd ed. Pittsburgh, PA: Hospice and Palliative Nurses Association; 2013. www.nationalconsensusproject.org/Guidelines_Download2.aspx. Accessed October 8, 2014.

24. The Joint Commission. *Facts about the Advanced Certification Program for Palliative Care.* 2014. www.jointcommission.org/facts_about_palliative_care/. Accessed September 26, 2014.

25. National Hospice and Palliative Care Organization (NHPCO). *Palliative Care: An Explanation of Palliative Care.* 2013. www.nhpco.org/palliative-care-0. Accessed November 20, 2013.

26. World Health Organization (WHO). *Cancer: WHO Definition of Palliative Care.* 2014. www.who.int/cancer/palliative/definition/en/. Accessed October 8, 2014.

27. Center to Advance Palliative Care. National Palliative Care Research Center. *A State-by-State Report Card on Access to Palliative Care in Our Nation's Hospitals.* 2011. www.capc.org/reportcard. Accessed October 8, 2014.

28. Center to Advance Palliative Care. Get Palliative Care. *Get Palliative Care Provider Directory.* 2012. www.getpalliativecare.org/providers/. Accessed October 8, 2014.

29. Center to Advance Palliative Care (CAPC). *Palliative Care in Hospitals Continues Rapid Growth Trend, According to Latest CAPC Analysis.* [Press Release] March 29, 2013. www.capc.org/news-and-events/releases/03-29-13. Accessed August 14, 2014.

30. American Acadamy of Hospice and Palliative Medicine (AAHPM). *Certification for Hospice and Palliative Medicine Specialists.* aahpm.org/education/certification. Accessed September 26, 2014.

INTERDISCIPLINARY COLLABORATIVE PRACTICE IN HOSPICE AND PALLIATIVE SETTINGS

Paula Larsen, LCSW, ACHP-SW
Sandra Jense, DNP, ACNP-BC

I. **Introduction**

    A. **A well-functioning palliative care team is essentially comprised of a physician, advanced practice or registered nurse, a master's level social worker, and a chaplain. Each member of the team has been certified to practice in the field of palliative care. Team members value and practice in a collaborative, respectful manner with each other and with other disciplines to meet the goal of exceptional patient and family care[1]**

II. **Palliative Nursing: Scope and Standards of Practice**

    A. **In accordance with Standard 13: Collaboration—"The hospice and palliative registered nurse collaborates with patient, family, interdisciplinary team, and others in the conduct of nursing practice"[2, p. 55]**

III. **Conceptual Models for End-of-Life Care**

    A. **Respectful Death[3]**

        1. A model designed to support the education of disciplines involved with providing end-of-life care

        2. Focuses on the therapeutic relationships with patients and families to facilitate the sharing of the patient and family's story, which is then integrated into the plan of care

        3. Nurses develop therapeutic relationships with patients and families to help establish open conversations about the death process

    B. **Whole Person Suffering (Dame Cicely Saunders)[4]**

        1. Four dimensions to suffering—physical, psychological, social, and spiritual

        2. Each area of suffering is addressed to achieve comfort at end of life

C. **Interdimensional Care Model[5]**

1. As multidimensional beings, each change in health status initiates changes in the multiple dimensions of the person—physical, spiritual, emotional, financial, functional, interpersonal, well-being, and transcendent

2. Care teams whose members possess expertise in these various dimensions and work in coordination with one another are well suited to aid the patient and family in adapting to these changes

D. **Tasks in Dying**

1. Dying involves the completion of developmental landmarks and task-work, to the extent chosen by and appropriate to the patient, family, and close others. Landmarks and task-work include completing worldly affairs by transferring financial and legal responsibilities and love of self by forgiving oneself[6]

2. Effective care teams provide a safe, encouraging, nurturing milieu to facilitate developmental task completion as the patient and family desires[5]

E. **Patient- and Family-Centered Care (serves as the basis for the National Hospice and Palliative Care Organization [NHPCO] family evaluation of care)[7]**

1. Providing dying persons with desired physical comfort

2. Helping dying persons control decisions about medical care and daily routines

3. Relieving family members of the burden of being present at all times to advocate for their dying family member/close other

4. Educating family members so they feel confident to care for their family member/close other at home

5. Providing family members with emotional support both before and after the patient's death

F. ***Clinical Practice Guidelines for Quality Palliative Care* from the National Consensus Project for Quality Palliative Care[8]**

1. The Clinical Practice Guidelines to improve the quality of palliative care in the United States are delineated by eight domains

    a) Structure and Processes of Care

    b) Physical Aspects of Care

    c) Psychological and Psychiatric Aspects of Care

    d) Social Aspects of Care

    e) Spiritual, Religious, and Existential Aspects of Care

    f) Cultural Aspects of Care

    g) Care for the Patient at the End of Life

    h) Ethical and Legal Aspects of Care

2. See Chapter XIII, *National Guidelines and RN Practice,* for more information about the *Clinical Practice Guidelines for Quality Palliative Care*

IV. Healthcare Teams

A. The Multidisciplinary Team

1. Team participants from other professional disciplines operate together, but also function on independent levels

2. Generally, there is limited coordination or consultation between the disciplines

3. Teams can be organized in a hierarchical manner, which can result in limited sharing of decisions and leadership

B. The Interdisciplinary Team[9]

1. In contrast to multidisciplinary teams, interdisciplinary teams (IDTs) have a collaborative approach to communication and function[10]

2. Considered a best or optimal practice and model of care

3. Five central elements

   a) Interdependence

   b) Recently organized expert exercises

   c) Flexibility

   d) Shared ownership of goals

   e) Review of process

4. Three attributes

   a) Problem-focused process

      i. An interpersonal process between team members, which is collaborative and focused on the challenges of patient and family care needs

   b) Sharing

      i. Collaborative sharing of responsibility, power, goals, and decisions to help secure unity and meeting a shared outcome related to patient care

      ii. Infers the nonhierarchical nature of interdisciplinary collaboration

   c) Working together

      i. Insinuates the ongoing cooperative nature of team members

      ii. Acknowledgment of the uniquely important contributions of each team member while also granting the joint donations to the process

C. Antecedents for Interdisciplinary Teams

1. Interprofessional education[11]

   a) In a less competitive environment, team professionals develop overlapping roles

   b) For both the team and the individual team member, overall functioning can be optimized with the implementation of interdisciplinary training programs

2. Role awareness

   a) Inclusive to the understanding of team members knowledge, skills, and perspectives

   b) Shared acknowledgement of the expertise and competence of team members

3. Interpersonal relationship skills

   a) Mutual trust and respect among team members

   b) Shared open communication that is noncontentious and nondominant in style

   c) Ability to effectively negotiate, handle conflicts, and manage respectful disagreements is essential

4. Deliberate action to effectively cultivate and maintain a sense of effort with practice is required

5. Support

   a) Team members must maintain a sense of support and commitment to a process of interdisciplinary collaboration

   b) The organization or administration support is critically important to the success of the collaborative interdisciplinary team

D. **Consequences**

1. Patient—strengthening of the quality of patient care with noted improved outcomes

2. Organization—cost containment through staff productivity and efficiency achieved improved coordination of patient care

3. Healthcare professional—improved sense of job satisfaction is most often noted as team members report improved morale and an improved sense of professionalism, particularly for nurses

E. **The Transdisciplinary Team**

1. The transdisciplinary approach to team building involves a blurring of roles and boundaries[10,12]

2. Team members are trained in the roles of other disciplines, and have similar responsibilities[10,12]

3. Transdisciplinary approaches can result in high quality care, but the concern is that the unique contributions of individual disciplines may be diluted[10]

V. **The Hospice and Palliative Care Interdisciplinary Team**

A. **Centers for Medicare & Medicaid Services (CMS) have identified core hospice requirements. These include the services of a physician, nurse, medical social worker, and counseling (including bereavement and spiritual).[13] Other common team members are hospice aides, volunteers, physical therapists, occupational therapists, and speech-language pathologists**

1. The practice of all members of the interdisciplinary team must be in accordance with state and federal regulations (e.g., states' nurse practice act)

B. Registered Nurse

1. All nurses practice primary palliative care as palliative care is embedded in nursing practice. Nurses who choose the specialty of palliative care, which includes hospice, are "expected to have a higher competence in pain and symptom management, communication skills, and coordination of interdisciplinary care"[2, p. 19]

2. The registered nurse (RN) or advanced practice registered nurse (APRN) assumes primary responsibility for the physical care of the patient providing expert pain and symptom management. In addition to their expertise in pain and symptom management, hospice and palliative nurses must also possess the skills necessary to recognize psychosocial and spiritual issues for patients and families. The RN or APRN generally serves as the service director or coordinator of the IDT

3. Core competencies of the RN include clinical judgment, advocacy and ethics, professionalism, collaboration, systems thinking, cultural competence, facilitation of learning, and communication[14]

C. Advanced Practice Nurse[2,15]

1. There are 2 roles of advanced practice palliative nursing—graduate-level prepared specialty nurses and advanced practice registered nurses (APRNs)

   a) Graduate-level prepared specialty nurses are essential to advanced palliative care roles other than direct care (e.g., educators, researchers, administrators)

   b) APRNs (i.e., clinical nurse specialist, nurse practitioner, nurse anesthetist, nurse midwife) "provide symptom management, optimize function, and enhance quality of life. In the process, they exercise a high degree of critical thinking, analysis, and independent judgment, within the framework of autonomous and/or collaborative interdisciplinary practice"[15, p. 4]

D. Licensed Practical/Vocational Nurse

1. The licensed practical/vocational nurse (LP/VN) "assists the RN by providing the necessary treatments, education, and documentation consistent with the plan of care. An integral member of the interdisciplinary team who provides excellent information to the team members ultimately responsible for the plan of care, the LP/VN monitors symptoms and changes, and reports these changes to the RN in charge of the patient's care. In essence, the RN is responsible for the act of assessment and the LP/VN is responsible for observing, monitoring, and reporting his/her observations"[16, p. 1]

E. Medical Director

1. The hospice or palliative medical director often assumes overall responsibility for the medical management of all patients on the team or service. As a member of the interdisciplinary team, the medical director assumes responsibility for medical care provided by the team or service and, in some programs, may also assume administrative duties. When the patient's physician remains involved, the medical director serves in an advisory/consultative role to him/her and to the interdisciplinary team

2. In palliative care, the role of the medical director varies widely, including, for example, in nurse practitioner-led teams where the medical director is an APRN

F.   Primary Provider

1.   The primary provider is responsible for oversight of care provided. He/she may continue to provide medical care for the patient should the patient desire

2.   The primary provider may be a physician or an APRN

3.   He/she provides medical care including prescribing medications, diagnostic exams, and procedures

G.   Psychosocial Professionals

1.   Psychosocial professionals are those members of the hospice and palliative care team primarily responsible for the provision of psychosocial assessment and treatment. Most often, they are social workers and counselors with expertise in grief and bereavement counseling. In addition to the provision of psychosocial assessment and treatment, they also support patients and families with concerns related to financial matters, legal issues, advance directives, and funeral arrangements

H.   Spiritual Care Professionals

1.   Spiritual care professionals, also known as chaplains, spiritual care counselors, or clergy, are primarily responsible for the provision of spiritual care that focuses on healing, forgiveness, and a sense of meaning

I.   Nursing Assistant (Hospice Aide, Home Health Aide, or Certified Nursing Assistant)

1.   The home health aide or certified nursing assistant is responsible for provision of basic personal care

2.   This personal care may include, but is not limited to, bathing, toileting, dressing, mouth care, skin care, and transfers

3.   Nursing assistants must be supervised by a nurse according to state practice acts

J.   Patient Care Volunteer[13,17,18]

1.   Patient care volunteers provide a variety of care and services to hospice (required by CMS) and palliative care patients

2.   Volunteers are members of the interdisciplinary team and may provide support, including companionship, making deliveries, and running errands

3.   Hospice volunteers must receive "orientation and training that is consistent with hospice industry standards"[17, p. 100]

K.   Consultative Members

1.   Consultative members of the interdisciplinary team represent a variety of disciplines that are involved on an as-needed basis

2.   These members include, but are not limited to, consulting physicians, pain specialists, pharmacists, nutritionists, psychiatrists, respiratory therapists, as well as physical, occupational, and speech therapists

3.   If the patient is a child, the team should include members with expertise in caring for children[8]

L. Patient and Family

  1. To maintain a patient-/family-centered focus, treatment plans should be developed in consultation with the patient and family, as they have a unique perspective in the care that will best suit them[19]

VI. Hospice and Palliative Care Nursing Collaborative Practice Issues

A. Interdisciplinary Group Meeting

  1. Palliative care, including hospice, is delivered by an interdisciplinary team, requiring frequent communication to review and revise the plan of care as needed, which is usually done via regularly scheduled team meetings.[8] Team meetings are attended by the core palliative care group along with ancillary members as needed. For hospice, that core group must include the physician, nurse, social worker, and chaplain. Most hospital and outpatient facilities follow a similar model

   a) For hospice—"The hospice interdisciplinary group (in collaboration with the individual's attending physician, if any) must review, revise, and document the individualized plan as frequently as the patient's condition requires, but no less frequently than every 15 calendar days"[17, p. 56]

   b) Hospital-based and outpatient palliative care do not have regulations regarding how often the plan must be reviewed and revised

  2. Patient and family attendance at team meetings

   a) Which persons are considered "family" is defined by the patient.[8] The patient also determines the extent of each family member's involvement

   b) Patient and family are encouraged to attend team meetings, though this is not required. If the patient and/or family are not attending the team meetings, they still need to be included in developing/updating the plan of care[17]

B. Facilitating Group Process

  1. How the palliative care team differs from the traditional medical team model[20]

   a) Patient and/or family are team members

   b) Physician is not the only leader and decision-maker

   c) Decision-making is coordinated by all members of the team

  2. Effective teams are able to work together as one cohesive unit with excellent communication. This develops over time by building on the strengths of each team member.[21] See Table 2-1 for behaviors of effective teams

  3. Conflict between team members

   a) Possible causes[22]

    i. Not agreeing with the plan of care

    ii. Not comfortable with the dying process

Table 2-1. Behaviors of Effective Teams[21]

• Communication in team meetings —Follow ground rules (e.g., allowing all to speak, how disagreements are communicated)
• Continuing improvement process in place (e.g., team listening skills); discuss team issues regularly
• Team meetings are —Scheduled regularly —Held in quiet places with minimal interruptions —Structured

        b)   Potential resolutions for team conflict[22]

            i.   Listen to a team member's concerns

            ii.   Use team meetings to address all issues and conflicts

            iii.   Establish goals and clarify goals as needed

            iv.   If team members do not agree on the goals, discover where the breakdown has occurred

            v.   Utilize organizational resources (e.g., ethics committee) as needed

C.   Advance Directives and the Advance Care Planning Process

    1.   Understand the applicable laws regarding advance directives

    2.   Educate the general and healthcare communities regarding the implication and uses of durable power of attorney for healthcare, living will, and the right to accept or refuse treatment in accordance with the Patient Self Determination Act of 1991

    3.   Based on the current literature regarding cardiopulmonary resuscitation (CPR), educate the general and healthcare communities on the appropriateness of "do not resuscitate" orders, allowing for patients and families to make informed decisions regarding resuscitation

    4.   Refer to Chapter IX, *Advance Care Planning and Goals of Care,* for a complete discussion of this topic

D.   Potential Clinician–Patient/Family Issues

    1.   Blurring of clinician–patient/family boundaries

        a)   Parentalism—making decisions for a patient who can make his/her own decisions thus infringing on his/her right to self-determination[23]

        b)   Deception—coercing or manipulating a patient to do what the clinician wants him/her to do via lying, avoiding answering questions, withholding details, imposing his/her beliefs on the patient, negative behaviors, and misleading body language[23]

        c)   Confidentiality—disclosing private information to people who are not involved in the care of the patient thereby not respecting the patient. Certain information (e.g., gunshot wounds, abuse, select diseases) is required to be reported by law. Instances in which a patient or family specifically ask that no one else be told something he/she told the clinician needs to be handled individually, based on the well-being of the person involved[23]

   i. A hospice patient is making a photo album for her children and does not want them to know until it is completed—the hospice nurse can tell her that this is important for the team to know, but he/she will not tell her children. In this case there is no concern for the woman's well-being

   ii. An elderly patient's heart disease has progressed to the point that he is no longer able to provide all of his personal care. He is refusing bathing assistance from outpatient palliative care because he does not want his wife to know that his condition has deteriorated, saying that "my wife [who is also elderly] can help me." His decision could affect the well-being of both husband and wife. In this case, it will be important to explore his decision and its effect on his elderly wife, as well as the probability that his wife already knows his condition has deteriorated

  d) Balancing obligations to the patient and family[23]—though palliative care is care of the patient and family,[8] there can be instances when clinicians may feel they have to "choose sides." It is common for patients and their families and between family members to disagree on aspects of care. For some of these conflicts, the team can assist the patient and family to resolve the conflict. For others, an additional team member may be needed. When a resolution to the conflict is not possible, the patient's wishes need to be followed

 2. Conflict between team members and the patient and/or family

  a) Possible reasons for conflict[22]

   i. Needed conversations have not happened

   ii. Patient and/or family is overwhelmed

   iii. Language barriers including too many medical terms

   iv. Cultural and/or religious differences[24]

   v. Unresolved interpersonal matters

  b) Potential methods of solving conflict[22]

   i. One key team member attempts to establish trust with the patient and/or family

   ii. Encourage the patient and family to attend family and team meetings

   iii. Identify unresolved interpersonal matters

   iv. Invite community or religious representative to assist with conflict resolution[24]

E. Consumer Education

 1. Participate in the development and review of media materials (e.g., print, audio, video) related to palliative care, ensuring information distributed is consistent with current standards of practice

  a) Evaluating educational materials—teach patients and families how to identify credible sources of information[25]

   i. Information should be current, based on scientific evidence, supported by facts, and list the original source

        ii.   Avoid printed materials and Internet information (e.g., websites, blogs, chat rooms) that

            (a)   Do not have a publisher, author, or date of publication

            (b)   Are primarily interested in selling a product or other conflicts of interest

            (c)   Do not have a date of publication or the date is more than 5 years old

            (d)   Claim "cures" or "miracles"

2.   Serve as a palliative care ambassador and resource to the general and healthcare communities via participation in community education classes and seminars

VII. Professional Development

A.   Participate in ongoing educational activities that increase knowledge, skill, and competence in palliative nursing

1.   All nurses are expected to have generalist level of competence in providing palliative care. The specialist hospice and palliative care nurse has additional education and experience in patterns of disease progression and pain and symptom management as well as caring for dying patients and their families[2,26]

2.   Continuing competence—"ongoing commitment of a registered nurse to integrate and apply the knowledge, skills, and judgment with the attitudes, values, and beliefs required to practice safely, effectively, and ethically in a designated role and setting"[27, p. 4]

B.   Serve as a role model, mentor, preceptor, and educator for professional colleagues, students, and other members of the healthcare community

1.   Role model—a passive method of supporting clinicians with less experience via direct observation with little to no interaction; a role model can also serve as a positive exemplar of the behavior and attitudes inherent in a role

2.   Mentor—a usually long-term relationship between an experienced person (mentor) and a less experienced person (mentee), in the example of a hospice and/or palliative care nurse, in which clinical and professional issues are discussed and dealt with

3.   Precepting—direct supervision provided to the clinician in hospice and palliative care. The precepting optimally should be in a one-on-one relationship with specific goals to learn information about the role

C.   Participate in Peer Reviews

1.   Peer review—a collegial, systematic, and periodic process by which clinicians are held accountable for practice and which fosters the refinement of one's knowledge, skills, and decision-making at all levels and in all areas of practice[2]

2.   Main reasons for peer review—maintain accreditation, observation of a clinician, and review of random cases or ones with poor outcomes for quality improvement.[28] Peer review can also be used for evaluation and promotion[29]

3.   Peer review should be done using set criteria

D. Seek and obtain status as a Certified Hospice and Palliative Nurse from the Hospice and Palliative Credentialing Center (HPCC)

    1. Certification is a voluntary process that validates and evaluates an individual's expertise in a specialty area. Initial hospice and palliative certification is validated via testing (see Table 2-2)[30,31]

    2. Benefits of certification

        a) Hallmark of professional competence[26,30,32,33]

        b) Improved quality of patient care[34,35]

        c) Improved patient outcomes[36]

        d) Improved job satisfaction[30,34,35]

        e) Improved collaboration with other members of the healthcare team[30,34]

        f) Improved sense of empowerment[34,37]

        g) Demonstrates commitment to profession and specialty[26]

E. Participate in the development and implementation of programs that increase knowledge of hospice and palliative nursing in the greater healthcare community

F. Seek membership and become involved in national organizations that support palliative nursing

    1. Professional organizations provide the opportunity for education (e.g., conferences, journals, publications, e-learning) and networking (e.g., national and local chapter meetings, online forums and list serves) with peers. Many professional organizations also support advocacy, research, and leadership efforts

    2. Hospice and Palliative Nurses Association (HPNA)—national and local chapters

        a) HPNA is the professional organization that represents palliative nursing. Members include hospice and palliative nurses and other members of the team. HPNA's mission is *to advance expert care in serious illness* through a focus on advancing expert communication skills, pain and symptom management, and coordination and transitions of care. HPNA seeks to support and engage members through the four pillars of education, advocacy, leadership, and research to achieve the vision of transforming the care and culture of serious illness

    3. American Nurses Association and state nursing associations

    4. Oncology Nursing Society (ONS), American Society of Pain Management Nursing (ASPMN), and other specialty organizations

    5. National Hospice and Palliative Care Organization

    6. State hospice and palliative care organizations

G. Self-Care

    1. Most common stressors in palliative care—communication problems with others in the system, team, administration, and patient/family; role conflict; the nature of the system; inadequate resources; unrealistic expectations of the organization; patient/family coping problems[38]

Table 2-2. Available Palliative Care Certifications for Interdisciplinary Team Members

Certification	Credential	Eligible Team Members	Certifying Body
Advanced Certified Hospice & Palliative Nurse	ACHPN®	• Clinical nurse specialists • Nurse practitioners	HPCC (hpcc.advancingexpertcare.org/competence/aprn-achpn/)
Certified Hospice & Palliative Nurse	CHPN®	• Registered nurses	HPCC (hpcc.advancingexpertcare.org/competence/rn-chpn/)
Certified Hospice & Palliative Licensed Nurse	CHPLN®	• Licensed practical/vocational nurses	HPCC (hpcc.advancingexpertcare.org/competence/lpvn-chpln/)
Certified Hospice & Palliative Nursing Assistant	CHPNA®	• Nursing assistants	HPCC (hpcc.advancingexpertcare.org/competence/na-chpna/)
Certified Hospice & Palliative Care Administrator	CHPCA®	• Administrators	HPCC (hpcc.advancingexpertcare.org/competence/admin-chpca/)
Certified in Perinatal Loss Care	CPLC®	• Chaplain • Child life specialist • Counselor • Physician • Psychologist • Registered nurse • Social worker	HPCC (hpcc.advancingexpertcare.org/competence/perinatal-loss-cplc/)
Hospice & Palliative Medicine	HPM	• Physicians	Multiple (www.aahpm.org/certification/subspecialty-certification)
Hospice Medical Director Certification	HMDC™	• Physicians	Hospice Medical Director Certification Board (www.hmdcb.org/)
Certified Hospice & Palliative Social Worker	CHP-SW	• Bachelor's level social worker	National Association of Social Workers (www.socialworkers.org/credentials/credentials/chpsw.asp)
Advanced Certified Hospice & Palliative Social Worker	ACHP-SW	• Master's level social worker	National Association of Social Workers (www.socialworkers.org/credentials/credentials/achp.asp)
Board Certified Chaplain—Hospice & Palliative Care Certification	BCC-HPCC	• Board certified chaplains	Board of Chaplaincy Certification Inc. (bcci.professionalchaplains.org/content.asp?pl=45&sl=42&contentid=48)

2. Burnout—chronic interpersonal stressors related to one's job exhibited by negative attitudes and behaviors resulting in decreased work performance[38]

a) There are 3 components of burnout

i. Emotional exhaustion—"feelings of being over-extended and depleted of one's emotional and physical resources"[38, p. 4]

ii. Cynicism and depersonalization—"negative, callous, or excessively detached response to various aspects of the job."[38, p. 4] It is closely related to exhaustion and both result in distancing oneself from work[38]

iii. Ineffectiveness and lack of personal accomplishment—"feelings of incompetence and a lack of achievement and productivity at work. [They] arise more clearly from a lack of resources to get the work done (e.g., lack of critical information, lack of necessary tools, insufficient time)."[38, p. 4] Ineffectiveness and lack of personal accomplishment may be experienced along with emotional exhaustion and cynicism[38]

b) Burnout can result from mismatch between the employee and their work environment in one or more of six areas of work life: workload, control, reward, community, fairness, and values[38]

3. Compassion fatigue—"almost identical to post-traumatic stress disorder, except that it applies to those emotionally affected by the trauma of another (usually a client or family member)"[38, p. 4]

4. Coping strategies[38]

a) Personal coping strategies (e.g., maintaining personal relationships, positive work attitude, in particular finding a healthy approach to working with patients who are dying, religious/spiritual practice, good work-life balance, participation in recreational activities and hobbies, exercise, humor and laughter, good nutrition, mindfulness practices)

b) Satisfaction with one's own career

c) Knowing one's self and how you deal with the difficult aspect of your job (e.g., change, grief)

d) Using positive emotions (e.g., compassion, forgiveness, love, hope, joy, faith/trust, awe, gratitude) can assist with your sense of purpose/self-determination, positive relationships as well as counteracting physical effects associated with negative emotions

VIII. Research

A. Participate in, conduct, and/or support research related to hospice and palliative care nursing

1. Direct care nurses are in a position to transform practice by identifying areas of needed research as well as collecting data[39]

B. Participate in the writing and reviewing of articles related to hospice and palliative nursing, submitting for publication when appropriate

C. Remain informed of current research and evidenced-based practice guidelines

CITED REFERENCES

1. Stark D. Teamwork in palliative care: an integrative approach. In: Altilio T, Otis-Green S, eds. *Oxford Textbook of Palliative Social Work*. New York, NY: Oxford University Press; 2011:415-424.

2. Dahlin CM, Sutermaster DJ, eds; Hospice and Palliative Nurses Association, American Nurses Association. *Palliative Nursing: Scope and Standards of Practice—An Essential Resource for Hospice and Palliative Nurses*. Silver Spring, MD: nursesbooks.org; 2014.

3. Wasserman LS. Respectful death: a model for end-of-life care. *Clin J Oncol Nurs*. 2008;12(4):621-626. doi: 10.1188/08.CJON.621-626.

4. Saunders C. The evolution of palliative care. *J R Soc Med*. 2001;94(9):430-432.

5. Egan City KA, Labyak MJ. Hospice palliative care for the 21st century: a model for quality end-of-life care. In: Ferrell BR, Coyle N, eds. *Oxford Textbook for Palliative Nursing*. 3rd ed. New York, NY: Oxford University Press; 2010:13-53.

6. Byock I. *Working Set of Landmarks and Developmental Taskwork*. 2014. www.dyingwell.org/landmarks.htm. Accessed July 17, 2014.

7. Teno JM, Casey VA, Welch LC, Edgman-Levitan S. Patient-focused, family-centered end-of-life medical care: views of the guidelines and bereaved family members. *J Pain Symptom Manage*. 2001;22(3):738-751.

8. National Consensus Project for Quality Palliative Care. *Clinical Practice Guidelines for Quality Palliative Care*. 3rd ed. Pittsburgh, PA: National Consensus Project for Quality Palliative Care; 2013.

9. Petri L. Concept analysis of interdisciplinary collaboration. *Nursing Forum*. 2010;45(2):73-82.

10. Parrott R, Kreuter MW. Multidisciplinary, interdisciplinary and transdisciplinary approaches to health communication. In: Thompson TL, Parrott R, Nussbaum JF, eds. *The Routledge Handbook of Health Communication*. 2nd ed. New York, NY: Routledge; 2011:3-17.

11. O'Connor M, Fisher C. Exploring the dynamics of interdisciplinary palliative care teams in providing psychosocial care: "everybody thinks that everybody can do it and they can't." *J Palliat Med*. 2011;14(2):191-196.

12. Dyer JA. Multidisciplinary, interdisciplinary and transdisciplinary educational models and nursing education. *Nursing Education Perspectives*. 2003;24(4):186-188.

13. Centers for Medicare & Medicaid Services (CMS). *Chapter 9—Coverage of Hospice Services Under Hospital Insurance. Hospice Benefit Policy Manual*. 2012. www.cms.gov/Regulations-and-Guidance/Guidance/Manuals/downloads/bp102c09.pdf. Accessed July 18, 2014.

14. Hospice and Palliative Nurses Association. *Competencies for the Generalist Hospice and Palliative Nurse*. 2nd ed. Pittsburgh, PA: Hospice and Palliative Nurses Association; 2010.

15. Dahlin C, ed. *Competencies for the Hospice and Palliative Advanced Practice Nurse*. Pittsburgh, PA: Hospice and Palliative Nurses Association; 2014.

16. Hospice and Palliative Nurses Association (HPNA). *Value of the Licensed Practical Vocational Nurse in Palliative Care*. [Position Statement] 2013. hpna.advancingexpertcare.org/education/position-statements/. Accessed October 20, 2014.

17. Centers for Medicare & Medicaid Services (CMS). *Appendix M—Guidance to Surveyors: Hospice*. 2014. www.cms.gov/Regulations-and-Guidance/Guidance/Manuals/downloads/som107ap_m_hospice.pdf. Accessed July 23, 2014.

18. Snider S, Byrne D. Hospice Medicare Benefit Administration. In: Snapp J, ed. *Core Curriculum for the Hospice and Palliative Administrator*. Pittsburgh, PA: Hospice and Palliative Nurses Association; 2010:69-83.

19. Haugen DF, Nauck F, Caraceni F. The core team and the extended team. In: Hanks G, Cherny NI, Christakis NA, Fallon M, Kaasa S, Portenoy RK, eds. *Oxford Textbook of Palliative Medicine*. 4th ed. New York, NY: Oxford University Press; 2010:167-176.

20. Sherman DW, Matzo M, Metheny T. The interprofessional practice of palliative care nursing. In: Matzo M, Sherman DW, eds. *Palliative Care Nursing: Quality Care to the End of Life*. 4th ed. New York, NY: Springer Publishing Company; 2015:3-20.

21. Otis-Green S, Finberg IC. Enhancing team effectiveness. In: Ferrell BR, Coyle N, eds. *Oxford Textbook of Palliative Nursing*. 3rd ed. New York, NY: Oxford University Press; 2010:1225-1235.

22. Boreale K, Richardson B. Communication. In: Panke JT, Coyne PJ, eds. *Conversations in Palliative Care: Questions and Answers with the Experts*. 3rd ed. Pittsburgh, PA: Hospice and Palliative Nurses Association; 2011:33-44.

23. Benjamin M, Curtis J. *Ethics in Nursing: Cases, Principles, and Reasoning*. 4th ed. New York, NY: Oxford University Press; 2010.

24. Garvin GS, Smith E, Astrow A. Spirituality. In: Panke JT, Coyne PJ, eds. *Conversations in Palliative Care: Questions and Answers with the Experts*. 3rd ed. Pittsburgh, PA: Hospice and Palliative Nurses Association; 2011:123-127.

25. University of California San Francisco (UCSF). *Evaluating Health Information*. 2014. www. ucsfhealth.org/education/evaluating_health_information/index.html. Accessed July 18, 2014.

26. Sherman DW. Nursing and palliative care. In: Hanks G, Cherny NI, Christakis NA, Fallon M, Kaasa S, Portenoy RK, eds. *Oxford Textbook of Palliative Medicine*. 4th ed. New York, NY: Oxford University Press; 2010:177-183.

27. American Board of Nursing Specialties (ABNS). Statement on Continuing Competence for Nursing: A Call to Action—National Board for Certification of Hospice and Palliative Nurses. 2011. *Statement on Continuing Competence for Nursing: A Call to Action*. nursingcertification.org/pdf/Statement%20 on%20Continuing%20Competence%20for%20Nursing%20June%2011%20FINAL.pdf. Accessed October 20, 2014.

28. Vyas D, Hozain AE. Clinical peer review in the United States: history, legal development and subsequent abuse. *World J Gastroenterol*. 2014;20(21):6357-6363. doi: 10.3748/wjg.v20.i21.6357.

29. Benner P. *From Novice to Expert: Excellence and Power in Clinical Nursing Practice. Commemorative edition*. Upper Saddle River, NJ: Prentice Hall; 2001.

30. Schmal BA, Derrevere SK. The vital role of professional certification. *J Hosp Palliat Nurs*. 2012; 14(3):177-181. doi: 10.1097/NJH.0b013e31824df12d.

31. Hospice and Palliative Credentialing Center (HPCC). *Why Certification?* 2014. hpcc.advancingexpert care.org/competence/why-certification/. Accessed July 18, 2014.

32. Horton JR, Indelicato RA. The advanced practice nurse. In: Ferrell BR, Coyle N, eds. *Oxford Textbook of Palliative Nursing*. 3rd ed. New York, NY: Oxford University Press; 2010:1121-1129.

33. Martinez JM. Hospice and palliative nursing certification: the journey to defining a new nursing specialty. *J Hosp Palliat Nurs*. 2011;13(65):S29-S34. doi: 10.1097/NJH.0b013e318234d54c.

34. Wade CH. Perceived effects of specialty nurse certification: a review of the literature. *AORN J*. 2009; 89(1):183-192. doi: 10.1016/j.aorn.2008.06.015.

35. Valente SM. Improving professional practice through certification. *J Nurses Staff Dev.* 2010;26(5): 215-219. doi: 10.1097/NND.0b013e31819b561c.

36. Kendall-Gallagher D, Aiken LH, Sloane DM, Cimiotti JP. Nurse specialty certification, inpatient mortality, and failure to rescue. *J Nurs Schol.* 2011;43(2):188-194.

37. Piazza IM, Donahue M, Dykes PC. Differences in perceptions of empowerment among nationally certified and noncertified nurses. *J Nurs Adm.* 2006;36(5):277-283.

38. Vachon MLS. Four decades of selected research in hospice/palliative care: have the stressors changed. In: Renzenbrink I, ed. *Caregiver Stress and Staff Support in Illness, Dying, and Bereavement.* New York, NY: Oxford University Press; 2011:1-24.

39. Hospice and Palliative Nurses Association (HPNA). *Role of Hospice and Palliative Nurses in Research.* [Position Statement] 2012. hpna.advancingexpertcare.org/education/position-statements/. Accessed July 18, 2014.

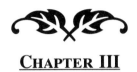

CHAPTER III

PATTERNS OF DISEASE PROGRESSION

Niki Koesel, ANP, ACHPN®, FPCN®
Marlene A. S. Foreman, RN, BSN, ACNS-BC, ACHPN®

I. **Cancer**

A. **Epidemiology**

1. Global cancer statistics[1]

    a) 12.6 million new cases of cancer diagnosed worldwide in 2008

    b) Most new cases of cancer are diagnosed in Eastern Asia with lung, stomach, and breast most frequently diagnosed

    c) Breast cancer is the most frequently diagnosed and is the leading cause of death from cancer in women worldwide

    d) Lung cancer is the most frequently diagnosed and the leading cause of death from cancer in men worldwide

2. National (United States) cancer statistics[2]

    a) More than 1.6 million estimated new cases of cancer in 2013 (excluding basal cell and squamous cell cancers of the skin)

    b) Breast cancer is the most frequently diagnosed cancer in women in the United States

    c) Prostate cancer is the most frequently diagnosed cancer in men in the United States

3. Cancer mortality[2]

    a) 580 350 Americans are estimated to have died in 2013 from a cancer diagnosis

    b) Cancer is the second most common cause of death in the United States following heart disease

    c) Lung cancer is the leading cause of death for men and women from cancer with a 16% survival rate for all stages combined[3]

    d) Breast cancer has the highest 5-year survival rate (all stages) of 89% while liver and pancreas have the lowest overall survival rate at 15% and 6%, respectively

4. Defining cancer

    a) Pathophysiology[2,4]

        i. Characterized by uncontrolled growth and spread of abnormal or mutated cells that can be caused by external and internal factors

        ii. Mutated cells have certain characteristics[4]

            (a) Can avoid apoptosis (cell death)

            (b) Resist normal aging process

            (c) Can replicate outside normal controlling mechanisms

            (d) Produce chemicals that dissolve surrounding tissue

            (e) Invade other parts of the body

            (f) Overcome the immune system

5. Staging criteria—TNM staging system[2]

    a) T—size and extent of primary tumor

    b) N—presence or absence of lymph node involvement

    c) M—presence or absence of distant metastases

    d) Stages 0 to IV are assigned based on TNM criteria with stage 0 being in situ and IV being most advanced disease

B. Process of Disease Progression[5]

1. Invasion—process where cells continue to divide and with increased bulk, pressure, and secretion of enzymes, cancer is spread locally or into surrounding structures

2. Angiogenesis—generation of blood vessels by the tumor site, which allows easier access for the tumor cells to enter the bloodstream; this increases risk of metastatic spread

3. Metastasis—the spread of cancer cells from a primary tumor site to distant sites in the body through one of several routes

    a) Direct invasion into an organ

    b) Seeding within a body cavity

    c) Spread through the lymphatic system

    d) Dissemination via capillaries and veins (most metastases occur this route)

4. Common sites for metastatic spread (see Table 3-1)

Table 3-1. Common Sites of Metastasis[6]

Cancer Type	Main Sites of Metastasis*								
	Adrenal Gland	Bone	Brain	Liver	Lung	Other Lung	Peritoneum	Skin/ Muscle	Vagina
Bladder		✓		✓	✓				
Breast		✓	✓	✓	✓				
Colorectal				✓	✓		✓		
Kidney	✓	✓	✓	✓	✓				
Lung	✓	✓	✓	✓		✓			
Melanoma		✓	✓	✓	✓			✓	
Ovary				✓	✓		✓		
Pancreas				✓	✓		✓		
Prostate	✓	✓		✓	✓				
Stomach				✓	✓		✓		
Thyroid		✓		✓	✓				
Uterus		✓		✓	✓		✓		✓

*In alphabetical order. Brain includes the neural tissue of the brain (parenchyma) and the leptomeninges (the 2 innermost membranes—arachnoid mater and pia mater—of the 3 membranes known as the meninges that surround the brain and spinal cord; the space between the arachnoid mater and the pia mater contains cerebrospinal fluid). Lung includes the main part of the lung (parenchyma) as well as the pleura (the membrane that covers the lungs and lines the chest cavity).

II. Genetics[7]

A. Hereditary Cancer Syndromes

1. Attributed to genes that are passed from either parent to their children

2. 5% to 10% of cancers are hereditary

3. Family history of maternal and paternal lineage is vital to determine those at risk and should include race/ethnicity, current health status, current age or age at death, types of primary cancer, age at diagnosis for each cancer, bilaterality of paired organs, environmental exposures

4. Hereditary syndromes that have evidence showing improved survival or benefit of early detection include hereditary breast and ovarian syndromes, hereditary colorectal syndrome, multiple endocrine neoplasia, Li-Fraumeni syndrome

5. Epigenetics leads to the reduced expression of the DNA repair genes and thereby contributes to genetic instability[8]

B. Features of Hereditary Cancers[9]

1. Early age of onset

2. Autosomal dominant inheritance pattern

3. Cancer in 2 or more close relatives

4. Bilaterally in paired organs

5. Multiple primary cancers in 1 person

C. Ethical and Social Issues Surrounding Genetic Testing

1. Autonomy—patients have the right to choose genetic testing or refuse testing regardless of their risk assessment

2. Survivor guilt of family members who did not inherit a genetic mutation

3. Transmitter guilt of a family member who passed on the genetic mutation

4. Increased anxiety and anticipatory grief in individuals who have or are determined to be at high risk for developing a malignancy, including higher risk of suicide potential

5. Stigmatization of the family members who are found with a genetic mutation

6. Potential for unethical practices by clinical researchers

7. Payer source discrimination for testing; increased risk for "dropping" patients if malignant trend identified in family

III. Treatment in Cancer

A. Types of Treatment[10]

1. Curative—the intention of the treatment is elimination of the tumor and cure of the patient from cancer

2. Adjuvant—a type of treatment that is used in addition to or after the primary therapy in order to aid in the principal treatment regimen and to lower the risk of cancer returning (e.g., radiation after surgical resection to minimize risk of local recurrence)

3. Neoadjuvant—a treatment given before the primary therapy (e.g., chemotherapy prior to surgical resection)

4. Palliative—a treatment that is intended to relieve or alleviate the symptoms or burden of the cancer and improve quality of life; not intended to cure

B. Treatment Modalities

1. Surgery—used for prevention (precancerous lesions), diagnosis, staging, curative therapy, or palliation[11]

    a) High potential for cure when disease is localized

    b) Requires acceptable performance status and ability to tolerate anesthesia

    c) Serves as primary mechanism for obtaining necessary tissue for pathologic diagnosis of cancer

    d) Approaches such as computed tomography (CT)-guided, stereotactic, and endoscopic interventions are being increasingly utilized to avoid open surgical procedures

        i. Restorative surgery is used to restore function, close open skin or wounds from surgical defects, restore cosmetic appearance, or promote quality of life

    e)   Palliative surgery can be used to promote comfort and quality of life without intention of cure (e.g., tumor debulking, malignant bowel obstruction, bone stabilization)[11]

2.   Radiation—approximately 60% of patients with cancer will receive radiation at some point of their treatment[12]

    a)   Teletherapy—delivery of radiation therapy from an external source

    b)   Brachytherapy—radioactive source is placed inside of or directly on the body

    c)   Curative—treatment regimens are typically lengthy and with a higher toxicity (e.g., early Hodgkin's disease or skin cancer)

    d)   Disease control—can provide results/disease control for months to years (e.g., recurrent breast cancer, lung cancer, soft tissue sarcomas)

    e)   Palliation—can provide relief of pain, prevention of pathologic fractures, return of function and mobility, treatment for oncologic emergencies, treatment of hemorrhage, obstruction, and ulcerations (e.g., painful skeletal lesions, superior vena cava syndrome, central nervous system [CNS] effects from brain lesions)

    f)   Prophylactic—a growing number of patients with small cell carcinoma are receiving prophylactic cranial irradiation given this cancer's high prevalence of brain metastasis[13]

    g)   Side effects can be acute, subacute, and late

        i.   Acute—site-specific, short-term effects such as mucositis, xerostomia, gastrointestinal distress, fatigue, or tissue ulceration; typically resolve at the conclusion of treatment

        ii.   Subacute—effects that appear within weeks to a few months after completion of treatment such as pneumonitis, rib fractures, renal damage

        iii.   Late—dependent on dose, volume, and length of radiation and can occur after 6 months following treatment such as small or large bowel injury, infertility, following abdominal treatment

    h)   Typical side effects—skin reaction, fatigue, weight loss, myelosuppression, alopecia, nausea and vomiting, mucositis, xerostomia[12]

3.   Chemotherapy—can be utilized for cure, control of disease, or palliation[14]

    a)   The cell-kill hypothesis is used to describe the effects of chemotherapy on a patient's cells—both tumor and normal cells—and response is based on cellular kinetics, cell cycle time, and disease burden

    b)   Most chemotherapies are cytotoxic to the reproductive cycle and normal functions of tumor cells, though now targeted therapies are being utilized to decrease the effects on normal tissue and focus the drug's effects upon the tumor cells (e.g., antiangiogenesis agents, monoclonal antibodies, tyrosine kinase inhibitors, hormonal agents)

    c)   Combination therapies (multiple agents) are often used to allow targeting of the disease at varying stages of the cell life cycle and growth[14]

    d)   Modes of administration

        i.   Oral

        ii.   Intravenous (peripheral or central venous access device)

iii.   Intramuscular

iv.   Intraarterial

v.   Intraperitoneal

vi.   Intrapleural

vii.   Intravesicular or intravesical (within the urinary bladder)

viii.   Intrathecal, epidural

ix.   Intralesional or intratumoral (directly into the lesion or tumor)

e)   Side effects of chemotherapy—incidence and severity are dependent on drug dosage, administration schedule, mechanism of action, comorbid conditions, performance status, utilization of prevention techniques[15]

    i.   Expected side effects should be prevented when possible and typically do not lead to discontinuation of regimen

        (a)   Stomatitis

        (b)   Alopecia

        (c)   Myelosuppression (e.g., neutropenia, anemia, thrombocytopenia)

        (d)   Nausea with and without vomiting, anorexia

        (e)   Diarrhea

        (f)   Fatigue

    ii.   Severe toxicities can often limit the treatment offered, may be life-threatening, and lead to long-term effects

    iii.   Long-term side effects/toxicities—occur weeks to months after administration

        (a)   Cardiotoxicity—toxicity to the cardiac system induced by chemotherapy is similar in presentation to congestive heart failure with dyspnea, cough, pedal edema, poor response to diuretics or digitalis (most common with anthracyclines)

        (b)   Neurotoxicity—if patient develops neurotoxicity during treatment, it may be necessary to hold the treatment, and consider a 50% dose reduction if the treatment resumes

            (i)   Typically caused by plant alkaloids, taxanes, and etoposide

            (ii)   Can occur in the periphery (extremities) or in the autonomic nervous system (e.g., constipation, ileus, impotence, urinary retention, postural hypotension)

            (iii)   Most common effect is present as chemotherapy-associated peripheral neuropathy (CAPN). CAPN is often reversible following the end of treatment but can persist long term in some circumstances. Presentation starts with a stocking and glove (which feels like the patient is wearing socks and/or gloves) distribution with report of burning, tingling, numbness, or vibratory sensations

    iv.   Pulmonary toxicity—typically irreversible and is progressive

        (a)   Presents as a drug-induced pneumonitis or restrictive lung disease with dyspnea, unproductive cough, basilar rales, tachypnea, and low grade fever

        (b)   Most common causative agent is bleomycin

    v.   Hepatotoxicity

        (a)   Presentation includes elevated hepatic enzymes and can progress to jaundice, hepatomegaly, encephalopathy, and abdominal pain

        (b)   High risk of reactivation with history of hepatitis B and C. Most hepatotoxicity is transient, though can lead to cirrhosis in a few patients

    f)   Nephrotoxicity—a dose-limiting toxicity for some chemotherapies, dependent on severity of renal dysfunction

        i.   Kidney damage can range from direct renal cell damage to obstructive nephropathy

        ii.   Cisplatin is known for mild-to-severe nephrotoxicity and can occur 3–21 hours after given; can persist for several years and may be irreversible[16]

4.   Complementary and alternative therapies (CAM)—term used that includes integrated approaches used in conjunction with conventional treatment, or alternative treatment when used in place of conventional therapies

    a)   Mind-body medicine (e.g., hypnosis, relaxation, imagery)—techniques to enhance the mind's ability to affect bodily functions

    b)   Biologically-based therapy (e.g., enzyme therapy, mistletoe, melatonin)—use of products from nature such as herbs, vitamins, and foods to assist in treatment and healing

    c)   Manipulative and body-based methods (e.g., chiropractor, reflexology, massage)—manipulation or movement of 1 or more body parts

    d)   Energy therapy (e.g., Reiki, healing touch)—use of energy fields to promote a bodily response

    e)   Acupuncture, trigger point injections

    f)   Spiritual therapy (e.g., prayer, spiritual healing)—treatment geared toward a connection with a higher power for healing[17]

IV. Prognostication

A. Clinical Indications of Poor Prognosis in Advanced Cancer[18]

1.   Poor performance status—a decline in functional status is the most important prognostic indicator and is a measure of how much a patient can do independently. In the cancer population performance status is typically measured by the Eastern Cooperative Oncology Group (ECOG) score, the Palliative Performance Scale (PPS), or the Karnofsky Index

2.   Malignant hypercalcemia (except in breast cancer or multiple myeloma)

3.   Malignant pericardial effusion

4. Carcinomatous meningitis

5. Multiple brain metastases

6. Malignant ascites

7. Malignant pleural effusion

8. Malignant bowel obstruction

9. Hemorrhage, disseminated intravascular coagulation (DIC)

10. Spinal cord compression

11. Superior vena cava syndrome

V. Major Cancer Diagnoses[19]

A. Lung Cancer

1. Leading cause of cancer death for women and men worldwide; average age of diagnosis is 71

2. Despite new efforts at prevention, 5-year survival rate (16%) has not improved over the past 10 years; cigarette smoking remains highest risk factor[2]

3. 50% of cases start in central structures of the chest and large airways and can present with hemoptysis; dyspnea; cough; hoarseness; atelectasis; harsh sounds with each breath; pain in chest, shoulder, or back unrelated to coughing; and postobstructive pneumonia

4. Common sites of metastases are brain, liver, bone, and adrenal glands

5. Risk factors—cigarette, cigar, or pipe smoking; radon gas exposure; occupational or environmental exposure to secondhand smoke, asbestos, certain metals, radiation, air pollution, diesel exhaust, and paint fumes; history of tuberculosis; positive family history

6. Associated symptoms—chest pain, fatigue, cough, dyspnea, anorexia/weight loss

7. Treatment is determined by stage and can include surgery, radiation, and chemotherapy

B. Breast Cancer[20]

1. Most frequently diagnosed cancer in women and leading cause of death due to cancer in women 20 to 59 years old

2. More than 50% occurs in women over age 61

3. Risk factors include hormone exposure, family or personal history, lifestyle factors, exposure to radiation; smoking; obesity; early menarche; late menopause; postmenopausal hormone therapy; excessive alcohol use; nulliparity;[21] 5% to 6% are associated with a genetic mutation (e.g., *BRCA1, BRCA2*)

4. Both surgery and chemoprevention are utilized to treat women with a family or personal history of breast cancer

5. Prognosis—younger women have a poorer prognosis related to hormone shifts and ovulation cycles; well-differentiated breast cancer cells have a better prognosis than undifferentiated cell types; hormone receptor status

6. Common sites of metastases are bone (most common), skin, lung, lymph nodes, liver, brain; and pleural effusion; many patients present with symptoms associated with metastatic site

7. Associated symptoms—lymphedema, pain, nausea, dyspnea, fatigue, anorexia, mental status changes

C. **Gastrointestinal Cancers**[2,22,23]

1. Pancreatic—less than 24% of patients survive longer than 1-year and 5-year survival is 6%; usually discovered in advanced stage; frequently resistant to chemotherapy and radiotherapy; fifth most common cause of cancer deaths in the United States

   a) Age is strongest risk factor and occurs between 60 and 80 years of age; other risk factors include smoking, environmental smoke exposure, chemical exposure

   b) Most common presentation includes weight loss and wasting; presentation will depend on location of tumor and will present earliest when in the head of the pancreas

   c) Associated symptoms—weight loss, pain, jaundice, nausea, fatigue

2. Colorectal—third-leading cause of cancer death in men and women; 5-year survival of those with distant spread is less than 10%

   a) Risk factors include genetic mutations, older age, poor diet, fecal carcinogens, bile acids, lifestyle, alcohol intake, inflammatory bowel conditions, cholecystectomy

   b) Associated symptoms—anemia, fatigue, partial or complete obstruction, pain, blood in the stool, fistula

3. Gastric (stomach)—significantly higher incidence in males, Caucasians to African-Americans (2:1)[22]; overall incidence has declined in the United States over the past 35 years[24]; third most common cause of cancer deaths globally[25]

   a) Risk factors—presence of helicobacter pylori (strongest risk factor); high amounts of salt, smoked, or pickled food in the diet; smoking; hereditary factors (e.g., Lynch syndrome); living in high risk areas including Japan and Korea; pernicious anemia

   b) Associated symptoms—dyspepsia, weight loss, anorexia, fatigue, epigastric pain, abdominal distention, gastrointestinal bleeding, bowel obstruction

4. Liver (hepatocellular carcinoma most common)[26]; most common solid tumor worldwide[27]

   a) Risk factors—chronic viral hepatitis, underlying liver disease, environmental and chemical toxin exposure, alcohol and smoking, nonalcoholic fatty liver disease, diabetes mellitus

   b) Death typically occurs from cachexia, gastrointestinal or esophageal varices bleeding, liver failure and coma, fatal hemorrhage

   c) Associated symptoms—pain, jaundice, pruritus, ascites, dyspnea, nausea/vomiting, early satiety, fatigue, weight loss

   d) Five-year overall survival rate 15% in the United States[2]

5. Esophageal—sixth leading cause of death from cancer and occurs most frequently in those over the age of 50[28]; overall 5-year survival rate in the United States is approximately 15%, with most people dying within the first year of diagnosis

a) Risk factors include smoking, high alcohol consumption, prior radiation to the chest, gastroesophageal reflux disease, Barrett's esophagus, and being male[29]

b) Associated symptoms—dysphagia, weight loss, diarrhea/constipation, excessive oral secretions, hemorrhage (tumors that invade vasculature), dumping syndrome (following esophagectomy)

D.   Genitourinary Cancers

1. Prostate—most common malignancy in males and second-leading cause of cancer death[30] with a 5-year survival rate approximately 99% in the United States[31]

   a) Risk factors—age, lifestyle, heredity, African-American ethnicity, fat consumption, smoking, increased alcohol consumption

   b) Most patients present with urinary dysfunction, symptoms of benign prostatic hypertrophy (BPH), nocturia; asymptomatic in early stages

   c) Associated symptoms—cachexia, weight loss, bone pain, leg or scrotal edema, erectile dysfunction, coagulation disorders, bladder or urethral obstruction

2. Bladder—median age at diagnosis is 65 years and men have 3 times higher incidence[32] with a 5-year survival rate approximately 77% in the United States[33]

   a) Smoking is the highest risk factor followed by occupational exposure to carcinogens and gene mutations

   b) Presenting symptoms include hematuria (most common), dysuria, urinary frequency, urinary tract infections

   c) Associated symptoms—sexual dysfunction (following removal of bladder), pain, vaginal dryness, decreased libido

3. Renal—localized disease is mostly curable and resectable; 5-year survival rate is 10% for those with stage IV disease[34]

   a) Risk factors—smoking, obesity, hypertension, regular use of nonsteroidal anti-inflammatory drugs (NSAIDs), faulty genes, hepatitis C[35-37]

   b) Associated symptoms—gross hematuria, costovertebral pain, weight loss, anorexia, pain, nausea/vomiting, fatigue

E.   Gynecological Cancers

1. Cervical—second-most common cancer in women worldwide and the human papillomavirus (HPV) is highest risk factor for the development of this cancer[38]

   a) Most cases are found during routine gynecologic examinations (usually asymptomatic in preinvasive stages) though can present with reports of intermenstrual bleeding, postcoital bleeding, or heavy menstrual flow

   b) Associated symptoms—pain, cachexia, bleeding/anemia, lymphedema, vaginal stenosis (secondary to treatment), ureteral obstruction

2. Ovarian—fifth leading cause of cancer deaths in women and most lethal of all gynecological cancers[39]; overall survival rate in the United States is 45% if discovered early

a) Risk factors—nulliparity, use of infertility drugs, pelvic inflammatory disease, use of talc, family history of breast or ovarian cancer, Lynch syndrome, Jewish descent, low serum gonadotropin, mutation present in the BRCA1 and BRCA2 genes

b) Associated symptoms—bloating, pelvic or abdominal pain, early satiety, urinary dysfunction, symptoms of intestinal obstruction, ascites, malnutrition, lymphedema, fistulas

c) Spread beyond the ovaries is found in 24% of women with stage I up to 73% of women with stage IV disease upon first surgery[40]

3. Endometrial—predominant cancer of the female genital tract and known as the most curable cancer when diagnosed early,[41] overall 5-year survival rate in the United States is greater than 80% if discovered early

a) Risk factors—postmenopausal state, obesity, nulliparity, late menopause, diabetes mellitus, polycystic ovarian syndrome, breast cancer, use of tamoxifen or unopposed estrogen, Lynch syndrome

b) Associated symptoms—structural-associated issues such as hematuria, bowel incontinence, pain, regional progression issues of ascites, bowel pattern changes, fistulas

F. Hematological Malignancies

1. Leukemia—includes both acute and chronic myelogenous and lymphocytic leukemias and myelodysplastic syndrome (acute myelocytic leukemia [AML] with lowest 5-year survival rate at 22%; chronic lymphocytic leukemia [CLL] with highest at 75%)[42]

a) Risk factors—antecedent hematological disorders, genetic predisposition, prior treatment for malignancy, chemical exposures, ionizing radiation, autoimmune diseases

b) Associated symptoms—fatigue, myelosuppression, thrombocytopenia, mucositis, gastrointestinal disturbances, tumor lysis syndrome

2. Lymphoma (Hodgkin's and non-Hodgkin's)—incidence has doubled since the 1970s; those with a T-cell origin are known to be most aggressive in progression; Hodgkin's is known as one of the most curable malignancies[43]

a) Lymphadenopathy is the most common presentation of both types of lymphoma

b) Associated symptoms—fatigue, myelosuppression, peripheral neuropathy (treatment related), organ toxicities related to treatments

3. Multiple myeloma—hallmarks of the disease include serum or urine monoclonal immunoglobulin, monoclonal plasmacytosis, bony lytic lesions[44]

a) Only risk factors identified include advanced age, African-American ethnicity, family history of monoclonal gammopathy of undetermined significance (MGUS)

b) Bone pain is most common presenting symptom (more than two-thirds of cases)

c) Associated symptoms—bone pain, symptoms of hypercalcemia and hyperuricemia, paraplegia (due to spinal cord compression), immunosuppression

G.   Head and Neck Cancer[45]

1.   Includes cancers of the oral cavity, pharynx, nasopharynx, oropharynx, hypopharynx, larynx, upper neck lymph nodes—is curable if diagnosed early though most cases found when advanced

2.   Risk factors include tobacco and alcohol use (all), HPV (oral cancers), Epstein-Barr virus, and inhalation of toxic chemicals and nitrosamines (nasopharynx)

3.   Associated symptoms—dysphagia, speech disorders, mucositis, xerostomia, loss of taste, trismus, pain, fatigue, constipation/diarrhea (from those requiring gastrostomy [G]-tube feedings)

H.   Malignant Melanoma[46]

1.   Worldwide incidence is rising faster than any other malignancy

2.   Tumor thickness is the most important factor to predict survival

3.   Risk factors—fair or light skin tone, presence of large congenital melanocytic nevi, a high number of nevi (moles), positive family history of melanoma, frequent and prolonged exposure to ultraviolet rays, living closer to the equator

4.   Associated symptoms—ulceration, pruritus, bleeding or pain to the malignant area, symptoms related to the site of metastases, fatigue, anorexia (related to treatment)

I.   Brain Tumors[47]

1.   Most prevalent central nervous system (CNS) malignancy is a metastatic brain tumor

2.   Five-year survival for primary brain tumors (most common is malignant glioma) range from 28% to 31%; however, for glioblastoma multiforme (GBM), survival is 12 to 15 months

3.   Associated symptoms (can range from focal effects, effects of increased intracranial pressure [ICP], and from displacement of brain structures)—decrease or loss of motor function, speech, seizures, memory and/or attention deficits, headaches, decreased level of consciousness, rapid change in vital signs/respiratory arrest (herniation)

VI.   Oncologic Emergencies

A.   Principles of Treatment

1.   Treatment of oncologic emergencies should be dependent on the patient's prognosis, functional status, and goals of treatment. Goals should be clarified upon initial assessment and upon the finding of the oncologic event

B.   Spinal Cord Compression[48,49]

1.   Vertebral metastases most commonly have spread from breast, lung, or prostate

2.   Compression is caused by direct pressure from the tumor mass or by displacement of bony fragments into the spinal canal

3.   Back pain is the most common presenting symptom of vertebral disease followed by lower motor neuron deficits (hypotonicity, hyperreflexia, paralysis), urinary dysfunction, and constipation

4. Mainstays of treatment (level of treatment will depend on goals of therapy)—dexamethasone, magnetic resonance imaging (MRI) or CT of spine, radiation therapy, and surgical evaluation

5. Outcomes and recovery are dependent upon tumor type (primary or metastatic), number of vertebrae involved, degree of neurologic impairment on presentation, oncologic status, and other medical conditions

C. **Syndrome of Inappropriate Secretion of Antidiuretic Hormone (SIADH)**

1. Definition—the inappropriate production and secretion of the antidiuretic hormone causing hyponatremia, urine osmolality higher than plasma osmolality, and elevated urinary sodium and is primarily associated with small cell lung cancer

2. Symptoms—headache, nausea, weakness, anorexia, fatigue, muscle cramps, changes in mental status, lethargy, psychosis (all associated with hyponatremia)

3. Treatment—treatment of underlying malignancy, free water restriction to correct hyponatremia, seizure precautions, hypertonic fluid administration if severe (rate of sodium correction should not exceed 8 mEq/L), daily weight and careful monitoring of fluid balance, demeclocycline (drug of choice) for chronic SIADH

D. **Cardiac Tamponade[50]**

1. Definition—result of excess accumulation of fluid in the pericardial sac causing compression of the heart and diminished blood flow to the ventricles. This occurs as an effect of treatment or disease within the pericardium (metastatic or primary)

2. Most commonly occurs in sarcomas, teratomas, mesotheliomas, breast, lung, or hematologic malignancies

3. Symptoms—tachycardia, cyanosis, oliguria/anuria, hypotension, anxiety, symptoms of shock, dyspnea, weakness, cough, dysphagia, peripheral edema, jugular venous distention, gastrointestinal disturbances

4. Treatment—stabilization of hemodynamic status with oxygen, fluid volume resuscitation, inotropic agents, bed rest, pericardiocentesis, pericardial window if other management not effective

E. **Superior Vena Cava Syndrome[51]**

1. A syndrome that develops from the obstruction or compression of the superior vena cava (the vessel that carries blood to the heart from the chest, arms, head, and neck) resulting in increased venous pressure and decreased cardiac output

2. Most common cause is a malignancy present in the mediastinal area (small cell lung cancer most common)

3. Symptoms—facial and neck swelling, magenta or bluish discoloration of skin, upper extremity swelling, dyspnea (most common), cough, dilated collateral chest wall veins

4. Treatment—radiation and/or chemotherapy (if indicated for that malignancy and chemosensitive), thrombolytic therapy (if cause is a catheter thrombosis), placement of an endovascular stent to bypass obstruction

F. Disseminated Intravascular Coagulation[52]

1. Definition—inappropriate and exaggerated overstimulation of normal coagulation when thrombosis, then bleeding occurs

2. Most commonly occurs in sepsis, acute leukemia, tumor lysis, massive tissue injury, obstetric complications, transfusion reactions[53]

3. Symptoms—focal ischemia, acrocyanosis, superficial gangrene, frank gangrene, altered sensation, ulceration of gastrointestinal system, jaundice, decreased urinary output, dyspnea, widespread thrombosis or bleeding

4. Treatment—management of underlying cause, oxygen, fluid replacement; consider blood products if appropriate, anticoagulant therapy

G. Septic Shock[54]

1. Definition—condition when overwhelming infection leads to hypotension, low blood flow, impaired coagulation, and impaired clot breakdown leading to poor tissue perfusion, cell ischemia, cell hypoxia, and organ failure

2. Patients with cancer show the highest rate of sepsis due to immunosuppression from chemotherapy, radiation, other treatment modalities, urinary tract infections, or vascular access catheters

3. Symptoms—fever, shaking chills, hypotension, tachycardia, tachypnea, dyspnea, mental status changes, increased white blood cell count, oliguria. In immunocompromised patients, presentation of septic shock may be atypical (e.g., low white blood cell count, hypothermia)

4. Treatment—immediate antibiotic therapy, hemodynamic support with volume replacement, blood products as appropriate, vasopressor/inotrope support, oxygen

H. Tumor Lysis Syndrome[55]

1. Definition—a metabolic response to tumor cells being killed rapidly resulting in hyperuricemia, hyperkalemia, hyperphosphatemia, hypocalcemia most frequently caused from chemotherapy, and most often in patients with hematological malignancies or poorly differentiated Burkitt's lymphoma

2. Symptoms—fatigue/lethargy, nausea, vomiting, anorexia, diarrhea, flank pain, cramps, muscle weakness, cloudy urine, increase in heart rate and blood pressure, neuromuscular symptoms as syndrome worsens (to include tetany or convulsions), sudden mental incapacity and emotional lability

3. Treatment—key is prevention 24 to 48 hours prior to treatment, frequent lab studies, aggressive hydration and diuresis, allopurinol, hemodialysis if abnormalities do not quickly reverse

VII. Common Psychosocial Issues in Cancer[56]

A. Quality-of-Life Issues

1. Both physical and psychosocial—affect both those with advanced cancer at diagnosis and those who are survivors from their cancer

a) Fear of recurrence

b) Depression

c) Finding meaning in their diagnosis

d) Financial stressors/employment changes or loss

e) Role clarification within their families (e.g., being unable to serve as a caregiver)

f) Cognitive impairment from treatments (e.g., "chemo brain")

g) Anticipatory grief

VIII. End-of-Life Care Considerations in Cancer

A. Decisions Related to Treatment in Advanced Disease[57]

1. Most patients are willing to seek treatment for even a 1-month extension of survival

2. Studies also show that patients continue to not be well-informed about prognosis and full benefits/burdens from antineoplastic therapies

3. Decisions about fluids, enteral feeding support, disabling defibrillator, code status

4. There is conflict for many who wish to participate in clinical trials and continue with curative treatment but also need support services such as hospice and/or palliative care since they may not be able to access both

5. Only 36.9% of hospice admissions were for a primary diagnosis of cancer in 2012[58]

6. Location of end-of-life care

B. Most Common Symptoms at the End of Life[59]

1. Fatigue

2. Pain

3. Noisy breathing/terminal secretions

4. Delirium

5. Dyspnea/cough

6. Urinary incontinence and/or retention

INTRODUCTION TO NON-CANCER CONDITIONS—Nonmalignant conditions tend to have a lengthy, chronic, and debilitating trajectory that can end in sudden death or a terminal phase. Due to the frequency of exacerbations and remissions, prognostication can be challenging. Persons with these conditions and their families may benefit from interdisciplinary palliative care from the time of diagnosis, and hospice care as they enter the final stages of illness.

The information in this chapter reflects current evidence-based disease progression, the role of palliative care, and guidelines for hospice eligibility. Persons with multisystem involvement may be eligible for hospice even if they do not meet specific criteria. "Adult Failure to Thrive" and "Generalized Debility" are no longer recognized as primary hospice diagnoses by the Centers for Medicare & Medicaid (CMS). However, they can be used for supporting evidence for hospice eligibility.

IX. Cardiac Conditions

A. Cardiac Disease

1. Leading cause of death in the United States for both women and men and the most costly in healthcare expenditures. It is also known as the most preventable disease process related to control of blood pressure, cholesterol, and diet.[60] Cardiac disease includes both cardiomyopathies and coronary artery disease, both of which impact quality of life by decreasing functional status due to progressive symptoms including dyspnea, hypoxia, and peripheral edema. Pain may occur due to cardiac ischemia, peripheral vascular disease, vascular occlusions, and other conditions such as osteoarthritis[61]

B. Pathophysiology

1. Heart failure can result from any structural or functional cardiac disorder that impairs the ability of the ventricle to fill with or eject blood, which can lead to cardiomyopathy. Reduced cardiac output and heart failure occur because of systolic dysfunction and diastolic dysfunction.[62] The development of cardiac disease is usually insidious and occurs over many years. Obesity, diabetes, and genetics are implicated in the development of cardiovascular disease. Persons with inflammatory diseases, autoimmune conditions, and exposure to toxins including chemotherapy may have higher incidence of cardiac diseases. Cardiac conditions include diseases of the valves, coronary arteries, conduction system, and heart muscle

2. Systolic dysfunction (left ventricular) is known for the inability to maintain adequate cardiac output, which leads to failure to oxygenate or perfuse organs and tissues and a decreased ejection fraction (pump failure). It can initially cause lung congestion as blood is not able to enter the left atrium and ventricle. This then leads to a hypertrophic left ventricle (cardiomyopathy) that weakens the muscle[63]

   a) Signs and symptoms

      i. Dyspnea, orthopnea, paroxysmal nocturnal dyspnea, cough

      ii. Fatigue and decreased exercise tolerance

      iii. Anxiety, restlessness, insomnia, depression

      iv. Tachycardia, palpitations

3. Diastolic dysfunction (right heart failure) is now being recognized as a separate or an additional component of heart disease, which is characterized by a preserved ejection fraction. Failure of the right ventricle leads to the inability to fill the ventricle appropriately. This can cause generalized systemic congestion with edema of extremities and hepatic system[61]

   a) Signs and symptoms

      i. Weight gain

      ii. Dependent peripheral edema, ascites

      iii. Weakness

      iv. Anorexia, nausea

C. Palliative Care in Heart Disease

1. The integration of palliative care in heart disease can be vital in supporting a patient's quality of life and treatment goals. Prognostication is difficult in heart disease due to the unpredictable nature of the disease process. It is important to understand the class or stage of the disease when assisting patients and families understand their options and quality-of-life needs (see Table 3-2). It is recommended that palliative care become part of the treatment plan once patients are New York Heart Association (NYHA) Class III–IV in order to begin the education and symptom management required to maintain quality of life. It is also vital to continue appropriate medical management to maximize symptom relief and minimize side effects. Along with cardiology specialists' input, pulmonology and nephrology consultations may be beneficial for symptom management assistance and the plan of care should be collaborative across disciplines[61,63]

Table 3-2. Stages and Classes of Heart Failure[adapted from 64,65]

ACC/AHA Stages in the Development of Heart Failure (heart failure stages C & D)		NYHA Classification of Heart Failure (all classes assume the presence of underlying cardiac disease)	
A	Patients at high risk of developing heart failure due to coronary artery disease (CAD), hypertension, diabetes, obesity, metabolic syndrome, cardiotoxin use or family history of cardiomyopathy	I	No limitation of physical activity
B	Patients with structural heart disease who have never had signs or symptoms of heart failure	II	Heart failure symptoms occur with ordinary physical activity, patient is comfortable at rest
C	Patients with current or prior heart failure symptoms associated with underlying structural heart disease	III	Heart failure symptoms occur with less than ordinary physical activity, but patient is comfortable at rest
D	Patients with advanced structural heart disease and refractory symptoms of heart failure requiring specialized interventions	IV	Symptoms occur with any activity and may occur at rest

2. Management of heart failure focuses on maximizing quality of life by prolonging survival, controlling symptoms, and promoting self-care (see Table 3-3)[63]

Table 3-3. Management of Heart Failure

• **Pharmacological** —Diuretics —Angiotensin-converting enzyme (ACE) inhibitors —Angiotensin II receptor blockers (ARBs) —Beta blockers —Aldosterone antagonists —Phophodiesterase-5 inhibition —Statins —Nitrates —Calcium channel blockers —Antiarrhythmics —Cardiac glycosides —Opioids, antianxiety agents	• **Nonpharmacological treatments** —Exercise conditioning —Stress reduction —Dietary changes —Supportive therapies including home health, physical therapy, occupational therapy • **Oxygen supplementation** • **Optimal management of comorbidities** • **Surgical procedures** —Pacemaker and/or automatic implantable cardioverter defibrillator (AICD) insertion —Left ventricular assist device (LVAD) insertion

D. **Hospice**

1. As the heart is further damaged and the body is unable to compensate due to increasing ischemia and edema, the patient and family need to review their goals of care with the provider to determine the most appropriate site of care, level of treatment, and any limitations they wish to place upon aggressive measures. Prognostication in heart disease is complicated and uncertain; therefore, the patient's goals are very important in the decisions related to hospice involvement. The eligibility guidelines are based on both pathophysiologic factors in addition to the frequency and severity of exacerbations and the effect upon the functional status (see Table 3-4)

Table 3-4. Hospice Eligibility Criteria for Heart Disease[66]

Patients are considered to be in the terminal stage of heart disease (life expectancy of 6 months or less) if they meet the following criteria. 1 and 2 should be present. Factors from 3 will add supporting documentation	
1. At the time of initial certification or recertification for hospice, the patient is or has been already optimally treated for heart disease or is not a candidate for a surgical procedure, or has declined a procedure. Optimally treated means that patients who are not on vasodilators have a medical reason for refusing these drugs (e.g., hypotension, renal disease). 2. The patient is classified as NYHA Class IV and may have significant symptoms of heart failure or angina at rest. (Class IV patients with heart disease have an inability to carry on any physical activity without discomfort. Symptoms of heart failure or of the anginal syndrome may be present even at rest. If any physical activity is undertaken, discomfort is increased.) Significant congestive heart failure may be documented by an ejection fraction of ≤ 20%, but is not required if not already available.	3. Documentation of the following factors will support but is not required to establish eligibility for hospice care a. Treatment resistant symptomatic supraventricular or ventricular arrhythmias b. History of cardiac arrest or resuscitation c. History of unexplained syncope d. Brain embolism of cardiac origin e. Concomitant HIV disease

2. Implanted devices

a) Pacemakers—the deactivation of a pacemaker is not typically done at the end of life as this device will not delay the dying process because the dying heart will not respond to signals

b) Automatic implantable cardioverter defibrillator (AICD)—address the deactivation of AICDs once a goal of comfort and a do not resuscitate (DNR) status is determined. Allowing the AICD to remain active at the time of death can cause unnecessary pain and distress to both the patient and family. This discussion and decision should include the patient, family, and cardiology team to ensure good communication and collaboration[67]

X. Neurologic Conditions

A. Many central and peripheral nervous system conditions that may progress to serious morbidity and death

1. Neurologic conditions include cerebrovascular accidents, trauma, and degenerative diseases, all of which can be difficult to prognosticate due to uncertain trajectories and common associated complications that may arise. The most common cerebral problems are ischemic and hemorrhagic stroke and brain injury from accidents or violence. Neurodegenerative diseases (e.g., multiple sclerosis, amyotrophic lateral sclerosis) usually have an insidious onset and progress very slowly over many years although some are more rapid

B. Strokes

1. Strokes can be classified as hemorrhagic or ischemic. Strokes are the fourth leading cause of death in the United States and more commonly occur in males. Hypertension is the strongest risk factor for a stroke, though atrial fibrillation is also a significant risk factor primarily in the elderly[68–71]

2. Pathophysiology

a) Ischemic stroke is the result of an occlusion that inhibits circulation to parts of the brain and is the cause of approximately 87% of strokes.[72] The specific area of the brain and the size of the area involved determine the deficits encountered and the degree of severity. The most common symptom is one-sided weakness or paralysis that will occur on the opposite side of the body from the side of the damage to the brain. Ischemic strokes can be caused by atrial fibrillation; septic embolus; embolus from the heart, aorta, or intracranial arteries; or microangiopathy from small vessel disease (due to diabetes or hypertension)[73,74]

b) Hemorrhagic strokes usually occur suddenly due to a rupture of a blood vessel, causing an intracranial bleed. Alterations in consciousness, headache, and nausea and vomiting are typical symptoms of a hemorrhagic stroke.[73] Subarachnoid hemorrhage from head trauma or an intracranial aneurysm is a cause of significant neurologic damage and death

3. Acute signs and symptoms—difficulty walking; aphasia (talking and understanding others); paralysis or numbness of face, arm, or leg; vision impairment; headache, which may be associated with vomiting

4. Chronic signs and symptoms—hemiparesis or hemi-weakness, dysphagia, expressive and/or receptive aphasia, apraxia, ataxia, and others

5. Palliative care—the initial response following a stroke is aimed at preserving as much brain function as possible, preventing complications, and rehabilitating the person to optimum functional level. However, in some cases, based on the extent of the stroke and the functional deficits associated, it may become evident that the person will not recover to a functional quality of life or even survive without artificial support. Many complications can also arise following a stroke, including aspiration pneumonias and severe infections from debility that may lead to the patient's eventual decline or death. Providers should discuss realistic goals for the patient with the family. If an advance directive was initiated, these guidelines should be followed when recovery is not expected or if the eventual outcome would not be considered an acceptable quality of life for the patient. Once goals of care are determined, treatments are aimed at maintaining comfort and preventing complications of immobility and debility

6. Medical management—dependent on goals of care

    a) Disease-specific therapy—anticoagulation, tissue plasminogen activator (must be given within 4.5 hours of stroke symptom presentation), corticosteroids, reduction of risk factors for recurrent stroke

    b) Opioids

    c) Antipsychotics and/or anxiolytics

    d) Anticholinergics

    e) Antidepressant therapy

    f) Surgical intervention

        i. Ischemic stroke

            (a) Intra-arterial thrombolysis—delivering medications directly to the brain using a catheter

            (b) Mechanical thrombectomy—using a device to break up or remove the clot

        ii. Hemorrhagic stroke

            (a) Surgical clipping

            (b) Endovascular embolization—coiling

            (c) Surgical arteriovenous malformation (AVM) removal

    g) Nonpharmacologic needs

        i. Speech language and pathology evaluation to determine communication and nutritional needs

        ii. Always expect that the person can hear you, so let them know when you are in the room, repositioning, or bathing them, etc.

        iii. Psychosocial support related to the loss of functional capabilities

C. **Hospice**

    1.   Specific findings may support poor prognosis based on location and size of defect. Strokes occurring with ischemia to the middle cerebral artery, basilar artery thrombosis, or brainstem or a severe intracerebral or subarachnoid hemorrhage are known to have a fatal outcome if the patient is unable to pursue aggressive surgical interventions. In addition, if the patient's goals are clear for a natural death and the patient has devastating functional loss from the stroke, prognosis will be based on the expected associated complications including pneumonia or infection from immobility. Discussions around the patient's wishes for artificial nutrition and mechanical ventilation/tracheostomy are typically necessary in this setting (see Table 3-5)[69,73]

Table 3-5. Hospice Eligibility Criteria for Stroke and Coma[66]

Patients will be considered to be in the terminal stage of stroke and coma (life expectancy of 6 months or less) if they meet the following criteria	

Stroke
 1. Karnofsky Performance Status (KPS) or Palliative Performance Scale of 40% or less
 2. Inability to maintain hydration and caloric intake with 1 of the following
   a. Weight loss > 10% in the last 6 months or > 7.5% in the last 3 months
   b. Serum albumin < 2.5 gm/dL
   c. Current history of pulmonary aspiration not responsive to speech language pathology intervention
   d. Sequential calorie counts documenting inadequate caloric/fluid intake
   e. Dysphagia severe enough to prevent the patient from receiving food and fluids necessary to sustain life, in a patient who declines or does not receive artificial nutrition and hydration
 	
 Coma (any etiology)
 Comatose patients with any 3 of the following on day 3 of coma
 a. Abnormal brainstem response
 b. Absent verbal response
 c. Absent withdrawal response to pain
 d. Serum creatinine > 1.5 mg/dL
	Documentation of the following factors will support eligibility for hospice care
	 Documentation of medical complications, in the context of progressive clinical decline, within the previous 12 months, which support a terminal prognosis
	 a. Aspiration pneumonia
	 b. Upper urinary tract infection (pyelonephritis)
	 c. Sepsis
	 d. Refractory stage 3–4 decubitus ulcers
	 e. Fever recurrent after antibiotics
	
	 Documentation of diagnostic imaging factors which support poor prognosis after stroke include
	 A. For nontraumatic hemorrhagic stroke
	   1. Large-volume hemorrhage on CT
	     a. Infratentorial: ≥ 20 mL
	     b. Supratentorial: ≥ 50 mL
	   2. Ventricular extension of hemorrhage
	   3. Surface area of involvement of hemorrhage ≥ 30% of cerebrum
	   4. Midline shift ≥ 1.5 cm
	   5. Obstructive hydrocephalus in patient who declines, or is not a candidate for, ventriculoperitoneal shunt
	 B. For thrombotic/embolic stroke
	   1. Large anterior infarcts with both cortical and subcortical involvement
	   2. Large bihemispheric infarcts
	   3. Basilar artery occlusion
	   4. Bilateral vertebral artery occlusion

D. **Neurodegenerative Conditions**

    1.   Many neurodegenerative and neuromuscular diseases can cause progressive decline, debility-related complications, malnutrition, and ultimately death. Patients and families experiencing these conditions require significant education and support and can benefit from both palliative care and hospice along their illness trajectory

2. Dementias—the prevalence of dementia is growing rapidly due to the aging of the population. Currently 1 of every 8 people over 65 years old have a diagnosis of dementia with 5.3 million having Alzheimer's dementia and 2 million having other types (vascular, Lewy body, frontotemporal)[75]

3. Pathophysiology—irreversible and progressive neurological disorder that results in impaired cognition, memory, and ultimately in physical functioning. Based on the type of the dementia the impaired function is due to degeneration of brain function within a variety of sites within the brain and can result in differing symptomatology during the course of the illness.[76] However, within the terminal stages of the disease process, these dementias tend to present similarly and require similar management for comfort

4. Palliative care—the role of palliative care is beneficial throughout the course of dementia. The trajectory can be complex and prognosis is difficult to determine prior to the final stages. Issues including behavior changes, nutritional deficits, pain, and functional decline are common among dementias, and patients and family will require assistance navigating their healthcare treatment choices.[75] Death due to this illness is a consequence from the associated complications and needs increase as the disease advances. Conversations related to artificial nutrition, mechanical ventilation, antibiotic therapy, and caregiving resources are necessary prior to the end of life to ensure that the patient's wishes are honored[76]

5. Treatment

   a) Disease-specific treatment—cholinesterase inhibitors (i.e., galantamine, donepezil, rivastigmine) are used for mild-to-moderate dementia; N-methyl-D-aspartate (NMDA) receptor antagonist (memantine) is used in moderate-to-severe dementia with reported benefit for slowing cognitive and functional decline[77]

6. Symptom management

   a) Pain management—recommend following the World Health Organization (WHO) ladder for pain management when initiating and titrating pharmacologic agents

   b) Constipation due to decreased mobility—high fiber diet, osmotic laxatives

   c) Behavior disturbances—antipsychotics or anxiolytics based on the stage of the disease, goals, and any contraindicating conditions or medications

7. Nonpharmacologic treatment—calm, consistent environment, provision of meaningful activities, prevention of pressure ulcers with optimal hygiene and self-care[76]

8. As any type of dementia progresses to end stage, the patient and family will need ongoing support in making end-of-life decisions. The Functional Assessment Staging Tool (FAST) assists in determining hospice eligibility (although only validated for Alzheimer's disease) in conjunction with other medical conditions and the patient's goals of care. See Table 3-6 for hospice eligibility

Table 3-6. Hospice Eligibility Criteria for Dementia Due to Alzheimer's Disease and Related Disorders[66]

Hospice eligibility dementia due to Alzheimer's disease and related disorders (not other types of multi-infarct dementia). Patients will be considered to be in the terminal stage of dementia (life expectancy of 6 months or less) if they meet the following criteria	
Patients with dementia should show all the following characteristics 1. Stage 7 or beyond according to the Functional Assessment Staging Scale 2. Unable to ambulate without assistance 3. Unable to dress without assistance 4. Unable to bathe without assistance 5. Urinary and bowel incontinence, intermittent or constant 6. No consistently meaningful verbal communication: stereotypical phrases only or the ability to speak is limited to 6 or fewer intelligible words	Patients should have had 1 of the following within the past 12 months 1. Aspiration pneumonia 2. Pyelonephritis or other upper urinary tract infection 3. Septicemia 4. Decubitus ulcers, multiple, stage 3–4 5. Fever, recurrent after antibiotics 6. Inability to maintain sufficient fluid and calorie intake with 10% weight loss during the previous 6 months or serum albumin < 2.5 gm/dL

E. **Other Neurodegenerative Disorders**

1. Parkinson's disease (PD) is a chronic degenerative disease of the central nervous system that often presents subtly and is normally characterized by pill rolling or a fine tremor at rest

   a) PD is not considered a fatal disease but people with this disease have a shorter life expectancy than the general population. Factors that are associated with a shorter life expectancy are as follows: older age upon diagnosis, scoring poorly on movement tests, experiencing psychotic symptoms, and developing dementia.[78] As PD progresses, deterioration in functional status and autonomic dysfunction are common along with dermatological issues and sensory deficits.[73] Levodopa/carbidopa is most commonly used to manage symptoms

2. Amyotrophic lateral sclerosis (ALS)—a motor neuron disease that causes gradual muscle weakness and wasting. Involvement of bulbar innervated muscles usually indicates a worse prognosis than the 5 or more years for those with motor neuron involvement. Typically life expectancy overall is approximately 3 years after symptom onset.[73] This disease is incurable and is managed with supportive therapies to assist with function, nutrition, and ventilation/oxygenation and with a multidisciplinary approach. Respiratory failure is the usual cause of death. Palliative care is beneficial across the trajectory of this disease process for symptom management and to assist patients and families in making end-of-life decisions. It is important to discuss issues around artificial nutrition and hydration, mechanical ventilation and tracheostomy, and attempts at cardiopulmonary resuscitation to avoid having to make these decisions in a crisis setting

3. Multiple sclerosis (MS)—a central nervous system disease that follows an exacerbation/ remission trajectory or in some persons may be progressive from the onset. Areas of destruction of the myelin sheath in the brain and spinal cord determine the pathology of any specific case. Muscle weakness, numbness, incontinence, and mental and visual difficulties may ensue. The disease is incurable and care is focused on support, optimization of quality of life, and function. Prognosis is variable and many patients with MS have a life span that is no shorter than otherwise expected[73]

4.   Palliative care for these neurodegenerative diseases should be an integral part of the treatment plan. The burden of care on the caregiver/family is high in this group of illnesses due to the unpredictability of the disease trajectory

    a)   These diseases often have a significant symptom burden and caregiving needs. Symptoms of agitation, fatigue, and constipation are all common in these disorders and management should be utilized across the trajectory in addition to disease-specific therapy as indicated by the patient goals. Medications need to be carefully titrated to achieve best results with minimal side effects. Due to the complex nature of these disorders and possible comorbid conditions, it is important to clarify goals and ensure careful medication review when treating the symptoms. It is important for the patient and family to review expectations, goals, and values with physicians prior to the onset of diminished cognition. Advance directives should be in place to assure that the patient's autonomy is preserved

    b)   Pharmacological treatments[74]

        i.   Opioids

        ii.   Bowel regimen to prevent constipation

        iii.   Psychostimulants—methylphenidate

        iv.   Antipsychotics/anxiolytics

        v.   Secretion management—glycopyrrolate

        vi.   Antispasticity—baclofen, tizanidine, gabapentin

    c)   Nonpharmacological treatments

        i.   Calm, consistent environment

        ii.   Communication assistance if needed (ALS)

        iii.   Speech and swallowing therapy

        iv.   Energy conservation techniques (physical therapy [PT]/occupational therapy [OT])

5.   Hospice eligibility guidelines—general guidelines for all neurodegenerative diseases are difficult to determine. Hospice physician's opinion and consultation with the attending provider may help with decision-making. During an exacerbation and rapid decline, the patient may be eligible for hospice care, but may need to be discharged if conditions improve significantly and a longer than 6-month life expectancy is anticipated (see Table 3-7 for ALS criteria)

    a)   Rapid progression of symptoms with decline of physical and mental functions as evidenced by Karnofsky and Palliative Performance Scales 50% or less, meaning the person requires considerable assistance in activities of daily living (ADLs) and other activities

    b)   Impaired breathing, shortness of breath, difficulty taking a deep breath with associated respiratory infections and increased secretions, refusal of ventilator assistance, or ineffectiveness of ventilator assistance

    c)   Difficulty achieving adequate nutritional intake, decreased efficiency, or refusal of medically administered nutrition and hydration with weight loss of more than 10% body weight in 6 months, albumin 2.5 gm/dL or less

d)   Infections, sepsis, wounds, repeated hospitalizations, deferring future hospitalizations, and willingness to seek comfort care only

Table 3-7. Hospice Eligibility Criteria for Amyotrophic Lateral Sclerosis[66]

General Considerations	Criteria—patients will be considered to be in the terminal stage of ALS (life expectancy of 6 months or less) if they meet the following criteria (should fulfill 1, 2, or 3)

• ALS tends to progress in a linear fashion over time. Thus, the overall rate of decline in each patient is fairly constant and predictable, unlike many other non-cancer diseases
• However, no single variable deteriorates at a uniform rate in all patients. Therefore, multiple clinical parameters are required to judge the progression of ALS
• Although ALS usually presents in a localized anatomical area, the location of initial presentation does not correlate with survival time. By the time patients become end stage, muscle denervation has become widespread, affecting all areas of the body, and initial predominance patterns do not persist
• Progression of disease differs markedly from patient to patient. Some patients decline rapidly and die quickly; others progress more slowly. For this reason, the history of the rate of progression in individual patients is important to obtain to predict prognosis
• In end stage ALS, 2 factors are critical in determining prognosis: ability to breathe and, to a lesser extent, ability to swallow. The former can be managed by artificial ventilation and the latter by gastrostomy or other artificial feeding, unless the patient has recurrent aspiration pneumonia. While not necessarily a contraindication to hospice care, the decision to institute either artificial ventilation or artificial feeding will significantly alter 6-month prognosis
• Examination by a neurologist within 3 months of assessment for hospice is advised, both to confirm the diagnosis and to assist with prognosis
	1. Patient should demonstrate critically-impaired breathing capacity
	— Critically-impaired breathing capacity as demonstrated by all the following characteristics occurring within the 12 months preceding initial hospice certification
	  • Vital capacity (VC) less than 30% of normal (if available)
	  • Dyspnea at rest
	  • Patient declines mechanical ventilation; external ventilation used for comfort measures only
	2. Patient should demonstrate both rapid progression of ALS and critical nutritional impairment
	— Rapid progression of ALS as demonstrated by all the following characteristics occurring within the 12 months preceding initial hospice certification
	  • Progression from independent ambulation to wheelchair to bed-bound status
	  • Progression from normal to barely intelligible or unintelligible speech
	  • Progression from normal to pureed diet
	  • Progression from independence in most or all ADLs to needing major assistance by caretaker in all ADLs
	— Critical nutritional impairment as demonstrated by all the following characteristics occurring within the 12 months preceding initial hospice certification
	  • Oral intake of nutrients and fluids insufficient to sustain life
	  • Continuing weight loss
	  • Dehydration or hypovolemia
	  • Absence of artificial feeding methods, sufficient to sustain life, but not for relieving hunger
	3. Patient should demonstrate both rapid progression of ALS and life-threatening complications
	— Rapid progression of ALS, see above
	— Life-threatening complications as demonstrated by 1 of the following characteristics occurring within the 12 months preceding initial hospice certification
	  • Recurrent aspiration pneumonia (with or without tube feedings)
	  • Upper urinary tract infection (e.g., pyelonephritis)
	  • Sepsis
	  • Recurrent fever after antibiotic therapy
	  • Stage 3 or 4 decubitus ulcer(s)

XI. Pulmonary Conditions

A. **Diseases of the pulmonary system are known as the third-leading cause of death in the United States and are rising in incidence[62]**

1. They are classified as obstructive or restrictive in nature, both with symptoms including dyspnea, cough, secretions, and pain. These disease states cannot be cured but their management can be optimized with disease-specific therapies and appropriate symptom management across the trajectory[79]

B. **Pathophysiology**

1. The result of these pulmonary conditions is increasing dyspnea initially on exertion followed by at rest, decreasing oxygenation, and increasing carbon dioxide retention, and functional impairments. The inability to mobilize secretions and prevent aspiration can lead to infection and often a terminal event

2. Obstructive lung disease—chronic obstructive pulmonary disease

   a) Type A: emphysema—causes distention of air spaces with destruction of alveolar walls. The use of accessory muscles for adequate breathing, barrel chest (anteroposterior diameter larger than lateral), diminished breath sounds, decreased ability to cough and expectorate, and weight loss are commonly-associated findings. The forced expiratory volume in 1 second (FEV_1) is typically used to assess severity of the disease and response to treatment[80]

   b) Type B: chronic bronchitis—causes increased mucus secretion and a productive cough. Adventitious breath sounds with resonance on percussion, central cyanosis are common exam findings and often patients may be overweight

3. Restrictive lung disease—these disease processes are characterized by a decrease in total lung capacity (TLC) and reduced lung volumes. Expiratory airflow is normal and airway resistance is normal, although gas transfer is reduced, leading to significant desaturation with activity. Examples of restrictive lung disease include interstitial lung disease, pneumonitis, sarcoidosis, idiopathic fibrotic disease, and connective tissue disease. Secondary causes of restrictive disorders are a result of extrapulmonary processes including neuromuscular diseases (e.g., ALS, myasthenia gravis)[81]

C. **Palliative Care**

1. Prognosis is difficult to determine in pulmonary disease due to an uncertain trajectory and the unpredictable course. Integrating palliative care across the course of care and then transitioning to hospice when eligible is critical in optimizing quality of life and symptom control for patients with both obstructive and restrictive disease. Factors including FEV_1, body mass index, comorbid conditions, degree of dyspnea, and activity tolerance assist patients and families to better understand the progression of disease and the need to clarify goals of care. The BODE (body mass index [BMI], exercise capacity, and subjective estimates of dyspnea) scale is helpful in predicting survival in patients with chronic obstructive pulmonary disease (COPD)[80]

D.   Pharmacological Treatment

1.   Opioids—gold standard for management of dyspnea[82]

2.   Anxiolytics

3.   Cough remedies including expectorants

4.   Secretion management, suctioning, tracheostomy

5.   Oxygen as needed, increasing to continuous; bilevel positive airway pressure (BiPAP), high flow nasal cannula

6.   Steroids—oral or inhaled

7.   Bronchodilators—oral, inhaled, or nebulized

8.   Antibiotics

9.   Antidepressants

E.   Nonpharmacological Management may include[82]

1.   Distraction, massage, aromatherapy

2.   Dietary changes

3.   Stress management

4.   Alternating activities with rest periods, naps

5.   Use of fan, air conditioner, light covers

6.   Upright or side lying position change

7.   Efforts to mobilize secretions

8.   Pulmonary rehabilitation

F.   Hospice

1.   As the disease progresses with increasing hospitalizations, pneumonia, exacerbations at home, and the maximizing of medical management, hospice should be discussed. It is difficult to predict the time frame in which death will occur, and hospice providers must use discretion when discussing this with patient and family. Many of the medications and treatments are needed even with hospice (see Table 3-8)

Table 3-8. Hospice Eligibility Criteria for Pulmonary Disease[66]

Patients will be considered to be in the terminal stage of pulmonary disease (life expectancy of 6 months or less) if they meet the following criteria. The criteria refer to patients with various forms of advanced pulmonary disease who eventually follow a final common pathway for end stage pulmonary disease. 1 and 2 should be present. Documentation of 3, 4, and 5 will lend supporting documentation

1. Severe chronic lung disease as documented by both a and b
  a. Disabling dyspnea at rest, poorly or unresponsive to bronchodilators, resulting in decreased functional capacity (e.g., bed to chair existence, fatigue, and cough). Documentation of forced expiratory volume in 1 second (FEV_1, after bronchodilator, less than 30% of predicted is objective evidence for disabling dyspnea, but is not necessary to obtain
  b. Progression of end stage pulmonary disease, as evidenced by increasing visits to the emergency department or hospitalizations for pulmonary infections and/or respiratory failure or increasing physician home visits prior to initial certification. Documentation of serial decrease of $FEV_1 > 40$ mL/year is objective evidence for disease progression, but is not necessary to obtain
 	
2. Hypoxemia at rest on room air, as evidenced by $Po_2 \leq 55$ mm Hg; or oxygen saturation $\leq 88\%$, determined either by arterial blood gases or oxygen saturation monitors (these values may be obtained from recent hospital records). OR hypercapnia, as evidenced by $Pco_2 \geq 50$ mm Hg. (This value may be obtained from recent [within 3 months] hospital records)
	3. Right heart failure (RHF) secondary to pulmonary disease (cor pulmonale) (e.g., not secondary to left heart disease or valvulopathy)
	4. Unintentional progressive weight loss of greater than 10% of body weight over the preceding 6 months
	5. Resting tachycardia > 100/min

XII. Renal Conditions

A. **Renal diseases have increased as obesity and diabetes incidences rise**

1. Multiorgan involvement increases the incidence of death from end stage renal disease. Hemodialysis has enabled individuals with renal failure to live longer and have a better quality of life. There is a time however when this treatment becomes difficult due to advancing age, comorbid conditions, or loss of access sites. At some point in the disease, dialysis fails to produce desired results and the individual may refuse to continue. It is estimated that approximately 60% of dialysis patients will die within 5 years. Several factors may influence prognosis—age, functional status, albumin level less than 3.5 g/dL. Some persons, especially those with serious conditions in other vital organs, may refuse to begin dialysis or attempt transplantation. It is important to consider the ethical and spiritual dimensions of aggressive therapy in view of continued physical decline

B.   Pathophysiology

1.   Acute kidney injury (AKI)—previously termed acute renal failure, is a condition with sudden and intermittent complete loss of renal function that can be caused by medications, metabolic conditions, infections, urine flow obstructions, and injury though the predominant underlying cause is hypovolemia or hypotension. This may be reversed by dietary management and short-term hemodialysis and is most common within the hospital setting and intensive care units. This condition may lead to oliguria though some patients retain some ability to maintain a urine output[83]

2.   Chronic renal failure (CRF)—also referred to as stage V of chronic kidney disease and is known as an irreversible state with less than 15% of function from the nephron and uremic symptoms are present. Uremia is diagnosed following persistent proteinuria and the retention of toxins occurs. CRF is most commonly caused by diabetes and hypertension and renal replacement therapy (dialysis) or transplant is typically offered and/or initiated at this stage. Clinical factors including fluid balance, electrolyte management, acidosis, and anemia must be monitored and treated as guided by the patient's goals[83]

C.   Palliative Care

1.   As renal failure progresses despite optimal medical management, it is imperative that patients and families have candid discussions regarding expectations of treatment and prognosis with their providers. This is a serious, life-limiting disease with many complications. As the disease progresses, patients may have cognitive impairment due to uremia that may limit their ability to participate in their own medical care. Providers may be reluctant to discontinue dialysis without advance directives and evidence shows that only 30% of patients with end stage renal disease have completed an advance directive. Symptom management is a large part of providing palliative care to this patient population due to prevalent symptoms of fatigue, neuropathy, xerostomia, pain, and pruritus[83,84]

D.   Treatment

1.   Disease-specific management

    a)   Fluid management—diuretics, weight monitoring

    b)   Management of underlying conditions (e.g., diabetes, heart disease)

    c)   Dietary restrictions

    d)   Dialysis

    e)   Transplant

    f)   Electrolyte management

    g)   Pruritus

2.   Symptom management

    a)   Opioids for pain and dyspnea[85]

        i.   Avoid morphine and codeine

        ii.   Hydromorphone and oxycodone with caution

        iii.   Fentanyl and methadone relatively safe, start low and titrate slowly

    b)   Antianxiety and neuroleptic agents for restlessness, delirium

      c)   Medications for pruritus

      d)   Facilitate discussions regarding discontinuing disease-specific treatment, including dialysis, when indicators suggest that burden outweighs benefit to patient and decision is collaborative between medical team and patient/family.[86] Symptom management at that time will center on patient-specific needs and assessment of present physical symptoms

      e)   If patient has discontinued dialysis, will need to prepare family for "days" rather than "weeks" and provide intensive support

E.   Hospice

    1.   Once the decision is made to discontinue dialysis, the patient is typically eligible for hospice (see Table 3-9). Medications should be reviewed, discontinued, or dosages changed, especially if dialysis is discontinued

Table 3-9. Hospice Eligibility Criteria for Renal Disease[66]

Patients will be considered to be in the terminal stage of renal disease (life expectancy of 6 months or less) if they meet the following criteria

Acute renal failure—1 and either 2 or 3 should be present. Factors from 4 will lend supporting documentation
1. The patient is not seeking dialysis or renal transplant or is discontinuing dialysis
2. Creatinine clearance < 10 mL/min (< 15 mL/min for diabetics) based on measurement or calculation; or < 15 mL/min (< 20 mL/min for diabetics) with comorbidity of congestive heart failure
3. Serum creatinine > 8.0 mg/dL (> 6.0 mg/dL for diabetics)
4. Comorbid conditions
   a. Mechanical ventilation
   b. Malignancy (other organ system)
   c. Chronic lung disease
   d. Advanced cardiac disease
   e. Advanced liver disease
   f. Sepsis
   g. Immunosuppression/AIDS
   h. Albumin < 3.5 gm/dL
   i. Cachexia
   j. Platelet count < 25,000/mm³
   k. Disseminated intravascular coagulation
   l. Gastrointestinal bleeding

Chronic renal failure—1 and either 2 or 3 should be present. Factors from 4 will lend supporting documentation
1. The patient is not seeking dialysis or renal transplant or is discontinuing dialysis
2. Creatinine clearance < 10 mL/min (< 15 mL/min for diabetics) based on measurement or calculation; or < 15 mL/min (< 20 mL/min for diabetics) with comorbidity of congestive heart failure
3. Serum creatinine > 8.0 mg/dL (> 6.0 mg/dL for diabetics)
4. Signs and symptoms of renal failure
   a. Uremia
   b. Oliguria (< 400 mL/24 hours)
   c. Intractable hyperkalemia (> 7.0 mEq/L) not responsive to treatment
   d. Uremic pericarditis
   e. Hepatorenal syndrome
   f. Intractable fluid overload, not responsive to treatment

XIII. Diabetes Mellitus

A. Diabetes Mellitus

1. Seventh leading cause of death in the United States[68]

2. Patients with cancer are more likely to have diabetes and diabetes has been linked to increased risk for cancer, though this may reflect the increasing numbers of undiagnosed diabetes in the adult population.[87,88] Having cancer with diabetes increases mortality[88]

3. Palliative patients with diabetes fall into 3 stages—active comorbid disease with stable diabetes, relatively stable diabetes with impending death or organ/system failure, and actively dying[87,89]

B. Pathophysiology

1. The most common types of diabetes are type 1 and type 2. Usually diagnosed in children, type 1 diabetes results from autoimmune loss of beta cells in the pancreatic islets leading to absolute insulin deficiency. Type 2 results from insulin resistance and decreased insulin secretion by beta cells. Treatment of both types focuses on maintaining as close to normal blood glucose levels as possible. Type 1 diabetes is treated with insulin, meal planning, exercise, and self-monitoring of blood glucose. Treatment of type 2 diabetes centers on meal planning, exercise, oral hypoglycemic agents, and weight loss if overweight[90]

C. Palliative Care

1. Ranges from preventing long-term complications to preventing osmotic symptoms and hypoglycemia.[88] The ongoing plan of care should evolve as the diabetes and comorbid diseases progress. Those with stable active diabetes will continue treatment plans if successful and modify those that are not[87]

2. Blood glucose monitoring

    a) Finger-stick glucose monitoring—as the patient's condition worsens, frequent finger-stick monitoring may not be needed.[89] While some feel finger-stick monitoring is uncomfortable,[88] others may consider it a part of their life.[91] Discontinuing monitoring may be seen as marking the progression of the diabetes and shorter life expectancy as well as a loss of control[89]

    b) Hemoglobin A_1C (the mean glucose levels over the past 1 to 2 months) may be able to be used to monitor the effectiveness of treatment instead of finger-sticks.[88] Though the American Diabetes Association recommends striving for a hemoglobin (Hb) A_1C of < 7%, "less stringent A_1C goals (such as < 8%) may be appropriate for patients with a history of severe hypoglycemia, limited life expectancy, advanced microvascular or macrovascular complications, and extensive comorbid conditions and in those with long-standing diabetes in whom the general goal is difficult to attain."[92] Though each situation should be treated individually, there is no consensus on diabetic palliative care; Table 3-10 gives general guidelines[89]

Table 3-10. General Guidelines for Palliative Diabetic Care[89]

Level	Finger-Stick Glucose Monitoring	Insulin and Oral Hypoglycemics	Diet
Active comorbid disease with stable diabetes	• Hb A₁C usually not needed • Type 1—continue if able • Type 2—only in specific situation (e.g., not able to report symptoms of hyper/hypoglycemia)	• Insulin—continue insulin with dose adjustments as needed; rapid acting insulin may decrease incidences of hypoglycemia seen with long-acting insulins • Oral hypoglycemics—continue if able to eat and recognize signs of hyper/hypoglycemia; caution with renal disease and liver failure	• Pleasure-based diet with decreased highly concentrated carbohydrates
Relatively stable diabetes with impending death or organ/system failure	• Type 1—only when a decision about management of diabetes is needed • Type 2— generally can be eliminated	• Insulin—decrease insulin administration, especially with renal or hepatic failure • Oral hypoglycemics—decrease or discontinue especially with poor caloric intake and renal or hepatic failure	• In the presence of anorexia and cachexia, liberalize diet as tolerated
Actively dying	• Discontinue	• Stop insulin and oral hypoglycemics	• Comfort only

D.   **Assessment and Treatment of Common Symptoms of Diabetes**

1.   Care goal discussions should include glycemic control, blood glucose monitoring, and treatment of hypoglycemic symptoms[87]

2.   Hypoglycemia

a)   Can lead to increased morbidity, decreased quality of life, and increased morbidity[87]

b)   Symptoms include tremors/shakiness, palpitations/tachycardia, diaphoresis, anxiety, nervousness, dizziness, weakness, headache, irritability, confusion and/or decrease consciousness[87,89] with seizures in extreme situations[89]

c)   Symptoms can be misinterpreted[87]

d)   Immediate care

i.   For alert patients who are able to swallow—give 1 cup of milk, half cup of orange juice, several pieces of hard candy to raise glucose levels, or 15 to 20 gm of glucose tablets or gels. Repeat within 15 minutes if symptoms persist and follow with a snack or meal[87]

ii. For nonalert patients and/or those with swallowing difficulties—administer intravenous dextrose; subcutaneous, intramuscular, or intravenous glucagon; or buccal glucose gel with oral stimulation to illicit a swallowing reflex. Glucagon is less likely to raise glucose levels in those with impaired glycogen stores or liver function[87]

e) Prevention

i. Know onset, peak, and half-life of insulins and oral hypoglycemic agents[70]

ii. Dosages of insulin and oral hypoglycemics may need to be reduced or discontinued[87]

iii. Assess for changes in renal and hepatic function, which can alter the pharmacokinetics of medications[87]

iv. Assess for symptoms that can decrease nutritional intake (e.g., nausea/vomiting, anorexia, food aversions)

v. Assess for an infection that could precipitate diabetic ketoacidosis[87]

3. Hyperglycemia

a) Symptoms include dry skin, drowsiness, blurred vision, nausea, polydipsia, and polyphagia. Except for polyphagia, the symptoms of hyperglycemia may be misinterpreted as general decline[87]

b) Risks of hyperglycemia includes presence of the hyperosmolar state and associated complications (e.g., osmotic diuresis, recurrent infection, poor wound healing)[89]

c) Assess for decreasing activity levels.[87] While exercise decreases postprandial blood glucose levels and insulin requirements, less activity without adjustment of insulin or oral hypoglycemics can lead to hyperglycemia[90]

d) Assess for drugs that may induce hyperglycemia (e.g., glucocorticoids, diuretics, octreotide)[87]

XIV. Liver Failure

A. Chronic Liver Disease

1. Twelfth leading cause of death in the United States and is caused by multiple conditions including cirrhosis, hepatitis, hepatorenal syndrome, and hepatobiliary malignancies. Liver disease can be classified as acute or chronic and can be treated and at times reversed prior to the development of liver failure

B. Pathophysiology

1. The liver is a large, complex organ with 4 lobes and many functions. It is active in amino acid, carbohydrate and fat metabolism, bile production, and detoxification of medications, alcohol, and other substances. It also has endocrine functions and excretion functions. The liver assists in keeping the body well by removing bacteria and other pathogens from the blood. It stores fat-soluble vitamins, minerals, and manufactures clotting factors

C. Diseases of the liver can cause widespread disorders within the body

1. Hepatitis is inflammation of the liver, usually due to exposure to infectious agents (hepatitis A, B, C, D, or E), toxins, or medications. Cirrhosis of the liver may be caused by alcohol and substance misuse or chronic viral hepatitis B or C, as well as primary biliary pathology. Damage to liver cells may be transient or permanent leading to liver failure and death. Hepatorenal syndrome typically is associated with a poor prognosis. Though transplant is the only definitive treatment, many patients with chronic liver disease are not candidates due to comorbid conditions or various host factors[93,94]

D. Signs and Symptoms

1. Hepatic encephalopathy, ascites, infections (e.g., spontaneous bacterial peritonitis), malnutrition and cachexia, jaundice, portal vein thrombosis, portal hypertension, pruritus, anorexia, nausea, liver capsule distention pain, malaise, and esophageal varices

E. Palliative Care

1. Given the symptom burden, the impact of liver disease upon a patient's quality of life is significant. These patients often experience malaise and fatigue, jaundice, refractory ascites, coagulopathy, malnutrition, infections (e.g., spontaneous bacterial peritonitis), and encephalopathy. Cognitive impairment can be problematic throughout the trajectory and can lead to disruptions in physical and mental well-being.[94] These patients can be at high risk from bleeding from esophageal varices or the gastrointestinal tract in late stage disease, which can lead to a terminal event. If transplantation is determined to not be an option, goals of care and advance care planning are critical[93]

F. Treatment

1. Weight monitoring/fluid balance

2. Avoid aspirin and other NSAIDs

3. Abstain/reduce alcohol intake

4. Fluid and sodium restriction

5. Dietary modifications, small frequent meals

6. Monitor for bleeding, prevention of bleeding (e.g., soft toothbrushes, electric razors, prevention of injury)

7. Paracentesis

8. Transjugular intrahepatic portosystemic shunt (TIPS)

9. Denver shunt

10. Transplantation

11. Pharmacological management[94]

    a) Diuretics and spironolactone for edema and ascites

    b) Lactulose or rifaximin to reduce ammonia levels and improve cognitive function

    c) Cholestyramine—pruritus if biliary obstruction ruled out

    d) Acetaminophen—mild pain, restrict to 1 g daily

e) Opioids (reduced dose) for pain and dyspnea management

    i. Fentanyl is considered the opioid of choice in end stage liver failure

f) Skin care to prevent wounds and injury

G. Hospice

1. Progressive malnutrition, muscle wasting, hepatitis, or noncompliance with medications and treatments may be presenting factors for inclusion in a hospice program (see Table 3-11)

Table 3-11. Hospice Eligibility Criteria for Liver Disease[66]

Patients will be considered to be in the terminal stage of liver disease (life expectancy of 6 months or less) if they meet the following criteria. 1 and 2 should be present; factors from 3 will lend supporting documentation	

1. The patient should show both a and b
  a. Prothrombin time prolonged more than 5 seconds over control, or international normalized ratio (INR) > 1.5
  b. Serum albumin < 2.5 g/dL
2. End stage liver disease is present and the patient shows at least 1 of the following
  a. Ascites, refractory to treatment or patient noncompliant
  b. Spontaneous bacterial peritonitis
  c. Hepatorenal syndrome (elevated creatinine and blood urea nitrogen (BUN) with oliguria (< 400 mL/day) and urine sodium concentration < 10 mEq/L
  d. Hepatic encephalopathy, refractory to treatment, or patient noncompliant
  e. Recurrent variceal bleeding, despite intensive therapy
	3. Documentation of the following factors will support eligibility for hospice care
	  a. Progressive malnutrition
	  b. Muscle wasting with reduced strength and endurance
	  c. Continued active alcoholism (> 80 g ethanol/day)
	  d. Hepatocellular carcinoma
	  e. HBsAg (hepatitis B) positivity
	  f. Hepatitis C refractory to interferon treatment
	
	Patients awaiting liver transplant who otherwise fit the above criteria may be certified for the Medicare Hospice Benefit, but if a donor organ is procured, the patient should be discharged from hospice

XV. Human Immunodeficiency Virus (HIV)/Acquired Immunodeficiency Syndrome (AIDS)

A. HIV Infection Leading to Late-Stage HIV (AIDS)

1. HIV has progressed from a terminal illness to a chronic illness over the last few years, following the development of antiretroviral therapy (ART) and currently statistics reflect that approximately 1.2 million people are living with HIV in the United States.[95] ART is recommended for all HIV-infected individuals to reduce the risk of disease progression and prevent transmission of HIV.[96] Timing of treatment and medication decisions is very important to improving the time interval from initial HIV infection to the development of late-stage HIV. The onset of opportunistic infections and comorbid conditions may impact life expectancy and present patients with the need for end-of-life care

B. Pathophysiology

1. HIV is transmitted by sexual intercourse, mother-to-child during childbirth, and parenterally. HIV specifically attacks the CD4 cells within the immune system through its RNA, which is converted to DNA within the host cell.[97] Primary infection is characterized by flu-like symptoms that occur a month or 2 after infection. Some persons do not have any symptoms; however, these asymptomatic individuals may infect others. The latent phase varies from months to years. As the virus multiplies, mild flu-like symptoms and swollen lymph nodes may be noted. Diarrhea, weight loss, cough, and shortness of breath may develop. If no treatment ensues, the disease will progress to late-stage HIV with a severely damaged immune system and onset of opportunistic infections

2. Diagnosis of late-stage HIV (AIDS) includes[97]

    a) Infection with HIV

    b) CD4 count of < 200 cells/mm^3

    c) Presence of AIDS-defining malignancies (e.g., Kaposi's sarcoma, invasive cervical cancer)

    d) Presence of opportunistic infections (e.g., tuberculosis, *Pneumocystis jiroveci* pneumonia)

3. HIV-1 and HIV-2 have been identified, with HIV-2 being limited mostly to Africa

C. Palliative Care

1. The role of palliative care in HIV has evolved as the life expectancy and ability to treat more patients has increased. Symptoms may be present across the continuum of the illness, which may include neuropathy, pain, gastrointestinal disturbances, candidiasis, or complications from opportunistic infections.[98–100] As the disease progresses, symptom burden, and functional decline will lead to increased care needs. In an effort to preserve the patient's autonomy and customize palliative care, emphasis should be placed on advance care planning, end-of-life wishes, and caregiving options

D. Treatment[97]

1. Disease-specific treatment

    a) Antiretroviral treatment (ART)

    b) Prophylaxis for opportunistic infections determined by specific CD4 count

2. Frequent communication to determine changing needs, goals, and the need for psychosocial or spiritual counseling

3. Symptom management

    a) Opioids

    b) Antidiarrheals

    c) Antidepressants and antianxiety agents

    d) Skin care, moisturizers, antipruritic creams

    e) Nutritional support for cachexia and diarrhea

E. **Hospice**

1. Many persons who are HIV infected are young and focused on living. Cure is not expected but prolonging life is always a hope. Factors affecting prognosis are age, failure of ARTs, opportunistic infections, complications, functional level, nutritional status, CD4 count, and viral load. Continue medications to prevent or treat cytomegalovirus retinitis, even when other antiretrovirals and antituberculin medications are discontinued. See Table 3-12

Table 3-12. Hospice Eligibility Criteria for HIV[66]

Patients will be considered to be in the terminal stage of their illness (life expectancy of 6 months or less) if they meet the following criteria. 1 and 2 should be present; factors from 3 will add supporting documentation	

1. CD4 count < 25 cells/mm³ or persistent (2 or more assays at least 1 month apart) viral load > 100 000 copies/mL, plus 1 of the following
  a. CNS lymphoma
  b. Untreated, or persistent despite treatment, wasting (loss of at least 10% lean body mass)
  c. Mycobacterium avium complex (MAC) bacteremia, untreated, unresponsive to treatment, or treatment refused
  d. Progressive multifocal leukoencephalopathy
  e. Systemic lymphoma, with advanced HIV disease and partial response to chemotherapy
  f. Visceral Kaposi's sarcoma unresponsive to therapy
  g. Renal failure in the absence of dialysis
  h. Cryptosporidium infection
  i. Toxoplasmosis, unresponsive to therapy
2. Decreased performance status, as measured by the Karnofsky Performance Status (KPS) scale, of ≤ 50%
	3. Documentation of the following factors will support eligibility for hospice care
	  a. Chronic persistent diarrhea for 1 year
	  b. Persistent serum albumin < 2.5 g/dL
	  c. Concomitant, active substance abuse
	  d. Age > 50 years
	  e. Absence of, or resistance to effective antiretroviral, chemotherapeutic, and prophylactic drug therapy related specifically to HIV disease
	  f. Advanced AIDS dementia complex
	  g. Toxoplasmosis
	  h. Congestive heart failure, symptomatic at rest
	  i. Advanced liver disease

CITED REFERENCES

1. American Cancer Society. *Global Cancer Facts & Figures.* 2nd ed. 2011. www.cancer.org/acs/groups/content/@epidemiologysurveilance/documents/document/acspc-027766.pdf. Accessed July 30, 2014.

2. American Cancer Society. *Cancer Facts & Figures 2013.* 2013. www.cancer.org/acs/groups/content/@epidemiologysurveilance/documents/document/acspc-036845.pdf. Accessed July 30, 2014.

3. National Cancer Institute (NCI). *Lung Cancer: Survival Rates and Prognosis.* 2012. www.cancer.gov/cancertopics/types/lung/cancer-survival-prognosis. Accessed October 6, 2014.

4. McIllmurray M. The medical treatment of cancer in palliative care. In: Hanks G, Cherny NI, Christakis NA, Fallon M, Kaasa S, Portenoy RK. *Oxford Textbook of Palliative Medicine.* 4th ed. New York, NY: Oxford University Press; 2010:513-525.

5. Virshup DM. Biology, clinical manifestation, and treatment of cancer. In: McCance KL, Huether SE, Brashers VL, Rote NS, eds. *Pathophysiology: The Biologic Basis for Disease in Adults and Children.* 6th ed. Maryland Heights, MO: Mosby Elsevier; 2010:360-395.

6. National Cancer Institute (NCI). *Metastatic Cancer.* 2013. www.cancer.gov/cancertopics/factsheet/Sites-Types/metastatic. Accessed August 19, 2014.

7. Loud JT, Hutson SP. Genetic risk and heredity cancer syndromes. In: Yarbro CH, Wujcik D, Gobel BH, eds. *Cancer Nursing: Principles and Practice.* 7th ed. Sudbury, MA: Jones and Bartlett Publishers; 2011:135-165.

8. Herman JG, Baylin SB. Epigenetic contributions to human cancer. In: Hong WK, Bast Jr. RC, Hait WN, Kufe DW, eds. *Holland-Frei Cancer Medicine.* 8th ed. Shelton, CT: People's Medical Publishing House-USA; 2010:170-174.

9. National Cancer Institute. *Cancer Genetics Overview (PDQ®).* 2014. Available at: www.cancer.gov/cancertopics/pdq/genetics/overview/healthprofessional. Accessed December 11, 2014.

10. American Cancer Society. The Goals of Chemotherapy. 2013. Available at: www.cancer.org/treatment/treatmentsandsideeffects/treatmenttypes/chemotherapy/chemotherapyprinciplesanin-depthdiscussionofthetechniquesanditsroleintreatment/chemotherapy-principles-goals-of-chemo. Accessed December 11, 2014.

11. Gillespie TW. Surgical therapy. In: Yarbro CH, Wujcik D, Gobel BH, eds. *Cancer Nursing: Principles and Practice.* 7th ed. Sudbury, MA: Jones and Bartlett Publishers; 2011:232-248.

12. Gosselin TK. Principles of radiation therapy. In: Yarbro CH, Wujcik D, Gobel BH, eds. *Cancer Nursing: Principles and Practice.* 7th ed. Sudbury, MA: Jones and Bartlett Publishers; 2011:249-268.

13. Baldini EH. Prophylactic cranial irradiation for patients with small cell lung cancer. *UpToDate.* 2014. www.uptodate.com/contents/prophylactic-cranial-irradiation-for-patients-with-small-cell-lung-cancer?source=search_result&search=prophylactic+small+cell+cranial+irradiation&selectedTitle=1%7E150. Accessed August 19, 2014.

14. Tortorice PV. Cytotoxic chemotherapy: principles of therapy. In: Yarbro CH, Wujcik D, Gobel BH, eds. *Cancer Nursing: Principles and Practice.* 7th ed. Sudbury, MA: Jones and Bartlett Publishers; 2011:352-389.

15. Wilkes GM. Chemotherapy: principles of administration. In: Yarbro CH, Wujcik D, Gobel BH, eds. *Cancer Nursing: Principles and Practice.* 7th ed. Sudbury, MA: Jones and Bartlett Publishers; 2011:390-457.

16. Camp-Sorrell D. Chemotherapy: toxicities and management. In: Yarbro CH, Wujcik D, Gobel BH, eds. *Cancer Nursing: Principles and Practice*. 7th ed. Sudbury, MA: Jones and Bartlett Publishers; 2011:458-503.

17. Decker G, Lee CO. Complementary and alternative medicine (CAM) therapies in integrative oncology. In: Yarbro CH, Wujcik D, Gobel BH, eds. *Cancer Nursing: Principles and Practice*. 7th ed. Sudbury, MA: Jones and Bartlett Publishers; 2011:626-654.

18. Weissman DE. Determining prognosis in advanced cancer, 2nd ed. *Fast Facts and Concepts*. 2009; 13. www.eperc.mcw.edu/EPERC/FastFactsIndex/ff_013.htm. Accessed July 30, 2014.

19. Eaby-Sandy B. Lung cancer. In: Yarbro CH, Wujcik D, Gobel BH, eds. *Cancer Nursing: Principles and Practice*. 7th ed. Sudbury, MA: Jones and Bartlett Publishers; 2011:1424-1457.

20. Foxson SB, Lattimer JG, Felder B. Breast cancer. In: Yarbro CH, Wujcik D, Gobel BH, eds. *Cancer Nursing: Principles and Practice*. 7th ed. Sudbury, MA: Jones and Bartlett Publishers; 2011:1091-1145.

21. Mayo Clinic. *Diseases and Conditions: Breast Cancer*. 2014. www.mayoclinic.org/diseases-conditions/breast-cancer/basics/definition/con-20029275. Accessed October 6, 2014.

22. Mickle M. Stomach cancer. In: Yarbro CH, Wujcik D, Gobel BH, eds. *Cancer Nursing: Principles and Practice*. 7th ed. Sudbury, MA: Jones and Bartlett Publishers; 2011:1683-1695.

23. Hogdin M. Pancreatic cancer. In: Yarbro CH, Wujcik D, Gobel BH, eds. *Cancer Nursing: Principles and Practice*. 7th ed. Sudbury, MA: Jones and Bartlett Publishers; 2011:1580-1608.

24. National Cancer Institute (NCI). *A Snapshot of Stomach Cancer*. 2013. www.cancer.gov/researchandfunding/snapshots/stomach. Accessed October 6, 2014.

25. World Health Organization (WHO). *Cancer*. 2014. www.who.int/mediacentre/factsheets/fs297/en/. Accessed October 6, 2014.

26. Grenon NN. Liver cancer. In: Yarbro CH, Wujcik D, Gobel BH, eds. *Cancer Nursing: Principles and Practice*. 7th ed. Sudbury, MA: Jones and Bartlett Publishers; 2011:1399-1423.

27. National Cancer Institute (NCI). *Adult Primary Liver Cancer Treatment (PDQ®)*. 2014. www.cancer.gov/cancertopics/pdq/treatment/adult-primary-liver/HealthProfessional. Accessed October 6, 2014.

28. Tsottles ND, Brynes HP. Esophageal cancer. In: Yarbro CH, Wujcik D, Gobel BH, eds. *Cancer Nursing: Principles and Practice*. 7th ed. Sudbury, MA: Jones and Bartlett Publishers; 2011:1295-1315.

29. National Cancer Institute (NCI). *Esophageal Cancer Treatment (PDQ®)*. 2014. www.cancer.gov/cancertopics/pdq/treatment/esophageal/Patient. Accessed October 6, 2014.

30. Kazer MW, Harmon AS. Prostate cancer. In: Yarbro CH, Wujcik D, Gobel BH, eds. *Cancer Nursing: Principles and Practice*. 7th ed. Sudbury, MA: Jones and Bartlett Publishers; 2011:1609-1633.

31. National Cancer Institute (NCI). *Prostate Cancer Treatment (PDQ®)*. 2014. www.cancer.gov/cancertopics/pdq/treatment/prostate/HealthProfessional. Accessed October 6, 2014.

32. Shelton G. Bladder cancer. In: Yarbro CH, Wujcik D, Gobel BH, eds. *Cancer Nursing: Principles and Practice*. 7th ed. Sudbury, MA: Jones and Bartlett Publishers; 2011:1080-1090.

33. National Cancer Institute (NCI). *SEER Stat Fact Sheet: Bladder Cancer*. 2014. seer.cancer.gov/statfacts/html/urinb.html. Accessed October 6, 2014.

34. Wood LS. Renal cancer. In: Yarbro CH, Wujcik D, Gobel BH, eds. *Cancer Nursing: Principles and Practice*. 7th ed. Sudbury, MA: Jones and Bartlett Publishers; 2011:1634-1649.

35. American Cancer Society. *What are the Risk Factors for Kidney Cancer.* 2014. www.cancer.org/cancer/kidneycancer/detailedguide/kidney-cancer-adult-risk-factors. Accessed October 6, 2014.

36. Choueiri TK, Je Y, Cho E. Analgesic use and the risk of kidney cancer: a meta-analysis of epidemiologic studies. *Int J Ca.* 2014;134(2):384-396. doi: 10.1002/ijc.28093. Epub September 23, 2013.

37. Gordon SC, Moonka D, Brown KA, et al. Risk for renal cell carcinoma in chronic hepatitis C infection. *Cancer Epidemiol Biomarkers Prev.* 2010;19(4):1066-1073. doi: 10.1158/1055-9965.EPI-09-1275. Epub March 23, 2010.

38. Martin VR, Temple SV. Cervical cancer. In: Yarbro CH, Wujcik D, Gobel BH, eds. *Cancer Nursing: Principles and Practice.* 7th ed. Sudbury, MA: Jones and Bartlett Publishers; 2011:1188-1204.

39. Martin VR. Ovarian cancer. In: Yarbro CH, Wujcik D, Gobel BH, eds. *Cancer Nursing: Principles and Practice.* 7th ed. Sudbury, MA: Jones and Bartlett Publishers; 2011:1546-1579.

40. National Cancer Institute (NCI). *Ovarian Epithelial Cancer Treatment (PDQ®).* 2014. www.cancer.gov/cancertopics/pdq/treatment/ovarianepithelial/HealthProfessional. Accessed October 9, 2014.

41. Cassidy LA. Endometrial cancer. In: Yarbro CH, Wujcik D, Gobel BH, eds. *Cancer Nursing: Principles and Practice.* 7th ed. Sudbury, MA: Jones and Bartlett Publishers; 2011:1281-1294.

42. Kurtin SE. Leukemia and myelodysplastic syndromes. In: Yarbro CH, Wujcik D, Gobel BH, eds. *Cancer Nursing: Principles and Practice.* 7th ed. Sudbury, MA: Jones and Bartlett Publishers; 2011:1369-1398.

43. Manson SD, Porter C. Lymphomas. In: Yarbro CH, Wujcik D, Gobel BH, eds. *Cancer Nursing: Principles and Practice.* 7th ed. Sudbury, MA: Jones and Bartlett Publishers; 2011:1458-1512.

44. Teriman JD, Faiman B. Multiple myeloma. In: Yarbro CH, Wujcik D, Gobel BH, eds. *Cancer Nursing: Principles and Practice.* 7th ed. Sudbury, MA: Jones and Bartlett Publishers; 2011:1513-1545.

45. Carr E. Head and neck malignancies. In: Yarbro CH, Wujcik D, Gobel BH, eds. *Cancer Nursing: Principles and Practice.* 7th ed. Sudbury, MA: Jones and Bartlett Publishers; 2011:1334-1368.

46. Mahon SM, Yackzan SG. Skin cancer. In: Yarbro CH, Wujcik D, Gobel BH, eds. *Cancer Nursing: Principles and Practice.* 7th ed. Sudbury, MA: Jones and Bartlett Publishers; 2011:1650-1682.

47. Armstrong T. Central nervous system cancers. In: Yarbro CH, Wujcik D, Gobel BH, eds. *Cancer Nursing: Principles and Practice.* 7th ed. Sudbury, MA: Jones and Bartlett Publishers; 2011:1146-1187.

48. Mehta R, Arnold R. Management of spinal cord compression. *Fast Facts and Concepts.* 2011; 238. www.eperc.mcw.edu/EPERC/FastFactsIndex/ff_238.htm. Accessed July 30, 2014.

49. Weinstein SM. Management of spinal cord and cauda equina compression. In: Berger AM, Shuster Jr JL, Von Roenn JH, eds. *Principles and Practice of Palliative Care and Supportive Oncology.* 3rd ed. Philadelphia, PA: Lippincott Williams & Wilkins; 2007:415-424.

50. Kaplow R. Cardiac tamponade. In: Yarbro CH, Wujcik D, Gobel BH, eds. *Cancer Nursing: Principles and Practice.* 7th ed. Sudbury, MA: Jones and Bartlett Publishers; 2011:915-927.

51. Brumbaugh HL. Superior vena cava syndrome. In: Yarbro CH, Wujcik D, Gobel BH, eds. *Cancer Nursing: Principles and Practice.* 7th ed. Sudbury, MA: Jones and Bartlett Publishers; 2011:995-1004.

52. Gobel BH. Disseminated intravascular coagulation. In: Yarbro CH, Wujcik D, Gobel BH, eds. *Cancer Nursing: Principles and Practice.* 7th ed. Sudbury, MA: Jones and Bartlett Publishers; 2011:928-938.

53. Levi M. Disseminated intravascular coagulation. In: Hoffman R, Benz Jr EJ, Silberstein LE, Heslop H, Weitz J, Anastasi J. *Hematology: Basic Principles and Practice.* 6th ed. Philadelphia, PA: Elsevier Saunders; 2013:2001-2012.

54. O'Leary C. Septic shock. In: Yarbro CH, Wujcik D, Gobel BH, eds. *Cancer Nursing: Principles and Practice.* 7th ed. Sudbury, MA: Jones and Bartlett Publishers; 2011:964-978.

55. Lydon J. Tumor lysis syndrome. In: Yarbro CH, Wujcik D, Gobel BH, eds. *Cancer Nursing: Principles and Practice.* 7th ed. Sudbury, MA: Jones and Bartlett Publishers; 2011:1014-1030.

56. Loerzel VW, Meneses K. Cancer survivorship: a critical aspect of care. In: Yarbro CH, Wujcik D, Gobel BH, eds. *Cancer Nursing: Principles and Practice.* 7th ed. Sudbury, MA: Jones and Bartlett Publishers; 2011:1743-1754.

57. Sun V. Palliative chemotherapy and clinical trials in advanced cancer: the nurse's role. In: Ferrell BR, Coyle N, eds. *Oxford Textbook of Palliative Nursing.* 3rd ed. New York, NY: Oxford University Press; 2010:969-982.

58. National Hospice and Palliative Care Organization (NHPCO). *NHPCO's Facts and Figures: Hospice Care in America.* 2013. www.nhpco.org/sites/default/files/public/Statistics_Research/2013_Facts_Figures.pdf. Accessed July 29, 2014.

59. Paice JA. Care during the final days of life. In: Yarbro CH, Wujcik D, Gobel BH, eds. *Cancer Nursing: Principles and Practice.* 7th ed. Sudbury, MA: Jones and Bartlett Publishers; 2011:1829-1842.

60. Centers for Disease Control and Prevention (CDC). *Heart Disease.* 2014. www.cdc.gov/heartdisease/index.htm. Accessed July 29, 2014.

61. McGavigan AD, Datta CL, Dunn FG. Palliative care for patients with end-stage heart disease. In: Hanks G, Cherney NI, Christakis NA, Fallon M, Kassa S, Portenoy RK. *Oxford Textbook of Palliative Medicine.* 4th ed. New York, NY: Oxford University Press; 2010:1257-1267.

62. Colucci WS. Overview of the therapy of heart failure due to systolic dysfunction. *UpToDate.* 2014. www.uptodate.com/contents/overview-of-the-therapy-of-heart-failure-due-to-systolic-dysfunction?source=search_result&search=heart+failure&selectedTitle=1%7E150. Accessed August 19, 2014.

63. Fahlberg BB, Panke JT; Coyne PJ, ed. *Compendium of End Stage Non-Cancer Diagnoses: Heart Failure.* 2nd ed. Pittsburgh, PA: Hospice and Palliative Nurses Association; 2011.

64. Criteria Committee of the New York Heart Association. *Nomenclature and Criteria for Diagnosis of Diseases of the Heart and Great Vessels.* 9th ed. Boston, MA: Little, Brown & Co; 1994:253-256.

65. Hunt SA, Abraham WT, Chin MH, et al. 2009 focused update incorporated into the ACC/AHA 2005 Guidelines for the Diagnosis and Management of Heart Failure in Adults: a report of the American College of Cardiology Foundation/American Heart Association Task Force on Practice Guidelines: developed in collaboration with the International Society for Heart and Lung Transplantation. *Circulation.* 2009;119:e391-e479. doi: 10.1161/CIRCULATIONAHA.109.192065.

66. Centers for Medicare & Medicaid Services (CMS). *Local Coverage Determination (LCD): Hospice Determining Terminal Status (L32015).* 2014. www.cms.gov/medicare-coverage-database/details/lcd-details.aspx?LCDId=32015&ContrId=236&ver=15&ContrVer=2&CntrctrSelected=236*2&Cntrctr=236&name=CGS+Administrators%2c+LLC+(15004%2c+HHH+MAC)&LCntrctr=236*2&bc=AgACAAIASAAAAA%3d%3d&. Accessed September 16, 2014.

67. Harrington MD, Luebke DL, Lewis WR, Aulisio MP, Johnson NJ. Implantable cardioverter-defibrillators at end-of-life. *Fast Facts and Concepts.* 2009; 112. www.eperc.mcw.edu/EPERC/FastFactsIndex/ff_112.htm. Accessed July 30, 2014.

68. Murphy SL, Xu J, Kochanek KD. Deaths: final data for 2010. *Natl Vital Stat Rep.* 2013;61(4):1-118.

69. Quill TE, Bower KA, Holloway RG, et al. *Primer of Palliative Care.* 6th ed. Glenview, IL: American Academy of Hospice and Palliative Medicine; 2014.

70. National Center for Chronic Disease Prevention and Health Promotion, Division for Heart Disease and Stroke Prevention. *Types of Stroke.* 2013. www.cdc.gov/stroke/types_of_stroke.htm. Accessed August 19, 2014.

71. Holloway RG, Ladwig S, Robb J, Kelly A, Nielsen E, Quill TE. Palliative care consultations in hospitalized stroke patients. *J Palliat Med.* 2010;13(4):407-412.

72. National Stroke Association. *Stroke 101: Fast Facts on Stroke.* 2014. www.stroke.org/stroke-resources/library/stroke-101. Accessed July 29, 2014.

73. Bowman ME; Coyne PJ, ed. *Compendium of Treatment of End Stage Non-Cancer Diagnoses: Neurological Diseases and Trauma.* 2nd ed. Pittsburgh, PA: Hospice and Palliative Nurses Association; 2013.

74. Borasio GD, Lorenzl S, Rogers A, Voltz R. Palliative care in non-malignant neurological disorders. In: Hanks G, Cherney NI, Christakis NA, Fallon M, Kaasa S, Portenoy RK, eds. *Oxford Textbook of Palliative Medicine.* 4th ed. New York, NY: Oxford University Press; 2010:1268-1279.

75. Gallagher M, Long CO. Advanced dementia care: demystifying behaviors, addressing pain, and maximizing comfort: research and practice: partners in care. *J Hosp Palliat Nurs.* 2011;13(2):70-78.

76. Volicer L. Palliative care in dementia. In: Hanks G, Cherney NI, Christakis NA, Fallon M, Kaasa S, Portenoy RK, eds. *Oxford Textbook of Palliative Medicine.* 4th ed. New York, NY: Oxford University Press; 2010:1375-1385.

77. Morrison LF, Liao S. Dementia medications in palliative care. *Fast Facts and Concepts.* 2007; 174. www.eperc.mcw.edu/EPERC/FastFactsIndex/ff_174.htm. Accessed July 30, 2014.

78. Forsaa EB, Larsen JP, Wentzel-Larsen T, Alves G. What predicts mortality in Parkinson disease?: a prospective population-based long-term study. *Neurology.* 2010;75(14):1270-1276. doi: 10.1212/WNL.0b013e3181f61311.

79. Campbell ML; Coyne PJ, ed. *Compendium of Treatment of End Stage Non-Cancer Diagnoses: Pulmonary.* 2nd ed. Pittsburgh, PA: Hospice and Palliative Nurses Association; 2011.

80. Childers JW, Arnold R, Curtis JR. Prognosis in end-stage COPD. *Fast Facts and Concepts.* 2009; 141. www.eperc.mcw.edu/EPERC/FastFactsIndex/ff_141.htm. Accessed July 30, 2014.

81. Caronia JR, Kanaparthi LK, Lessnau KD. Restrictive lung disease. *Medscape.* 2014. emedicine.medscape.com/article/301760-overview. Accessed July 30, 2014.

82. Brennan CW, Mazanec P. Dyspnea management across the palliative care continuum. *J Hosp Palliat Nurs.* 2011;13(3):130-139.

83. Gorman LM; Coyne PJ, ed. *Compendium of Treatment of End Stage Non-Cancer Diagnosis: Renal.* 2nd ed. Pittsburgh, PA: Hospice and Palliative Nurses Association; 2011.

84. Owens DA. Palliative care and end stage renal disease. *J Hosp Palliat Nurs.* 2006;8(6):318-319.

85. Arnold R, Verrico P, Davison S. Opioid use in renal failure. *Fast Facts and Concepts.* 2009; 161. www.eperc.mcw.edu/EPERC/FastFactsIndex/ff_161.htm. Accessed July 30, 2014.

86. Davison SN, Rosielle DA. Withdrawal of dialysis: decision-making. *Fast Facts and Concepts.* 2008; 207. www.eperc.mcw.edu/EPERC/FastFactsIndex/ff_207.htm. Accessed July 30, 2014.

87. Scheufler JM, Prince-Paul M. The diabetic hospice patient: incorporating evidence and medications into goals of care. *J Hosp Palliat Nurs.* 2011;13(6):356-365. doi: 10.1097/NJH.0b013e3182330edc.

88. Kondo S, Kondo M, Kondo A. Glycemia control using A1C level in terminal cancer patients with preexisting type 2 diabetes. *J Palliat Med.* 2013;16(7):790-793. doi: 10.1089/jpm.2012.0471.

89. Angelo M, Ruchalki C, Sproge BJ. An approach to diabetes mellitus in hospice and palliative medicine. *J Palliat Med.* 2011;14(1):83-87.

90. Jones RE, Brashers VL, Huether SE. Alterations of hormonal regulation. In: McCance KL, Huether SE, Brashers VL, Rote NS, eds. *Pathophysiology: The Biologic Basis for Disease in Adults and Children.* 6th ed. Maryland Heights, MO: Mosby Elsevier; 2010:727-780.

91. Savage S, Duggan N, Dunning T, Martin P. The experiences and care preferences of people with diabetes at the end of life. *J Hosp Palliat Nurs.* 2012;14(4):293-302. doi: 10.1097/NJH.0b013e3182 bdb39.

92. American Diabetes Care. Standards of medical care in diabetes—2014. *Diabetes Care.* 2014;37(1 suppl):S14-S80. doi: 10.2337/dc14-S014. care.diabetesjournals.org/content/37/Supplement_1/S14.full. Accessed October 1, 2014.

93. Bobb BT; Coyne PJ, ed. *Compendium of Treatment of End Stage Non-Cancer Diagnoses: Hepatic.* 2nd ed. Pittsburgh, PA: Hospice and Palliative Nurses Association; 2012.

94. Cox-North P, Doorenbos A, Shannon SE, Scott J, Curtis JR. The transition to end-of-life care in end-stage liver disease. *J Hosp Palliat Nurs.* 2013;15(4):209-215.

95. Centers for Disease Control and Prevention (CDC). *Today's HIV/AIDS Epidemic.* 2013. www.cdc.gov/nchhstp/newsroom/docs/HIVFactSheets/TodaysEpidemic-508.pdf. Accessed July 30, 2014.

96. Panel on Antiretroviral Guidelines for Adults and Adolescents. *Guidelines for the Use of Antiretroviral Agents in HIV-1-Infected Adults and Adolescents.* 2014. aidsinfo.nih.gov/contentfiles/lvguidelines/adultandadolescentgl.pdf. Accessed July 30, 2014.

97. Whitehead P; Coyne PJ, ed. *Compendium of Treatment of End Stage Non-Cancer Diagnoses: HIV/AIDS.* 2nd ed. Pittsburgh, PA: Hospice and Palliative Nurses Association; 2013.

98. Wilner LS, Arnold R. Cannabinoids in the treatment of symptoms in cancer and AIDS, 2nd ed. *Fast Facts and Concepts.* 2009; 93. www.eperc.mcw.edu/EPERC/FastFactsIndex/ff_093.htm. Accessed July 30, 2014.

99. Alderman J. Diarrhea in palliative care, 2nd ed. *Fast Facts and Concepts.* 2009; 96. www.eperc.mcw.edu/EPERC/FastFactsIndex/ff_096.htm. Accessed July 30, 2014.

100. Groninger H, Schisler RE. Capsaicin for neuropathic pain. *Fast Facts and Concepts.* 2012; 255. www.eperc.mcw.edu/EPERC/FastFactsIndex/ff_255.htm. Accessed July 30, 2014.

CHAPTER IV

PAIN MANAGEMENT

Judith A. Paice, PhD, RN

I. Introduction

    A. Overview

        1. Prevalence

            a) The prevalence of pain varies by diagnosis, stage of disease, and setting of care

                i. Approximately one-third of patients with cancer experience pain at the time of diagnosis, while two-thirds with metastatic disease report pain[1]

                ii. Less is known about the prevalence of pain in those with diagnoses other than cancer

                iii. Higher pain intensity and pain interference are associated with impaired quality of life, and in some cases, increased risk of hastened death.[2] Nurses must screen all patients for the presence of pain and conduct a more thorough pain assessment when any pain is present; this process must be ongoing as pain can occur at any phase of care

    B. Barriers to Pain Assessment and Treatment

        1. Barriers exist to pain assessment and pain treatment. Nurses who are aware of these obstacles can work to overcome these, both in their individual encounters with patients/families, but also in making systems changes. Barriers are often categorized as those related to healthcare providers, those related to the system, and those related to patients/families[3]

            a) Barriers related to healthcare providers

                i. Instruction regarding pain during basic education remains inadequate in many programs

                ii. Assessment of pain using only a simple screening such as a 0–10 scale is insufficient

                iii. Fears regarding addiction, tolerance, and adverse effects related to analgesics, particularly opioids, persist

b) Barriers related to the healthcare system

    i. Inadequate time and reimbursement, along with a low priority given to pain and symptom management in some systems

    ii. Restrictive regulations, poor reimbursement, and lack of availability of treatments—especially opioids but also access to other therapies

c) Barriers related to patients and family members

    i. Reluctance to report pain, often related to stoicism; concern about distracting healthcare providers from treatment of the underlying disease; belief that pain is an expected outcome of the disease, or admission that the disease is worse

    ii. Patients and/or family members may also fear addiction and/or tolerance along with adverse effects, limiting their compliance with the analgesic regimen

    iii. Myths held by patients, family members, and the public persist

        (a) *Good* patients do not complain

        (b) Pain is inevitable with aging

        (c) Strong medicine only comes in an injectable form

        (d) Bearing the pain is better than bearing the side effects of pain medicine

        (e) Addiction to pain medicine is common

        (f) Strong pain medicine should only be used for very severe pain

        (g) Morphine and other opioids are used as a last resort and only when one is imminently dying

        (h) Morphine and other opioids hasten death

d) Nursing role in overcoming barriers

    i. Review one's own learning needs on an ongoing basis as symptom science continues to advance; encourage educational offerings related to pain through one's employment setting and professional organizations

    ii. Evaluate the strengths and weaknesses within one's setting of care for opportunities to improve pain control; engage management and team members in this process to have the necessary buy-in to make these changes

    iii. Assess patient barriers, validate fears, provide reassurance and empathy, along with cognitive interventions such as verbal, print, or video education

C. Definitions

1. Pain is a complex biopsychosocial phenomenon

a) Pain is an unpleasant sensory and emotional experience associated with actual or potential tissue damage or described in these terms[4]

b) Pain is whatever the patient says it is[5]

 c) The subjectivity surrounding pain often leads to tension in the patient–provider relationship. Because there are no definitive laboratory or imaging tests that reveal what an individual might be feeling, providers may question the validity of a patient's report. This is compounded by misperceptions that someone should demonstrate outward signs of pain. "He does not look like someone who has an '8' on a 0–10 scale; in fact, I just saw him talking on the telephone" may reveal that distraction is important to this patient who believes his pain is severe. Strong assessment skills are warranted to discern the underlying etiology of pain along with the contribution of emotional or other components to the sensory experience. Believing the patient's report is an important aspect of empathic care but it does not mean an automatic increase in analgesic doses. The interdisciplinary team is crucial in addressing the biopsychosocial aspects of pain in advanced disease

2. Misuse—use of a medication other than as directed or as indicated; whether willful or unintentional, and whether harm results or not. Examples may include the use of pain medications for sleep rather than pain control; can also include diversion of medications to others for use or sale

3. Addiction—"a primary, chronic, neurobiological disease with genetic, psychosocial, and environmental factors influencing its development and manifestations. It is characterized by behaviors that include one or more of the following: impaired control over drug use, compulsive use, and continued use despite harm and craving"[6, p. 165]

4. Tolerance—"a state of adaptation in which exposure to a drug induces changes that result in a diminution of one or more of the drug's effects over time"[6, p. 165]

5. Physical dependence—"a state of adaptation that is manifested by a drug class-specific withdrawal syndrome that can be produced by abrupt cessation, rapid dose reduction, decreasing blood level of the drug, and/or administration of an antagonist"[6, p. 165]

 a) Signs and symptoms of abstinence syndrome (withdrawal) include anxiety, irritability, lacrimation, rhinorrhea, sweating, nausea, vomiting, diarrhea, abdominal cramps, insomnia, tachycardia, elevated blood pressure, and rarely multifocal myoclonus (multiple sites of mild to severe muscle twitching)

  i. Appearance of abstinence syndrome is a function of the elimination half-life of the opioid; for example, abstinence symptoms appear between 6 and 12 hours and peak between 24 and 72 hours following the last dose of a medication with a short (2–3 hours) half-life (e.g., morphine)

  ii. Conversely, with medications with a longer half-life, the appearance of abstinence symptoms are delayed, for example, with methadone, as much as 36–48 hours after the last dose, although this can be quite variable

6. Opioid pseudoaddiction—iatrogenic syndrome in which patients develop certain behavioral characteristics of psychological dependence as a consequence of inadequate pain treatment. Patients with this syndrome must continually demonstrate their need for analgesics and are often described as difficult patients, chronic complainers, drug seekers, and/or "addicts." Patients will often resort to bizarre or dramatic behavior (acting out) in an attempt to prove their pain is real so analgesics are provided[5,7]

7. Double effect—an ethical principle that permits an action, intended to have a good effect, when there is a risk of also causing a harmful effect, ONLY when the intention was to produce the good effect

    a) Double effect, as a principle guiding care, is complex, but nonetheless erroneously applied to end-of-life care, especially pain and symptom management. Misunderstandings regarding this principle enhance beliefs that opioids are responsible for shortening life, when data do not support these beliefs. Adequately controlling symptoms at end of life does not shorten life; there is a growing research literature that demonstrates opioids are not associated with a shortened survival period in people at end of life[8-10]

    b) An analysis of the potential benefits of a therapy weighed against the possible risks should be conducted when considering any therapy

II. Assessment of Pain—Effectiveness of Pain Management Is Directly Related to Assessment

A. Assessment Parameters[5]

1. Site—have patient point on themselves or on a diagram, identify and assess all sites as well as sites of radiation; the patient may have more than one site of pain

2. Character—use the patient's own words; a careful description will lead to the diagnosis of pain type and therefore use of appropriate adjuvant analgesics (i.e., tingling, burning, sharp, shooting describe neuropathic pain syndromes); refer to the section, "Types of Pain" for additional, in depth descriptions

3. Onset—when did it start? Did (or does) a specific event trigger the pain?

    a) Carefully distinguish between new and preexisting pain (e.g., arthritis, chronic low back pain syndromes)

    b) Assess for breakthrough pain (i.e., transient flares of pain in patients with chronic pain syndromes)

    c) Breakthrough pain can be incidental (e.g., associated with movement), idiopathic (i.e., the cause is not known), or can occur as end-of-dose failure (e.g., the pain recurs prior to the next dose of pain medication)

4. Duration and frequency—how long has the pain persisted? Is it constant or does it come and go (intermittent)? Pain is often categorized as acute (e.g., postsurgical pain), chronic (e.g., postherpetic neuropathy), or acute on chronic (e.g., pain crisis in sickle cell disease in a patient with persistent joint/bone pain)

5. Intensity—pain intensity is an important component of pain assessment as it directly correlates with interference with the patient's quality of life. Commonly defined on a scale, the intensity rating method must be adapted to each patient. The most common intensity rating method for adults is the 0–10 numerical scale. Record pain intensity now, at its worst, at its least, and on an average. Verbal descriptors, such as no pain, mild, moderate, or severe, can be used when pain cannot be conceptualized as a number

    a) Pain rating scales for cognitively impaired or nonverbal patients are available, but caregivers (be they family or staff in a care facility) can often give valuable information to add to the pain assessment

b) A change in the patient's behavior is considered the *gold standard* for measuring effectiveness of pain interventions and determining a patient's level of discomfort. Changes in functional ability and alterations in the patient's normal routine are two behaviors that may aide in identifying severity of pain

c) One indicator of the presence of pain in patients who are unable to respond is the furrowed brow

d) Relief of the furrowing is often seen when pain is relieved; likewise, response to treatment can be considered part of the assessment

6. Exacerbating factors—what times, activities, or other circumstances make the pain worse?

7. Associated symptoms—what other symptoms occur before, with, or after the pain?

8. Alleviating factors—what makes the pain better? What treatments (including nonpharmacological interventions) have been successful in the past and what have been unsuccessful? Include a thorough medication history that includes adverse effects that have occurred with previous exposure to pain medications

9. Medication history—what medication(s) have been ordered? What medication(s) is the patient currently taking? If there is a disparity, examine the underlying reasons (e.g., cost, adverse effects, fear of addiction or tolerance). What medication(s) worked in the past for unrelated pain episodes? What are the patient, family, and caregivers' beliefs about opioids?

10. Impact on quality of life—what does the pain mean to the patient and family? How has this pain affected them and their quality of life? Does it keep the patient from doing things he/she wants to do? How much do the patient and the family know about pain? Do they have the expectation that it can be relieved? Are there emotional or spiritual components to the pain? Does unrelieved pain lead to increased fear or anxiety or to fears that death is imminent?

11. Physical examination—observe the site of the pain and validate with the patient the pain's location; note skin color, warmth, irritation, integrity, swelling, and any other unusual findings; utilize other physical assessment techniques, for example, palpation, percussion, and auscultation, as appropriate; be mindful that persons with chronic pain often have no changes in vital signs or facial expression

12. Values—what are the patient's goals for pain management? What is the patient's self-identified threshold? What are the cultural aspects of pain for this patient?

B. **Etiology of Pain[3]**

1. Cancer pain syndromes

a) Pain associated with direct tumor involvement

i. Examples include metastatic bone disease, nerve compression or infiltration, or hollow viscus involvement

b) Pain associated with cancer therapy

i. Any pain that occurs in the course of or as a result of surgery, chemotherapy, radiation therapy, hematopoietic stem cell transplant, hormonal, or other treatments (e.g., mucositis, chemotherapy-induced peripheral neuropathy, phantom pain syndromes, extravasation of vesicant chemotherapy, arthralgia from aromatase inhibitors, graft versus host disease)

c) Pain unrelated to cancer or cancer therapy (e.g., arthritis, migraine headache, low back pain, fibromyalgia, or any other pain syndromes present among the general population)

2. Pain syndromes common in selected medical conditions seen in palliative care

   a) Human immunodeficiency virus (HIV) infection

      i. HIV pain is often categorized in a manner similar to cancer—pain associated with the virus (e.g., direct involvement of the virus in the sensory neurons that transmit pain), pain associated with the treatment (e.g., neuropathy due to antiretroviral drugs), or pain unrelated to HIV or its treatment (e.g., musculoskeletal pains after exercise)

      ii. The most common pain syndrome seen in HIV disease is now peripheral neuropathy that occurs from both the virus and the treatment. Late-stage HIV is often associated with infectious processes that can produce pain (e.g., headaches from acute and chronic meningitis, chest pain from *Pneumocystis* pneumonia)

   b) Other disorders

      i. As palliative care moves upstream and assists patients earlier in the course of the disease, patients will be cared for with diagnoses other than cancer including cardiovascular disorders, neurologic syndromes, sickle cell disease, and other disorders

         (a) Cardiovascular disorders

            (i) Chest pain—can range from an acute coronary syndrome to more chronic stable angina pectoris; differential diagnosis includes respiratory syndromes, gastroesophageal reflux disease, or panic attacks, among many possibilities

            (ii) Peripheral vascular disease—can range from mild muscular discomfort to debilitating claudication of hip/leg/calves; may be accompanied by painful sensations in the feet/toes due to decreased circulation

         (b) Neurologic syndromes

            (i) Central pain or post stroke pain—may occur immediately after stroke or may be delayed for several years after the stroke; accompanied by decreased temperature sensation; may be superficial or deep; often severe in intensity and accompanied by hyperalgesia (increasing pain)[6] and allodynia (pain from a stimulus that does not usually cause pain such as touch)[11]

            (ii) Spinal cord injury—central pain may occur from an injury at any level of the spinal cord

            (iii) Multiple sclerosis (MS)—paroxysmal trigeminal neuralgia, optic neuritis, and periorbital pain, painful spasms, as well as extremity pain, including dysesthesia, allodynia, and painful electric shock sensations

            (iv) Amyotrophic lateral sclerosis (ALS)—painful syndromes may be associated with deconditioning and loss of muscle mass, as well as spasticity and muscle fasciculation (muscular twitching involving the simultaneous contraction of contiguous groups of muscle fibers)

    (c) Hematologic disorders

        (i) Sickle cell disease—pain is severe and acute; focal (bone, joint, and muscle) and visceral pain from ischemia and infarction[12]

C. Types of Pain

1. Acute pain versus chronic[13,14]

    a) Acute pain—usually has a clear cause; may see observable signs (e.g., increased pulse rate, increase in blood pressure; nonverbal signs and symptoms, such as facial expressions, tense muscles); can serve the purpose of being a warning sign; examples: myocardial infarction, postoperative pain, acute appendicitis

    b) Chronic pain—etiology may be unclear; does not serve purpose; often associated with decreased social interaction, insomnia, depressed affect; examples: persistent cancer pain, chronic back pain

2. Quality of pain

    a) Nociceptive pain (or somatic and visceral pain)

      i. Somatic pain—well-localized; often described as deep, dull ache; musculoskeletal in nature; examples: bone metastasis, inflammation of soft tissue, tumor invasion of soft tissue

      ii. Visceral pain—poorly localized; cramping, deep ache, pressure, often referred to distant dermatomal sites; examples: bowel obstruction resulting in bowel spasms, cholecystitis, primary or metastatic tumors in the liver

      iii. Referred pain common in visceral pain syndromes

        (a) Pain from tumor involvement of the pancreas, lower esophagus, stomach or retroperitoneal area may be referred to the back

        (b) Gallbladder or liver disease may produce referred pain in the back or right shoulder (suprascapular)

        (c) Rectosigmoid involvement may result in pain to sacrum or rectal area

    b) Neuropathic pain—sharp, burning, shooting, shock-like; examples: spinal nerve root compression, tumor invasion of nerves, post-herpetic neuralgia, surgical interruption of nerves, central pain syndromes occurring after stroke, phantom limb pain

      i. Opioids relieve neuropathic pain but higher doses usually indicated; adjuvant analgesics warranted. Non-opioids (e.g., acetaminophen, nonsteroidal anti-inflammatory drugs [NSAIDs]) are rarely beneficial

D. Biopsychosocial Model of Pain[5]

1. Numerous variables influence the experience of pain—pain is experienced by the patient *and* family in keeping with the model of *total pain* and includes physical, psychological, social, and spiritual effects; when adequate assessment and management of controllable symptoms precede psychological, social, and spiritual assessment and intervention, overall outcomes often improve

2. Common effects of pain

a) Physical effects—biological factors leading to pain as well as decreased functional ability, including ability to walk and perform other basic activities of daily living (ADLs), decreased strength and endurance, nausea, anorexia, insomnia, and impaired immune response

b) Psychological variables—increased fear and anxiety, depression, hopelessness, despair, loss of control; if pain uncontrolled, consideration of suicide or physician-assisted suicide

c) Social effects—alteration in social and close relationships (e.g., roles and responsibilities, intimacy, sexual function), isolation, inability to work; diminished leisure, loss of self-esteem, self-worth; increased caregiver burden, further disruption of important social supports for both patient and family

d) Spiritual and existential issues—increased suffering, reevaluation and perhaps doubt regarding past religious foundations and beliefs; questioning the meaning of suffering

e) Financial effects—inability to work and earn income, loss of caregiver income, issues of workplace discrimination and having to apply for governmental assistance leading to decreased income and loss of health insurance coverage

f) Cultural issues—ethnic minority, female, and elderly persons often receive less than optimal pain management in all settings[5]

   i. Consider the patient's family of origin, their manner of expressing pain, and how suffering is valued

   ii. Explore perceptions of pain, end of life, afterlife, bereavement, and other aspects of palliative care as they can vary widely by ethnicity and within ethnicities

   iii. Assess specific aspects of culture when caring for patients in pain, such as ethnic identity, gender, age, differing abilities, sexual orientation, religion and spirituality, financial status, place of residency, employment, and educational level

III. Pharmacological Intervention

A. Nonopioids[15]

1. Acetaminophen

a) Actions—analgesic, antipyretic, no anti-inflammatory effect

b) Adverse effects—hepatotoxicity in larger doses or with hepatic dysfunction (acetaminophen overdose is the leading cause of acute liver failure in the United States); can also compromise renal function; formerly the limit on the total amount of acetaminophen that can be given in a 24-hour period was considered to be 4 gm a day, but because this was not based on longitudinal studies, lower doses (3000 mg/day) recommended for chronic use, including in older/debilitated individuals, alcoholic patients, people with HIV, patients with liver metastasis, or those with active liver disease. Dose escalation is limited by the quantity of acetaminophen in combination medications (e.g., oxycodone/acetaminophen [Percocet®], hydromorphone/acetaminophen [Vicodin®], over-the-counter cold medications)[1]

2.   Nonsteroidal anti-inflammatory drugs (NSAIDs)

  a)   Actions—analgesic, antipyretic, anti-inflammatory

  b)   Includes nonselective and selective cyclo-oxygenase 2 (COX-2) inhibitors

     i.   Nonselective NSAIDs include aspirin, ibuprofen, naproxen, and others

     ii.   Celecoxib is the only COX-2 that remains on the market, but it has black box warnings regarding the increased risk of cardiovascular events and gastrointestinal bleeds[1]

  c)   Adverse effects

     i.   Gastrointestinal distress—no relation between symptoms and seriousness of gastrointestinal effects; concomitant administration of misoprostol or proton pump inhibiter can prevent gastropathy

     ii.   Renal insufficiency—elderly and dehydrated patients are at increased risk

     iii.   Inhibiting platelet aggregation

     iv.   Cardiovascular effects, including myocardial infarction and stroke; individuals with risk factors for these events are at higher than average risk and should avoid NSAIDs

     v.   Hypersensitivity reactions (not allergic reactions); symptoms include urticaria, bronchospasm, severe rhinitis, and shock

        (a)   Adverse effects are often labeled by patients/caregivers as *allergies* (e.g., nausea, vomiting)

        (b)   These are not absolute contraindications to using the drug

     vi.   Central nervous system (CNS) effects—dizziness, tinnitus, decreased hearing, headache

     vii.   Dose escalation is limited by analgesic ceiling and the appearance of side effects

B.   Opioid Medications[16]

1.   Types of opioids

  a)   Pure agonists

  b)   Partial agonists (e.g., buprenorphine); same precautions as pure opioids

  c)   Mixed agonist-antagonists (e.g., pentazocine, butorphanol, nalbuphine); not recommended for the treatment of chronic pain due to analgesic ceiling, psychomimetic actions, precipitation of withdrawal when given to patients on pure mu opioid agonists such as morphine, oxycodone, and hydromorphone

  d)   Action—bind to receptors in the brain, spinal cord, and in peripheral nervous system

  e)   Adverse effects of opioids

     i.   Sedation, sometimes, but rarely confusion

     ii.   Dizziness, dysphoria

     iii.   Nausea

iv. Constipation; tolerance does not develop—*must be prevented and treated aggressively.* See the section on constipation in Chapter V, *Symptom Management*

v. Itching and urticaria

vi. Respiratory depression

(a) Feared and misunderstood

(b) Clinically significant respiratory depression is extremely rare when patients in severe pain receive opioids, especially in patients who are currently receiving opioids and when doses are titrated upward in appropriate steps; patients who are at risk are those who are opioid naïve, have obstructive sleep apnea, concomitantly taking other sedating drugs (e.g., benzodiazepines, antihistamines), first night after surgery

(c) Respiratory rate alone is not an indicator of respiratory depression; some patients may have a respiratory rate of 7 breaths/min, while alert and well perfused; other factors that must be considered are the level of sedation, the depth of respiration, and the adequacy of perfusion of oxygen in the tissues as determined by examining nail beds for changes in color. In the acute setting, obtaining an oxygen saturation level or pulse oximetry may be warranted in some circumstances, yet intermittent pulse oximetry may produce higher levels due to deep inspiration on being awakened, and changes are often late signs of respiratory change

(d) Mechanism of opioid induced respiratory depression—opioids render the CO_2 receptors less sensitive to increasing CO_2 levels

(e) True respiratory depression is unusual in the palliative care population. When this occurs, it is best treated by slow infusion of dilute naloxone rather than a bolus dose, which will completely block binding of all opioids, resulting in rapid onset of abstinence syndrome and return of pain. This cannot be treated until the effects of the antagonist wears off, often in several hours

vii. Opioid active metabolites

(a) Meperidine—should not be used in any pain management; it does have an active metabolite that is converted to a long-lived, centrally acting excitatory metabolite (normeperidine) causing shaky feelings, tremors/ twitches, and myoclonus/grand mal seizures

(b) Morphine and hydromorphone also have active metabolites (morphine 6-glucuronide [M6G], morphine 3-glucuronide [M3G] and hydromorphone 6-glucuronide [H6G], hydromorphone 3-glucuronide [H3G]), which are excreted by the kidneys. These metabolites can accumulate in elderly patients and in those with diminished renal function (although myoclonus has been observed without renal dysfunction); has strong analgesic and respiratory depressant properties; M3G and H3G may produce central nervous system hyperexcitability and possibly myoclonus, while elevated M6G and H6G levels appear to cause sedation. Small amounts of hydration (intravenous fluids at 30–50 mL/hour) may help to clear these metabolites and relieve opioid toxicity

f) Routes of administration[11]

 i. Oral—most preferred for comfort, convenience, and cost effectiveness; many forms available: immediate release tablets, sustained release tablets, and liquids

  (a) Sublingual and buccal administration of opioids such as morphine, hydromorphone, or oxycodone is similar in dose to the oral route, as the majority of the dose is absorbed via the gastrointestinal tract rather than the oral mucosa

 ii. Rectal—useful for patients who are not to have anything by mouth or have nausea and vomiting; contraindicated with anal lesions, diarrhea, thrombocytopenia, or neutropenia; family caregivers and some cultures will have varying comfort levels with the rectal route for medication administration. Bioavailability of rectally administered opioids varies as there is a high degree of interindividual absorption[17]

 iii. Parenteral delivery

  (a) Intravenous administration is more common in inpatient settings, but can be provided at home, especially when patient has an existing port or other type of vascular access; doses can be delivered by bolus or basal rate (e.g., patient controlled, programmed intermittent, or continuous infusion)

  (b) Subcutaneous infusions (via bolus or basal) can be used in most settings when venous access not possible or the oral route is no longer effective/safe. Subcutaneous infusions can also be maintained in the home; useful for pain requiring rapid titration of medication, particularly when there is concern about absorption through the gastrointestinal tract. Expense of home parenteral infusions to hospice programs is a barrier to use. Subcutaneous delivery is a reasonable alternative although absorption may be erratic in patients with third-space fluid retention and generalized edema

  (c) Intramuscular injections should be avoided—injections are painful, unnecessary, and absorption is not reliable

 iv. Transmucosal—employs buccal or sublingual delivery, provides rapid onset of action when product is lipophilic (i.e., fat soluble such as fentanyl); currently requires prescriber to obtain additional education (Transmucosal Immediate Release Fentanyl [TIRF]—Risk Evaluation Mitigation Strategy [REMS]) if prescribing these agents for patients except those in hospital, hospice, or in nursing home facilities

 v. Transdermal delivery

  (a) Fentanyl is most commonly employed transdermal system for patients with stable pain; delayed onset of action (12–24 hours) with first patch application and with each dose change, some patients require a patch change every 48 hours; should not be given to opioid naïve patients. A study of cachectic patients receiving a fentanyl patch revealed that plasma levels tended to be lower when compared to patients of normal weight, but the drug was still absorbed.[18] Thus, these individuals may require a higher dose; as with other pharmacologic therapies, assessment is crucial

  (b) Buprenorphine, a partial agonist, has been used as part of an opioid maintenance program instead of methadone and is now available as a 7-day patch approved for moderate to severe pain

vi.   Spinal—via indwelling catheters into the epidural or intrathecal space; an implantable pump should be used in only carefully selected patients after appropriate consultation; cost, care issues, and potential adverse effects should also be carefully weighed; can dramatically improve some patients quality of life, especially with severe pain in lower extremities

C.   Adjuvant Analgesics (see Table 4-3 at the end of the chapter)[3,14]

1.   Antiepileptic drugs

   a)   Because newer antiepileptic drugs do not have the severe adverse effects associated with earlier agents, these are often first line therapies for many people with neuropathic pain

   b)   Major adverse effects

      i.   Gabapentin—sedation, ataxia, dizziness, dependent edema, side effects generally less than with others; less costly now that generic form is available

      ii.   Pregabalin—similar to gabapentin with similar mechanisms of action; may provide an effect equivalent to gabapentin at lower doses

      iii.   Carbamazepine—bone marrow suppression, vertigo, confusion, sedation; requires serum monitoring; costly

      iv.   Phenytoin—ataxia, rash, hepatotoxicity; requires serum monitoring

      v.   Valproic acid—nausea, vomiting, sedation, ataxia, tremor, thrombocytopenia, neutropenia, hepatotoxicity; requires serum monitoring

        (a)   Clonazepam—sedation, physical dependence; not as effective as an analgesic; useful for anxiety associated with pain

2.   Antidepressants

   a)   Tricyclic antidepressants—desipramine and nortriptyline are recommended over amitriptyline, which has more anticholinergic effects (e.g., cardiovascular changes, dry mouth, constipation, cognitive changes, especially in older adults)

      i.   Start with a low dose (e.g., desipramine 10–25 mg orally or nortriptyline 10–25 mg at bedtime); these drugs may cause sedation and enhance sleep

      ii.   Increase dose by 10–25 mg increments every few days based upon the patient's response

      iii.   Response may be delayed by 3–7 days

      iv.   Monitor adverse effects

      v.   Maximum dose of nortriptyline and desipramine is 75–100 mg/day

      vi.   Adverse effects—sedation, orthostatic hypotension, anticholinergic side effects (including urinary retention), cardiac effects

   b)   Serotonin selective reuptake inhibitors (SSRIs) appear to have limited analgesic effect, despite being very effective antidepressants

      c) Serotonin-norepinephrine reuptake inhibitors—venlafaxine and duloxetine, both used for treating depression, hot flashes, and neuropathy

  3. Local anesthetics

      a) Lidocaine patch 5%—approved for topical relief of postherpetic neuropathy but also used for persistent postthoracotomy or postmastectomy pain syndromes; unlikely to be beneficial for deeper pains

         i. The patches should be placed over intact skin only

         ii. Up to three patches can be used to cover the painful area; package insert instructs to apply for 12 hours and then remove for 12 hours, but is safe to leave in place for 18–24 hours

         iii. Adverse effects are uncommon and include pain with removal of the patch

         iv. Patients with sensitivity to touch (also called allodynia) often report relief

      b) Lidocaine infusions are used in palliative care for management of refractory neuropathic pain

         i. Adverse effects include dizziness, lightheadedness, lowered blood pressure, sensory disturbances and tremor, seizures at high doses, nausea, and vomiting

  4. Corticosteroids—used in metastatic bone pain (can produce significant pain control, along with increased energy, enhanced mood and improved appetite). Also useful to relieve pain associated with liver metastases (right upper quadrant pain as well as referred right shoulder pain) and other visceral pain syndromes

  5. Other medications—see Table 4-3 at the end of the chapter

D. Opioid Equianalgesic Conversions

  1. Converting from one opioid to another opioid (i.e., opioid rotation) is needed when adverse effects (e.g., myoclonus, hyperalgesia) are interfering with the analgesic effect and adherence, decrease in effectiveness of the opioid, or a route change is needed. Opioid conversion uses a chart with approximate equianalgesic doses.[17] Doses listed in each row have the same approximate potency; likewise for columns. Table 4-1 is just one example of an equianalgesic chart. Refer to the chart accepted by your organization. See Table 4-2 for the process and an example

Important Note—if converting from one drug to another *and* the patient's pain is well controlled, many experts recommend reducing the dose by 25% to account for incomplete cross tolerance. If converting from the oral to the intravenous route and it is not clear the patient has had reasonable absorption of the drug through the gastrointestinal system, reduce the dose by 25%. However, if you are converting from one drug to another *and* the patient is in severe pain, dose reduction is often not necessary. Throughout the process of conversion, ensure frequent reassessment and provision of breakthrough doses.

Table 4-1. Approximate Equianalgesic Doses of Most Commonly Used Opioid Analgesics[adapted from 14]

Drug	Parenteral Route	Enteral Route
Morphine[†]	10 mg	30 mg
Codeine	130 mg	200 mg (not recommended)
Fentanyl[‡ ††]	50–100 mcg	TIRF[‡]
Hydrocodone	Not available	30 mg
Hydromorphone[§]	1.5 mg	7.5 mg
Levorphanol[¶]	2 mg acute, 1 mg chronic	4 mg acute, 1 mg chronic
Methadone[¶*]	Unknown	Unknown
Oxycodone[**]	Not available	20 mg

[†]Available in continuous and sustained-release pills and capsules, formulated to last 12 or 24 hours.

[‡]Also available in transdermal and transmucosal immediate release fentanyl (TIRF), see package insert materials for dose recommendations.

[§]Available as a continuous-release formulation lasting 24 hours.

[¶]These drugs have long half-lives, so accumulation can occur; close monitoring during first few days of therapy is very important.

[**]Available in several continuous-release doses, formulated to last 12 hours.

[††]Fentanyl 100 mcg patch ≈ 2–3 mg intravenous morphine/hour.[17]

[*]Because equipotent ratios for methadone are unknown, many recommend starting the oral dose at 2.5–5 mg every 8 hours (half-dose for elderly or severe renal or liver disease: 1.25–2.5mg)[19] regardless of the previous opioid dose; do not titrate any more frequently than every 3–7 days; provide sufficient immediate release opioids for breakthrough pain. Methadone can prolong the QT interval. The general guideline is to avoid methadone if QT is approaching or exceeding 500. The frequency of electrocardiogram monitoring depends on the patient's goals of care.

Table 4-2. Equianalgesic Conversion Process

Process	Example
Step 1	
Add up the total amount of the current drug given in 24 hours • Remember to add in both the scheduled and breakthrough or rescue doses • Calculate separately if more than one drug used	Converting oral hydrocodone to hydromorphone: the patient is taking 2 tablets of acetaminophen in combination with hydrocodone 5 mg every 4 hours (6 doses/day). Because each tablet contains 5 mg of hydrocodone, 2 contain 10 mg 6 doses × 10 mg = 60 mg/day of hydrocodone
Step 2	
Divide current 24-hour total by the equianalgesic value for the current drug and route of administration (see Table 4-1)	60 mg of hydrocodone divided by 30 mg (equivalent value for hydrocodone) = 2
Step 3	
Multiply the Step 2 number by the equianalgesic value for the new drug and route • This will give you the new 24-hour dose	2 × 7.5 mg (equivalent value for oral hydromorphone) = 15 mg (or 15 mg of hydromorphone in 24 hours)

Table 4-2. Equianalgesic Conversion Process (continued)

Process	Example
Step 4	
Determine how many doses the patient will take each day and divide this number into the total 24-hour dose • This gives the amount of medication needed per dose	Hydromorphone can be given every 4 hours, which is 6 doses a day; divide the 24-hour dose by 6 doses 15 divided by 6 = 2.5 2.5 mg hydromorphone every 4 hours; as hydromorphone comes in 2-, 4-, and 8-mg tablets, round the dose down to 2 mg, have the appropriate breakthrough medications ordered and carefully monitor the patient for the need to increase the dose

2. Calculating breakthrough or rescue doses

    a) A rescue dose is always ordered with long-acting opioids; it is preferable to match the breakthrough medication with the long-acting opioid (e.g., immediate release morphine with sustained release morphine)

    b) Doses should increase commensurate with increases in the scheduled doses

    c) Guidelines recommend using 10% to 20% of the 24-hour oral dose, given every 1–2 hours as needed[20]

    d) For parenteral administration (intravenous or subcutaneous), the breakthrough dose is 50% to 100% of the hourly rate; since the peak effect is in 15 minutes, boluses may be given safely in the majority of patients every 15 minutes

    e) Increase baseline dose of long-acting opioid if more than 3 rescue doses are used in 24 hours

    f) Example—a patient is taking 120 mg morphine extended release every 12 hours; the appropriate breakthrough dose of MSIR (immediate release morphine) is 24–48 mg (10% to 20%) every 2 hours as needed

IV. Nonpharmacological Interventions

A. Can be used concurrently with medications and other modalities to relieve pain and can often be taught to patients and/or family members. The use of nonpharmacological interventions should never preclude appropriate use of medications, including opioids. The most common nonpharmacological interventions are listed below[6]

1. Physical modalities

    a) Physical therapy (PT) and occupational therapy (OT) consults

    b) Heat, cold

    c) Exercise (with limitations based on physical condition), passive or active range of motion

      d)   Transcutaneous nerve stimulation (efficacy controversial may be useful in patients with mild pain)

      e)   Acupuncture, acupressure

      f)   Massage, healing touch

      g)   Therapeutic touch (a structured and standardized healing practice performed by practitioners trained to be sensitive to the receiver's energy field that surrounds the body)

      h)   Reiki (a Japanese technique for stress reduction and relaxation that also promotes healing. It is administered by "laying on hands" and is based on the idea that an unseen "life force energy" flows through us and is what causes us to be alive)

2.   Cognitive behavioral interventions

      a)   Relaxation and guided imagery

      b)   Pet therapy

      c)   Mindfulness

      d)   Distraction

      e)   Creative arts (e.g., music and art therapy)

      f)   Reframing

      g)   Patient and family education

      h)   Hypnosis

      i)   Counseling (e.g., social worker, counselors, chaplains) for existential pain and suffering

      j)   Prayer

      k)   Spiritual reflection or meditation

3.   Anticancer therapy

      a)   Palliative radiation

            i.   May be used to relieve symptoms of patients with advanced disease, (e.g., pain, bleeding), compression of vital organ systems (e.g., the brain, ulcerating skin lesions), and metastasis to weight bearing bones susceptible to fracture

            ii.   Radiation therapy is the treatment of choice for spinal cord compression, bone pain, and is frequently used in superior vena cava syndrome and symptomatic brain metastases

           iii.   While external beam radiation is the modality commonly used for palliative radiation therapy, Strontium-89, an intravenous radionuclide that emits beta radiation at the bony metastatic site, is sometimes used to treat areas of painful skeletal metastasis; newer radionuclides are currently under study that may not produce the painful flair that occurs when Strontium-89 is given

b) Palliative chemotherapy—may improve or enhance comfort when neither cure nor control is possible

    i. Antineoplastic therapy may produce tumor shrinkage, relieving pressure on nerves, lymphatics, and blood vessels, and reducing organ obstruction, thus relieving pain

c) Bisphosphonates are useful in treating pain related to multiple myeloma and metastatic bone disease[14]

V. Pain During the Final Days of Life

A. Pain Assessment

1. Patients may become nonverbal in the final days of life[14]

    a) A furrowed brow or other nonverbal behaviors indicating discomfort may be a sign of pain

    b) Guarding and vocalization during turning or dressing changes may suggest pain

    c) A therapeutic trial of an opioid should be considered to determine if these behaviors change with the use of an analgesic

2. If the patient had pain prior to becoming unresponsive, assume pain is still present; continue treatment of pain with adjustments as required (e.g., in the route of administration)

B. Pharmacological Management[14]

1. As organ system dysfunction increases, particularly renal clearance, drugs or their metabolites are cleared from the body less efficiently and sedation may increase

    a) Therefore, a therapeutic trial of opioid dose reduction may be indicated if sedation is not a desired effect

    b) In some cases, patients may become more alert and responsive

    c) If any signs of pain return, the dose should be returned to its previous level

2. Rapid discontinuation of opioids, benzodiazepines, or other agents can result in abstinence syndrome; whenever possible, gradual reduction in dose of these drugs is indicated

3. Sedation (also called palliative sedation) at the end of life is an option for patients with intractable pain and suffering[6]

    a) There are numerous medications that can be used

        i.   Benzodiazepines

        ii.   Opioids

        iii. Barbiturates

        iv. Ketamine

        v.   Propofol

    b)   Therapy is based on obtaining initial relief of symptoms followed by ongoing sedation to maintain the effect

    c)   All other options should be employed prior to considering palliative sedation

    d)   The patient (if feasible) and the family provide consent; the interdisciplinary team is convened to offer support and care

    e)   At times, the dose may be reduced if lightening of sedation is desired, such as when a family member arrives from out of town; in some cases, this allows the patient to say goodbye. However, if pain or other symptoms return, the dose is returned to the previous level to resume relief and sedation

VI. Summary of Principles of Pain Management in Palliative Care

A. Conduct a complete pain assessment and document findings to ensure continuity of care

1.   Ongoing evaluation of pain and the effect of interventions should be conducted in a timely manner, in accordance with expected pharmacological peak action or when the nonpharmacological intervention is completed

2.   Ongoing evaluation should include

    a)   Pain intensity, type, duration, etc.

    b)   Medication side effects, interactions, or complications

    c)   Patient, family, and caregiver satisfaction with method(s) of pain relief

B. Select an appropriate pharmacological and nonpharmacological regimen based on the assessment findings, past experience, and patient preference

1.   Select a route of administration appropriate to the patient and setting of care

    a)   The oral route is used whenever possible

    b)   If the patient is unable to take oral medications, buccal, sublingual, rectal, and transdermal routes are considered before parenteral routes

    c)   Intramuscular route is avoided

    d)   Intravenous or subcutaneous route can be used for any patient that cannot tolerate above choices or when pain is rapidly escalating and severe. Subcutaneous route is a useful alternative in the home setting when reliable intravenous access is not possible

2.   Constant pain requires treatment with an around-the-clock scheduled long-acting opioid and a short-acting medication for breakthrough pain

    a)   Only one long-acting opioid is ordered for constant pain

    b)   Doses of opioids are increased commensurate with the patient's report of pain

    c)   Equianalgesic conversions are used when changing opioids and/or routes

3.   Breakthrough pain

    a)   Only one opioid analgesic is ordered for breakthrough pain

    b)   Use an adequate rescue dose for breakthrough pain; rescue dose recommendations are 10% to 20% of the 24-hour dose every 2 hours as needed; always increase the rescue dose when the baseline dose is increased

c)   In general, increase the baseline dose if the patient needs more than 3 rescue doses in 24 hours unless pain is related to a specific activity or if patient becomes sedated with increased around-the-clock opioid dosing

d)   To calculate rescue dose when transdermal fentanyl is used, multiply the total patch dose by 2; this is the approximate 24-hour oral morphine equivalent dose. If using morphine for breakthrough, calculate 10% to 20% of that dose to obtain the morphine immediate release breakthrough dose. If using an alternate opioid, convert from morphine to the other opioid

e)   Educate patients (and families) to take the medication when the pain is first perceived or in anticipation of a painful activity, not when it has become severe or unbearable

4.   Nonpharmacological approaches are always a part of any pain management plan

5.   An appropriate preventative bowel regimen is ordered with a stimulant laxative and stool softener to correct the effects of the opioid. See Chapter V, *Symptom Management*

C.   **Nursing knowledge and compassion are critical skills when relieving pain; caring presence is an essential intervention**

Table 4-3. Adjuvant Analgesics[adapted from 14]

Drug Class	Daily Adult Starting Dose* (Range)	Routes of Administration	Adverse Effects	Indications
Antiepileptic	Clonazepam 0.5–1 mg • Bedtime, 2–3 times a day	PO	• Sedation	• Neuropathic pain
	Carbamazepine 100 mg • Every day or 3 times a day	PO	• Sedation • Aplastic anemia (rare)	
	Gabapentin 100 mg • 3 times a day	PO	• Sedation • Dizziness	
	Pregabalin 50 mg • 2–3 times a day	PO	• Sedation • Dizziness	
Antidepressants	Nortriptyline 10–25 mg • Once a day	PO	• Anticholinergic effects	• Neuropathic pain
	Desipramine 10–25 mg • Once a day	PO	• Nausea • Dizziness	
	Venlafaxine 37.5 mg • Twice a day	PO	• Nausea • Dizziness	
	Duloxetine 30 mg • Once a day	PO	• Nausea	

(continued)

Table 4-3. Adjuvant Analgesics[adapted from 14] (continued)

Drug Class	Daily Adult Starting Dose* (Range)	Routes of Administration	Adverse Effects	Indications
Corticosteroids	Dexamethasone 2–20 mg • Every day • May give up to 100 mg intravenous bolus for pain crises	PO/IV/SC	• "Steroid psychosis" • Dyspepsia	• Cerebral edema • Spinal cord compression • Bone pain • Neuropathic pain • Visceral pain
	Prednisone 15–30 mg • 3 times a day	PO		
Local anesthetics	Lidocaine 1–5 mg/kg • Hourly	IV or SC	• Lightheadedness, arrhythmias	• Neuropathic pain
	Lidocaine 5% patch • On 12 hours/ off 12 hours	Topical	• Rare skin reactions	
N-Methyl-D-aspartate antagonists	Dextromethorphan • Effective dose unknown	PO	• Confusion	• Neuropathic pain
	Ketamine bolus dose 0.1 mg/kg; infusion 0.015 mg/kg/min	IV	• Hallucinations • Frightful dreams • Increased secretions	• Pain crisis • SC and IM routes possible • Advisable to medicate with a benzodiazepine to mitigate side effects even if the patient is moribund
Bisphosphonates	Pamidronate 60–90 mg over 2 hrs • Every 2–4 weeks	IV	• Pain flare	• Osteolytic bone pain
Calcitonin	25 IU/day	SC/Nasal	• Hypersensitivity reaction • Nausea	• Neuropathic pain • Bone pain
Capsaicin	0.025% to 0.075% • 4 times a day	Topical	• Burning	• Neuropathic pain
Baclofen	10 mg once a day or • 3 times a day	PO	• Muscle weakness • Cognitive changes	• Muscle spasm/ spasticity
Calcium channel blockers	Nifedipine 10 mg • 3 times a day	PO	• Bradycardia • Hypotension	• Ischemic pain • Neuropathic pain • Smooth muscle spasms with pain

*Pediatric doses for pain control are not well established.

Key: IV = intravenous; PO = orally; SC = subcutaneous

CITED REFERENCES

1. American Pain Society. *Principles of Analgesic Use in the Treatment of Acute Pain and Cancer Pain.* 6th ed. Glenview, IL: American Pain Society; 2008.

2. Azoulay D, Jacobs JM, Cialic R, Mor EE, Stessman J. Opioids, survival, and advanced cancer in the hospice setting. *J Am Med Dir Assoc.* 2011;12(2):129-134. doi: 10.1016/j.jamda.2010.07.012. Epub October 16, 2010.

3. Paice JA, Ferrell B. The management of cancer pain. *CA Cancer J Clin.* 2011;61(3):157-182. doi: 10.3322/caac.20112. Epub May 4, 2011.

4. International Association for the Study of Pain (IASP). *IASP Taxonomy.* 2012. www.iasp-pain.org/Education/Content.aspx?ItemNumber=1698&navItemNumber=576. Accessed August 22, 2014.

5. McCaffery M, Herr K, Pasero C. Assessment. In: Pasero C, McCaffery M, eds. *Pain Assessment and Pharmacological Management.* St. Louis, MO: Mosby Elsevier; 2011:13-176.

6. Paice JA. Pain at the end of life. In: Ferrell BR, Coyle N, eds. *Oxford Textbook of Palliative Nursing.* 3rd ed. New York, NY: Oxford University Press; 2010:161-185.

7. Haddox JD, Weissman DE. Opioid pseudoaddiction—an iatrogenic syndrome. *Pain.* 1989;36(3):363-366.

8. Portenoy RK, Sibirceva U, Smout R, et al. Opioid use and survival at end-of-life: a survey of hospice population. *J Pain Symptom Manage.* 2006;32(6):532-540.

9. Sykes N, Thorns A. Sedative use in the last week of life and implications for end-of-life decision making. *Arch Intern Med.* 2003;163(3):341-344.

10. Thorns A, Sykes N. Opioid use in last week of life and implications for end-of-life decision-making. *Lancet.* 2000;356(9227):398-399.

11. Pasero C, Quinn TE, Portenoy RK, McCaffery M, Rizos A. Opioid analgesics. In: Pasero C, McCaffery M, eds. *Pain Assessment and Pharmacological Management.* St. Louis, MO: Mosby Inc.; 2011:277-622.

12. Benjamin LJ, Dampier CD, Jacox A, et al. *Guideline for the Management of Acute and Chronic Pain in Sickle-Cell Disease. APS Clinical Practice Guideline Series No 1.* Glenview, IL: American Pain Society; 1999.

13. Pasero C, Portenoy RK. Neurophysiology of pain and analgesia and the pathophysiology of neuropathic pain. In: Pasero C, McCaffery M, eds. *Pain Assessment and Pharmacologic Management.* St. Louis, MO: Mosby Inc.; 2011:1-12.

14. Paice JA. Pain at the end of life. In: Ferrell B, Coyle N, eds. *Oxford Textbook of Palliative Nursing.* 4th ed. New York, NY: Oxford University Press. 2015:in press.

15. Pasero C, Portenoy RK, McCaffery M. Nonopioid analgesics. In: Pasero C, McCaffery M, eds. *Pain Assessment and Pharmacologic Management.* St. Louis, MO: Mosby Inc., 2011:177-276.

16. Caraceni A, Hanks G, Kaasa S, et al. Use of opioid analgesics in the treatment of cancer pain: evidence-based recommendations from the EAPC. *Lancet Oncol.* 2012;13(2):58-68.

17. McPherson ML. *Demystifying Opioid Conversion Calculations: A Guide for Effective Dosing.* Bethesda, MD: American Society of Health-System Pharmacists; 2010.

18. Heiskanen T, Mätzke S, Haakana S, Gergov M, Vuori E, Kalso E. Transdermal fentanyl in cachectic cancer patients. *Pain.* 2009;144(1-2):218-222. doi: 10.1016/j.pain.2009.04.012. Epub May 12, 2009.

19. Quill TE, Holloway RG, Shah MS, Caprio TV, Olden AM, Storey CP. *Primer of Palliative Care.* 5th ed. Glenview, IL: American Academy of Hospice and Palliative Medicine; 2010.

20. Swarm RA, Abernethy AP, Anghelescu DL, et al. Adult cancer pain. *J Natl Compr Canc Netw.* 2013; 11(8):992-1022.

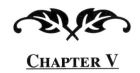

CHAPTER V

SYMPTOM MANAGEMENT

Amy Z. McDevitt, MSN, ANP, ACHPN®
Margaret Donegan, MSN, APRN, NP-BC, ACHPN®
Sandra Muchka, MSN, RN, APNP, ACNS-BC, ACHPN®, FPCN®

I. **Principles**

    A.   Palliative care, which includes hospice, is "patient and family-centered care that optimizes quality of life by anticipating, preventing, and treating suffering."[1, p. 9] Palliative care can be given in any setting anytime during the illness trajectory. Hospice care in the United States is bound by the Medicare Hospice Benefit[2]

    B.   Application of the nursing process (using assessment, diagnosis, outcomes/planning, implementation, evaluation)[3] is essential for symptom management and care at the end of life

    C.   Care at the end of life is multidimensional with emphasis on quality of life as the patient and family define it, with respect for, support, and education of patient and family

    D.   Understanding of expectations, goals of treatment, end-of-life goals. Issues must be clarified with patient and family, taking into account the patient's position on the disease trajectory. Recommendations for symptom management will vary depending on individual goals of care which reflect the patient and family's stated values and what is meaningful to them

    E.   The interdisciplinary team (IDT) is the framework for hospice and palliative care

    F.   The patient and family are the unit of care in hospice and palliative care and are included in the assessment, planning, decision-making, and evaluation of interventions

        1.   Options and expected or possible outcomes are discussed with patient and family to inform their decision-making; the IDT is responsible for giving them information regarding the benefits and the burdens of any treatment that is proposed

        2.   Patients and families require time, opportunity for clarification, and review in anticipation of making decisions

G. **The end of life can be a time of growth, reconciliation, peace, joy, and hope for patients and families; appropriate symptom management can facilitate this process by maximizing patient comfort**

H. **Patients may experience a variety of symptoms. Those covered in this chapter are some of the most often experienced by individuals with serious or life-threatening illness**

I. **See Chapter III, *Patterns of Disease Progression*, for further information on specific conditions**

J. **See Chapter IV, *Pain Management*, for further information on pain assessment and management**

II. **Neurologic**

A. **Dysphagia**

1. Definitions

   a) Dysphagia—difficulty in swallowing

   b) Odynophagia—pain on swallowing

2. Prevalence

   a) The exact prevalence of dysphagia is unknown. Epidemiological studies indicate prevalence may be as high as 22% in those over 50 years of age[4]

   b) Approximately 10 million Americans are evaluated each year with swallowing difficulties[5]

   c) Prevalence with stroke—an estimated 42% to 73% of stroke patients have dysphagia[6,7]

   d) Prevalence with head and neck cancer—an estimated 60% to 70% of patients who undergo radiation therapy for head and neck cancer have dysphagia[8,9]

   e) Prevalence in Parkinson's and other neurological diseases—an estimated 20% to 40% of patients have dysphagia[5]

   f) Prevalence in the elderly—suggests that up to 60% of nursing home residents experience some degree of dysphagia[10]

3. Etiologies

   a) Types

      i. Obstructive

         (a) Cancer of esophagus and other head and neck cancers; benign peptic stricture; history of gastroesophageal reflux disease (GERD); compression of vessels or mediastinal nodes

         (b) This type of dysphagia is intermittent, usually occurring when eating or drinking; meat and bread are most difficult foods to swallow; some patients can tolerate only liquids

          ii.   Motor

             (a)   Neuromuscular, esophageal dysfunction (stasis) related to smooth muscle hypertonia or dystonia (e.g., cardiospasm)

  b)   Diseases/other causes

      i.   Stroke and other cerebral vascular accidents

      ii.   Traumatic head injury

      iii.   Spinal cord injury

      iv.   Meningitis

      v.   Cancer—brain tumors; head and neck cancers and their treatments

      vi.   Neuromuscular diseases—Parkinson's disease; multiple sclerosis; amyotrophic lateral sclerosis (ALS); polymyositis; muscular dystrophy; myasthenia gravis

      vii.   Weakness due to overall disease progression

      viii.   Cognitive impairment[11]

      ix.   Inflammatory process—candidiasis; compromised cellular immunity (human immunodeficiency virus [HIV], leukemia, chemotherapy)

      x.   Dry mucous membranes (xerostomia)

      xi.   Poor fitting dentures

      xii.   Poor oral hygiene

4.   Assessment

  a)   Etiology of dysphagia or odynophagia will direct intervention plan

  b)   Assessment of swallowing

      i.   Oral hygiene

      ii.   Gag reflex; ability to manage secretions

      iii.   Airway protection

      iv.   Choking on fluids

      v.   Protracted meal times

      vi.   Nasal regurgitation of fluids

      vii.   Regurgitation or emesis after swallowing

      viii.   Difficulty getting swallow started

      ix.   Dry mouth

      x.   Solid materials (e.g., food, pills) caught in throat

      xi.   Pain on swallowing

  c)   Swallowing studies

      i.   Used to evaluate a patient's ability to safely ingest oral food and oral secretions. The role of swallowing studies to facilitate optimal care near the end of life is not clear[12,13]

      ii.   Potential indications for swallowing studies

         (a)   Acute stroke or other neurological condition affecting oral motor function

         (b)   Tracheostomy or recent endotracheal extubation

         (c)   Changes to oropharyngeal anatomy secondary to tumor, surgery, trauma, etc.

         (d)   Observed difficulty swallowing food or fluid

         (e)   Reduced oral intake; unexplained weight loss

      iii.   Contraindications for swallowing evaluation[12]

         (a)   Death expected within weeks from any progressive terminal illness

         (b)   Reduced level of arousal (e.g., coma/obtunded)

      iv.   Types of swallowing studies

         (a)   Bedside exam—performed by a speech pathologist at the bedside. Small volumes of food or water are given to the patient and he/she is observed for signs of dyspnea, aspiration, poor coordination of muscles, facial weakness, coughing or clearing throat, and changes in voice quality after swallowing

         (b)   Instrumental assessments (NOTE—requires patient to be alert and cooperative, and able to follow simple commands); also performed by a speech pathologist or other specialist

           (i)   Video fluoroscopy study (VFS)

           (ii)   Fiberoptic endoscopic evaluation of swallowing (FEES)

           (iii)   Fiberoptic endoscopic evaluation of swallowing with sensory testing (FEESST)[5]

5.   Interventions

   a)   If dysphagia/odynophagia are due to a known etiology, treat underlying cause (e.g., candidiasis, mucositis, GERD) with standard interventions

   b)   Referral to a speech-language pathologist

   c)   Dietary—appropriate food consistencies; cut food into bite sizes; provide small, frequent meals; encourage patient to chew thoroughly and to remain upright for 15 minutes after eating

   d)   Positioning of head and neck

   e)   Timing of meals and family involvement

   f)   Placement of a feeding tube for medically-administered nutrition may be considered depending on the patient's place on the disease trajectory, current nutritional and functional status, and goals of care

6.   Patient and family education

   a)   Teach importance of excellent oral hygiene

   b)   Avoid nicotine, alcohol, and caffeine, which increase esophageal vasospasm and have mucosal drying effects

      c)   Cool, nonirritating foods and liquids may be better tolerated

      d)   Mealtimes

          i.   Encourage patient to chew food well and to avoid large boluses of meat or bread

          ii.   Remove distractions at mealtimes

          iii. Proper positioning of the patient

          iv. Provide proper feeding utensils

      e)   Anticipated medication effects and potential side effects

B. Myoclonus

    1.   Definition—a movement disorder described as focal or multifocal, sudden, brief, shocklike, involuntary movements caused by muscle contractions arising from the central nervous system[14]

    2.   Prevalence

      a)   Risk factors—patients on medications listed below, especially in the setting of liver, renal impairment, or dehydration[15]

      b)   Higher doses of medications that cause myoclonus more frequently result in myoclonus, but the dose relationship is variable[15]

      c)   Can occur with all routes of administration

    3.   Etiologies

      a)   Medications cause[14,16]

          i.   High dose opioid therapy—related to increased levels of the 3-glucuronide opioid metabolites, which are the most likely cause of the neuro-excitatory side effects

          ii.   Antiepileptic—gabapentin, phenytoin, valproate, lamotrigine, phenobarbital

          iii. Tricyclic antidepressants and selective serotonin reuptake inhibitors (SSRIs)

          iv. Contrast dye

          v.   Anesthetics

          vi. Antibiotics—penicillins, cephalosporins, imipenem, and quinolones

          vii. Cannabinoids

      b)   Metabolic disturbances—uremia, hypercalcemia, liver or renal failure

      c)   Inflammatory or degenerative central nervous system (CNS) diseases—Jakob-Creutzfeldt, subacute sclerosing panencephalitis, end stage Alzheimer's disease

    4.   Assessment

      a)   Onset, duration of myoclonus, and its impact on patient and patient's functional status

      b)   Interruption of sleep, rest

    c)   Frequency of myoclonic jerks

        i.   Observe patient for 30–60 seconds. Watch and count the number of uncontrolled jerking movements

    d)   New or worsening delirium—complete a mental status exam or delirium assessment

    e)   Hydration status

    f)   Estimated prognosis—a longer prognosis may call for a more definitive change in treatment (depending on patient/family goals of care)

    g)   Chart review for

        i.   Recent opioid analgesic history

        ii.   Current medication list for potentially exacerbating drugs—haloperidol, phenothiazines

        iii.   Recent laboratory studies—renal and liver function; low magnesium, glucose, or sodium levels

5.   Interventions

    a)   Correct exacerbating factors (e.g., hypercalcemia could be treated with pamidronate)

    b)   Observation—if patient/family are satisfied with current therapy, explaining cause/progression of symptoms may be all that is necessary[15]

    c)   Pharmacological interventions

        i.   Opioid reduction—symptom may resolve over a few days with a decrease in opioid dose

        ii.   Do not reduce the opioid solely to control myoclonus at the expense of good pain control

        iii.   Adjuvant and other analgesic therapy may allow for opioid reduction, without compromising analgesic effect (e.g., gabapentin for neuropathic pain)

        iv.   Muscle relaxants and other drugs (benzodiazepines) may reduce myoclonus without alteration in the opioid dose, BUT can cause increased sedation

        v.   "Gentle" hydration by intravenous (IV), subcutaneous (SC), or hypodermoclysis may also be an option if the patient is unable to take fluids orally to clear metabolites

    d)   Nonpharmacological interventions[17]

        i.   Local heat/cold applications

        ii.   Gentle massage

        iii.   Relaxation

        iv.   Position patient for comfort

6.   Patient/family education

    a)   Discuss possible etiologies and recommended interventions

    b)   Discuss medication effects and potential side effects

c)   Educate patient/family regarding use of nonpharmacological interventions such as heat, gentle massage, and relaxation to decrease anxiety

d)   Monitor patient safety either if patient is ambulatory or bedbound due to muscular jerking movements

C.   Seizures

1.   Definitions

a)   Seizure—usually intermittent tonic/clonic movements; convulsions caused by a large number of neurons discharging abnormally

b)   Primary (generalized)—involves large parts of the brain and includes grand mal and petit mal types

i.   Usually loss of consciousness

ii. General muscle contraction/twitching that may last 1–2 minutes

iii. May exhibit biting, incontinence, difficulty in breathing

c)   Focal (partial)—involves specific regions of the brain with symptoms that reflect the location of the disturbance

i.   May have sensory, motor, or vision disturbances

ii. May remain conscious or can experience loss of consciousness

2.   Prevalence

a)   Primary brain tumors

i.   Up to 40% of patients with brain tumors have a seizure at the time of diagnosis[18]

ii. Another 20% of patients with brain tumors develop seizures during the course of the illness[18]

b)   Brain metastases

i.   15% to 20% of patients with brain metastases present with a seizure[19]

ii. Another 10% will develop seizures during the course of their illness[19]

c)   Tumor location is the most important predictive factor of seizure occurrence[19]

3.   Etiologies

a)   Primary or metastatic brain cancer

b)   Stroke

c)   Toxic/metabolic—hypoglycemia, hyponatremia, hypercalcemia, hypomagnesemia, hypoxemia

d)   Preexisting seizure disorder, missing dose(s) of antiepileptic medication

e)   Increased intracranial pressure

f)   Metabolites from normeperidine and propoxyphene

g)   Preservatives—sodium bisulfate

    h) Medications that lower seizure threshold—phenothiazines, butyrophenones, tricyclic antidepressants, tramadol

    i) Miscellaneous—infection, hemorrhage, paraneoplastic syndromes, drug toxicity, drug withdrawal

4.   Assessment

    a) Chart review for

        i. Medical history

        ii. Disease process

        iii. Current medications

        iv. History of trauma or recent fall

        v. Differentiate from myoclonus

    b) Question patient/family to determine

        i. Onset and type of seizure

        ii. Presence of aura

        iii. Headache

        iv. Nausea

        v. Projectile vomiting

    c) Check for treatable causes

    d) Check drug levels if patient was previously taking antiepileptic

    e) Electroencephalogram (EEG) if warranted

5.   Interventions

    a) For single seizure—work up for treatable causes

        i. If no reversible cause is found, consult the provider about antiepileptic medication, especially if the patient is expected to survive more than a few weeks

    b) For actively seizing patients

        i. Assess airway, breathing, circulation, and ensure adequate airway

           (a) Airway protection may be needed for patients who are seizing continuously for 15 minutes or longer[17]

           (b) Suction, if available, as needed to prevent aspiration

        ii. Protect patient from harm and ensure safety

        iii. Maintain patient in neutral, supine, or decubitus position[17]

        iv. Model calm behaviors for the patient and family; acknowledge how difficult this is to witness for the family

        v.   Medical therapy may include

           (a)   IV, subcutaneous, or sublingual (SL) lorazepam

           (b)   Rectal or IV diazepam

           (c)   Oral clonazepam

           (d)   Initiation of antiepileptic therapy as needed and depending on the goals of care

        vi.   Determine potentially treatable etiologies and treat

           (a)   Hypoglycemia—glucose oral/IV or glucagon as indicated

           (b)   Hyponatremia—fluid restrictions; IV sodium chloride (NaCl), adjustment of diuretics

           (c)   Hypercalcemia—increase fluids oral/IV; pamidronate may be appropriate depending on goals of care and life expectancy

           (d)   Hypoxemia—supplemental oxygen

           (e)   Hypomagnesemia—supplemental magnesium

           (f)   Infectious process—antibiotics as indicated and according to life expectancy and goals of care

           (g)   Substance abuse—support withdrawal; consult substance abuse specialist

6.   Patient and family education

   a)   Educate patient and family regarding side effects of antiepileptic medications—sedation

   b)   Provide seizure medication kit at home and establish a plan for acute seizures

   c)   Review seizure safety

   d)   Do not put anything in the patient's mouth

   e)   Provide for safe environment[20,21]

        i.   Cover hard or sharp surfaces with soft objects such as pillows or thick blankets

        ii.   Keep nearby or overhanging objects at a safe distance

        iii.   Provide a fan, cold compress, or cool damp washcloth if patient is febrile and/or diaphoretic

D.   Extrapyramidal Symptoms (EPS)

1.   Definition

   a)   EPS—involuntary movements, which may not respond to reversal therapies

   b)   Akathisia—inability to sit still, pacing, agitation, restless movement

   c)   Dystonia—slow, retarded movements

   d)   Tardive dyskinesia (TD)

        i.   Movement disorder characterized by involuntary movements in limbs, trunk, and/or respiratory system[22]

ii.   Most clinicians in psychiatry view TD as an antipsychotic-related side effect and unrelated to the underlying disease for which the antipsychotics are prescribed[22]

2. Prevalence

a)   All dopamine D-2 receptor antagonists have the potential to cause EPS[23]

b)   Second-generation antipsychotics are associated with a reduced risk of EPS-related, treatment-emergent events compared with first generation antipsychotics[23]

3. Etiologies

a)   Iatrogenic drug-induced from

i.   Neuroleptics and butyrophenones (haloperidol)

ii.   Phenothiazines (chlorpromazine)

iii.   Prokinetics (i.e., stimulate motility of the upper gastrointestinal tract; metoclopramide)

iv.   Opioids

b)   Parkinson's disease

c)   Cerebral lesions

4. Assessment

a)   Etiology of EPS and medication review will direct intervention plan

b)   Assess possible iatrogenic response to a medical therapy used to treat a symptom

c)   Assess patient safety with ambulation and activities of daily living (ADLs)

d)   Assess patient/family anxiety related to EPS and their understanding of medication effects and side effects

5. Interventions

a)   For phenothiazine toxicity

i.   Stop phenothiazine

ii.   Benztropine mesylate, trihexyphenidyl, diphenhydramine

b)   For akathisia

i.   Benzodiazepines

ii.   Beta-blockers

c)   For dystonia

i.   Physical or occupational therapy may be an adjunct if appropriate

d)   Review medications for those that may cause EPS. If symptom remains present, discuss with medical team regarding alternative medications to control symptom

6. Patient/family education

    a) Educate regarding reason for stopping medication(s) that may be contributing to EPS

    b) Educate regarding medication effects and side effects

    c) Monitor patient safety

III. Cardiovascular

A. Edema

1. Definition—palpable swelling produced by expansion of the interstitial fluid volume that can occur both diffusely throughout the body or locally

2. Etiologies[24]

    a) Localized edema can occur in the setting of a deep vein thrombosis, lymphatic obstruction (lymphedema following mastectomy)

    b) Generalized edema is most common in heart failure, end stage renal and hepatic diseases

    c) Superior vena cava syndrome (SVCS) caused by compression and obstruction of blood flow from a tumor mass

    d) Medications—arteriolar vasodilators, nonsteroidal anti-inflammatory drugs (NSAIDs), certain diabetic medications

    e) Malignant ascites

    f) Shock

3. Assessment

    a) History of edema and correlating disease process may direct interventions

    b) Peripheral edema—pitting, weeping, erythema, pain, palpable pulses

    c) Pulmonary edema (respiratory distress, pink, frothy sputum) versus pleural effusion (can be asymptomatic, slower onset, dyspnea, chest pain especially when breathing deeply [pleuritic pain], fever, cough)

    d) Abdominal ascites—size, pain, associated dyspnea, anorexia (see section on Ascites)

    e) SVCS may present as facial, neck, and upper extremity edema

    f) Patient and family distress

4. Interventions

    a) Diuretics should be given with caution, except in cases of acute pulmonary edema[24]

        i. Monitor for potential side effects of resulting volume deficits such as weakness, fatigue, postural dizziness, and lethargy or confusion

    b) Abdominal ascites—diuresis should be done slowly to avoid volume loss

        i. Combination of furosemide and spironolactone balance potassium loss with retention and may reduce need for frequent labs

        ii. Fluid can be removed with paracentesis and/or drain placement

        c)   SVCS may be treated with chemotherapy, radiation, or vascular stenting[25]

             i.   Potential life-threatening event if accompanied by airway obstruction[26]

        d)   Lymphedema—usually not responsive to diuretics and may lead to volume depletion[27]

             i.   Confer with physical or occupational therapists for recommendations—compression devices and/or lymphatic massage as appropriate

        e)   Lower extremity edema

             i.   Elevate legs as tolerated—"toes above the nose"

             ii.   Compression stockings applied in the morning and removed in the evening

                 (a)   Check for circulation, pedal pulses, and skin temperature to avoid compressing a limb with compromised circulation

             iii.   Consider soft stockinette for more comfortable support

             iv.   May wrap with ace bandages during the day

             v.   Provide meticulous skin care and keep skin moisturized

    5.   Patient and family education

        a)   Correlate factors for peripheral edema in specific disease entities

        b)   Use of nonpharmacological strategies to manage extremity edema

             i.   How to use compression hose or ace wraps

        c)   Review role of fluid and salt restrictions (if appropriate) in patients with heart, renal, and liver failure

        d)   Review natural dying trajectory, including expected decline in oral intake and risks of IV fluid and tube feedings

---

Teaching Tip

YouTube.com has videos on many procedures including applying compression hose and ace wraps. Be sure to review, though, before suggesting them to a patient or family.

B. Angina

    1.   Definition—chest pain or discomfort from inadequate blood flow to the heart muscle[28]

        a)   Typical angina includes constricting discomfort in the anterior chest (e.g., tight, heavy, squeezing), neck, shoulders, jaw, and or arms; it can be precipitated by physical exertion; and is usually relieved by rest or nitroglycerine in 5 minutes[29]

        b)   Atypical angina—having 2 of the 3 symptoms of typical angina[29]

    2.   Prevalence

        a)   Angina is a symptom of heart disease; heart disease is the leading cause of death in the United States (nearly 597689/year)[30]

        b)   Angina is experienced by over 0.5% of 20–39 year olds, 7.2% of 40–59 year olds, 14.7% of 60–79 year olds, and 21.1% of those 80 years of age and older[28]

3. Etiology

    a) Angina is a symptom of coronary heart disease. Plaque accumulates in areas of damaged atrial walls and impedes blood flow to the heart[31]

4. Assessment—extent of diagnostic investigation depends on goals of care

    a) History of heart disease, hypertension, smoking, diabetes, obesity, limited physical activity, and older age are risk factors for coronary heart disease[31]

    b) Exacerbating factors, quality (e.g., heaviness, tightness), frequency, severity, and duration of angina as well as any referred pain (e.g., arm, jaw)[31]

    c) Diagnostic test can include electrocardiogram, chest x-ray, stress test, computed tomography angiography (CTA), blood tests (e.g., cholesterol, glucose, albumin, C-reactive protein, hemoglobin, and cardiac enzymes if a myocardial infarction is suspected).[31] Coronary arteriography is only recommended for patients eligible for revascularization[32]

    d) Interventions—guided by goals of care

        i. Underlying coronary heart disease is treated on an individual basis[31]

           (a) Life style changes (e.g., diet, exercise, stress reduction, stopping smoking)

           (b) Pharmacological—beta-blockers, calcium channel blockers, angiotensin converting enzyme (ACE) inhibitors, angiotensin II receptor blockers (ARBs), antiplatelet drugs, anticoagulants, nitrates

               (i) Acute angina is treated with sublingual or buccal nitroglycerine with caution as it can cause hypotension

           (c) Surgical—angioplasty, coronary artery bypass graft

    e) Patient and family education

        i. Signs and symptoms of angina along with causes of coronary heart disease

        ii. Correct administration and side effects of medications

        iii. Include in plan of care when and who to call for persistent angina

IV. Respiratory

A. Cough

1. Definition—normally protective function to remove mucus and foreign bodies from the respiratory tract[33]

2. Prevalence—one of the most common symptoms with dyspnea and fatigue in patients with advanced heart failure, cancer, and chronic obstructive pulmonary disease (COPD)[34,35]

3. Etiologies

    a) Acute cough—infections, allergies, exacerbation of COPD, pulmonary embolism, pleural effusion, pericardial effusion, invasive tumor[36]

    b) Chronic cough—cancer and cancer treatments, gastroesophageal reflux disease (GERD), drug induced (e.g., acetylcholinesterase inhibitors [ACEIs]), chronic bronchitis, smoking, and COPD[36]

4. Assessment

    a) History and physical exam to determine underlying etiology and direct next steps

    b) Production of sputum versus dry, hacking cough

    c) Medication review

        i. Proper use of metered-dose inhalers, spacers

    d) Alleviating and exacerbating factors—time of day, positioning, exertion

    e) Contributing to dyspnea, fatigue, pain, nausea/vomiting, and/or insomnia

    f) Intensity of emotional distress for patient and family

5. Interventions

    a) Over-the-counter cough products—vast array of combination products with no clear evidence to support one over another[33]

    b) Antitussives

        i. Centrally acting in the brain

            (a) Opioids (e.g., codeine, morphine, hydrocodone)

            (b) Opioid derivatives—dextromethorphan[33]

        ii. Peripherally acting

            (a) Syrups—sugar stimulates saliva and soothes the oropharynx

            (b) Benzonatate—anesthetizes respiratory passage, lung, and pleural stretch receptors reducing cough reflex

            (c) Nebulized lidocaine—refractory cough[36]

            (d) Gabapentin—refractory cough[37]

    c) Expectorants—to thin secretions and ease expectoration

        i. Nebulized saline

        ii. *N*-acetylcysteine—given via nebulizer

        iii. Guaifenesin—often found in over-the-counter products

    d) Corticosteroids—reduces inflammation following chemotherapy or radiation induced pneumonitis, immunosuppression for COPD exacerbations[25]

        i. Dexamethasone

        ii. Prednisone

    e) Antibiotics—for bacterial pneumonia

    f) Proton pump inhibitors (e.g., dexlansoprazole, esomeprazole, lansoprazole, omeprazole, pantoprazole)—for treatment of GERD

6. Patient and family education

    a) Environmental factors that may be exacerbating cough (e.g., secondhand smoke, wood-burning stove or fireplace, allergens, pollution, perfumes)

    b) Rationale for medications and proper use

    c) Room humidifier

B. Dyspnea

1. Definitions

    a) Subjective sensation of shortness of breath that can only be perceived by the person experiencing it[38]

    b) Occurs in response to sensory information from the respiratory system activating regions of the brain that produce breathing-related distress[38]

2. Prevalence

    a) One of the most common symptoms reported by patients with advanced illnesses[39]

    b) Affects up to 50% of patients receiving end-of-life care and most patients imminently dying in the last 3 days of life[40]

3. Etiologies

    a) Pulmonary obstructive diseases—COPD, reactive airways, cough/secretions, tumors, SVCS

    b) Pulmonary restrictive diseases—fibrosis, effusions, infections, kyphosis, obesity

    c) Perfusion/oxygenation mismatch—anemia, pulmonary hypertension, heart failure, pulmonary embolism

    d) Pneumothorax

    e) Weakness and fatigue—multiple sclerosis, ALS, cancer fatigue, frailty

    f) Positioning—slumped, flat

    g) Complex biopsychosocial etiologies may exacerbate perception[39]

        i. **D**epression, sadness

        ii. **Y**earning (peace, rest, forgiveness)

        iii. **S**ocial issues (family, community)

        iv. **P**hysical problems

        v. **N**onacceptance or spiritual distress

        vi. **E**conomic or financial distress

        vii. **A**nxiety (often creates a vicious cycle with dyspnea), anger

---

Teaching Tip

There are many Internet sites that offer printable guides and online tools to help patients and their caregivers quit smoking (e.g., American Cancer Society [www.cancer.org/healthy/stayawayfrom tobacco/guidetoquitting smoking/index], American Lung Association [www.quitterinyou.org/]). Be sure to review before providing them to the patient and family.

4. Assessment

    a) Patient description is the most important measurement tool[41]

        i.   Listen for words patients use to describe their dyspnea (e.g., shortness of breath, can't catch my breath)

    b) Physical exam—respiratory and heart rate, pulse oximetry, lung auscultation

    c) Check oxygen source for liter flow/tubing kink

    d) Assess for fluid overload from artificial nutrition and hydration or excess oral intake in setting of heart failure

    e) Effect on ability to complete ADLs and functional status

    f) Heart failure patients—ask about medication compliance, daily weights, salt and fluid intake, and edema[42]

    g) Nonverbal/imminently dying patients—observe for restlessness, accessory muscle use, paradoxical breathing pattern, grunting, nasal flaring, and look of fear[43]

    h) Level of emotional distress for patient and family

    i) Depression is common in COPD and heart failure and coping skills should be assessed in all patients[39]

5. Interventions

    a) Investigate reversible causes while pursuing comfort measures

    b) Position for comfort and optimal lung expansion (e.g., head of bed elevated, tripod position)

    c) Cognitive-behavioral interventions may be appropriate for first-line treatment but may not be sufficient for refractory or severe dyspnea[44]

        i.   Guided imagery

        ii. Bio feedback

    d) Suctioning is rarely indicated and may increase secretions by irritation of mucous membranes

    e) Dyspnea management in heart failure includes optimizing medications, which can increase quality of life and prolong life. Include interdisciplinary team and address underlying psychosocial and spiritual or existential issues

    f) Goals of care and prognosis may determine appropriate treatment, including antibiotics and high-flow oxygen options

    g) Refractory dyspnea at the end of life may require inpatient management for rapid up-titration of medications and palliative sedation if necessary

    h) High-flow oxygen can be life-prolonging, and should the goals of care lead to discussions of withdrawal, a plan needs to be in place to treat worsening dyspnea (i.e., opioid infusion)

    i) Noisy respirations in the actively dying patient may not cause respiratory distress to the patient, though family may feel distress, but should be minimized using repositioning and antisecretory agents (e.g., scopolamine patches, atropine drops, glycopyrrolate)[45,46]

j) See Tables 5-1 and 5-2 for pharmacological and nonpharmacological interventions for dyspnea

Table 5-1. Pharmacological Interventions for Dyspnea[39,40,47]

Class	Dosages	Additional Information
Opioids[48]	• Morphine (most common) 2.5–5 mg PO every 2–4 hours, 1–2 mg IV or SC every 5–7 min.	• If taking for pain, use same drug/dose • Should be titrated for relief • All opioids work similarly—it is not necessary to use morphine if taking another opioid for pain
Oxygen[47]	• 2–6 L via nasal cannula	• In hypoxic patients, may provide comfort and prolong life • No proven benefit for dyspnea without hypoxemia • Noninvasive support with BiPAP or CPAP may be appropriate
Anxiolytics[49]	• Lorazepam 0.5–2 mg PO/SL every 4–6 hours as needed • Midazolam 2.5–10 mg SC every 4–6 hours as needed	• Benzodiazepines address anxiety • Topical formulations are not sufficiently absorbed to provide relief • Caution on use with opioids
Antidepressants/ selective serotonin reuptake inhibitors (SSRIs)[40]	• Fluoxetine 20 mg PO every day • Paroxetine 20 mg PO every day SSRI selection will vary based on patients' unique characteristics	• Antidepressant effects may take weeks • Neurostimulants may provide more timely relief, used short-term depending upon goals of care • Treating depression may help with coping but will not improve symptom of dyspnea
Diuretics[39,42,50]	• Furosemide 20–40 mg PO/IV/SC	• Used in heart failure with evidence of fluid overload • Heart failure patients can develop diuretic resistance requiring much larger doses and SC route • Insufficient evidence to support nebulized route
Corticosteroids[48]	• Dexamethasone 2–4 mg • Prednisone 5–20 mg PO, IV, or inhalers/nebulizers	• Reduce inflammation associated with mass effect, COPD, inflammation, infection, SVCS • May disrupt sleep if given late in the day
Antibiotics	• Varies with infection	• May significantly reduce dyspnea with infection
Blood transfusions for anemia	• 1–2 units of packed red blood cell—dependent upon hemoglobin	• Burden of coming in to facility and risk of fluid overload needs to be balanced with potential benefit

(continued)

Table 5-1. Pharmacological Interventions for Dyspnea[39,40,47] (continued)

Class	Dosages	Additional Information
Bronchodilators	• Albuterol/Proventil HFA 90 mcg/spray MDI—2 puffs inhaled every 4–6 hours (max 12 puffs/day) • Ipratropium 17 mcg/spray MDI—2 puffs inhaled 4/day (max 12 puffs/day) • Salmeterol 50 mcg/blister DPI—1 puff inhaled every 12 hours (max 1 puff every 12 hours)	• Quick-acting rescue inhaler or nebulizer every 4 hours as need • Anticholinergic • Beta adrenergic • Long-acting inhaler or nebulizer 2 times/day • Combination inhalers may also contain steroids • Use for bronchospasm, wheezing, COPD, asthma

Key: BiPAP = bilevel positive airway pressure; COPD = chronic obstructive pulmonary disease; CPAP = continuous positive air pressure; IV = intravenous; min. = minutes; PO = orally; SC = subcutaneous; SL = sublingual

Table 5-2. Nonpharmacological Interventions for Dyspnea

Intervention	Additional Information
Low salt diet and fluid restriction[42]	• May provide symptom relief in heart failure patients • Stopping IV fluids/TPN/tube feedings may be appropriate for imminently dying patients
Cardiac and pulmonary rehabilitation[42]	• May improve exercise capacity • May not be appropriate in advanced illness states
Fans[51]	• Study used handheld fans directed at face
Explore relaxation strategies[52]	• Distraction, music, yoga, prayer as appropriate • Supporting evidence is mixed but probably helpful for some people
Thoracentesis/drain placement[40]	• To remove fluid in the lung caused by pleural effusions
Acupuncture[48]	• Mixed evidence to support and may not be covered by insurance
Positioning[53]	• Sitting at side of bed with upper body resting on bedside table • Pursed lip controlled breathing for patients with COPD

Key: COPD = chronic obstructive pulmonary disease; IV = intravenous; TPN = total parenteral nutrition

6. Patient/family education

   a) Medication management strategies and clarification of goals

   b) Instruction on appropriate nonpharmacological strategies, energy conservation, and safety

   c) Give realistic expectations for symptom trajectory with reassuring education on continued management strategies to allay fears

   d) Role of low sodium diet and fluid restriction in heart failure patients

   e) Clarify goal for use of opioids to manage dyspnea

Teaching Tip

Many Patient/Family Teaching Sheets, including Shortness of Breath, can be found at hpna.advancing expertcare.org/education/ position-statements/. Most are also in Spanish and Chinese.

    f)   Explain expected changes in breathing patterns in actively dying patients if appropriate

    g)   Noisy respirations are probably more distressing to family than patient who likely is not perceiving respiratory distress[46]

    h)   Review benefits and burdens of intravenous fluids at end of life

C. Pleural Effusions

1.   Definition—disparity between secretion and absorption of fluid in the pleural space secondary to increased secretion, impaired absorption, or both, resulting in excessive fluid collection[54]

    a)   Transudative—occurs when the balance of forces influencing formation and absorption alters to favor pleural fluid accumulation—most common in cardiac failure[55]

    b)   Exudative—develops when either the pleural surface or the local capillary permeability is altered—most common in malignancy[55]

2.   Prevalence—more than 150 000 cases are diagnosed annually in the United States[54]

3.   Etiologies[54]

    a)   Parapneumonic disease (e.g., pneumonia, hypoalbuminemia, atelectasis)—most common followed by

    b)   Malignant disease

        i.   Breast, ovarian, and lung cancer plus lymphomas account for over 75%, followed by ovarian and gastric cancer (in order of decreasing frequency)

        ii.   Almost half of patients with metastatic disease will experience a pleural effusion sometime during their disease

4.   Assessment[55]

    a)   Detailed history-taking, including medications

        i.   Medications that can cause pleural effusions—amiodarone, beta-blockers, methotrexate, nitrofurantoin, phenytoin

    b)   Thorough physical examination

        i.   Exam will likely reveal decreased breath sounds on auscultation on the affected side, reduced transmission of the voice to the chest wall (vocal fremitus), and stony dullness on percussion

    c)   Discussion of other medical history, smoking habits, and employment

    d)   Details of potential asbestos exposure

5.   Interventions

    a)   Remove/treat etiologic factor if known

        i.   Fluid may resolve as underlying disease is treated, for example, following chemotherapy for lymphoma[55]

b) Nonpharmacologic

  i.   Relaxation techniques

  ii. Positioning

  iii. Oxygen as appropriate

c) Thoracentesis

  i.   Inserting a large bore needle into the effusion and drain into a vacuum container

  ii. Relief of symptoms can be achieved rapidly though fluid tends to reoccur quickly, usually within 3–4 days[54]

  iii. Current recommendations are that large pleural effusions are drained gradually with a maximum of 1.5 L being removed at 2-hour intervals to prevent associated complications such as pain, cough, or vasovagal symptoms (e.g., tachycardia, hypotension, fainting)[55]

  iv. May require concomitant infusion of albumin due to hypotension, depending on goals of care

d) Tube thoracostomy (chest tube) and pleurodesis[54]

  i.   Drains the pleural cavity completely, expands the lung fully, and instills a chemical agent into the cavity

  ii. Known to be a very painful procedure thus using intrapleural bupivacaine or epidural and IV conscious sedation is recommended

e) Pleurodesis[54,55]

  i.   Artificially synthesizing visceral and parietal pleural surfaces

  ii. Instillation of sclerosing agents (i.e., bleomycin, tetracycline, iodized talc) that cause inflammation and subsequent fibrosis into the pleural cavity to produce long-term adhesion of the visceral and parietal pleural surfaces. The goal is to prevent reaccumulation of the fluid

    (a) Talc has been shown to be the most effective

  iii. Can be quite painful for the patient and manifests pyrexia (fever)

f) Thoracoscopy[55]

  i.   Recommended approach for patients with symptomatic exudative pleural effusions without a diagnosis

  ii. Useful in patients with poor respiratory function or who are at high risk for general anesthesia

  iii. Inside of the chest and pleural surfaces are visualized using a thoracoscope

    (a) Allows visual examination of hemithorax

    (b) Biopsies may be taken

    (c) Mechanical or chemical pleurodesis with improved distribution of the sclerosing agent

    (d) Assess potential for full lung re-expansion under positive pressure ventilation

g)   In malignant pleural effusions

    i.   Insertion of an indwelling pleural catheter that allows for intermittent drainage into a vacuum bottle

        (a)   Patient and family may be taught to perform the drainage, which is relatively simple

        (b)   Ideal in a terminal setting as frequent clinic and medical provider visits for drainage are not necessary

        (c)   Positive quality of life impact as evidenced by improvement in symptoms, improved mobility, and may cause spontaneous pleurodesis

6.   Patient and family education

a)   Dyspnea and anxiety management strategies, both pharmacological and nonpharmacological

b)   Intervention-specific education

    i.   Reviewing expectation, management, and maintenance of thoracostomy tubes, indwelling catheters, etc.

    ii.   Pain management strategies

    iii.   Review side effects and complications that may occur

c)   Signs and symptoms of fluid accumulation

    i.   At the end of life, education of symptoms related to approaching death rather than accumulation of fluid should be done

d)   Risk versus benefit ratio of interventions

e)   Prognosis

V.   Gastrointestinal

A.   Constipation

1.   Definitions

a)   Infrequent, difficult passage of small, hard stools

b)   Associated symptoms can include inability to defecate at will, pain and discomfort when defecating, straining, unproductive urges, flatulence or bloating, or a sensation of incomplete evacuation[56]

c)   Obstipation—severe constipation due to an obstruction

d)   Impaction—too much feces in the bowel to allow passage of the feces

2.   Prevalence[57]

a)   Approximately 10% of general population

b)   Incidence can be as high as 50% to 78% in the ill adult

3. Etiologies

   a) Medication side effects

      i. Opioids

      ii. Antacids

      iii. Antiepileptics

      iv. Antiemetics—5-HT$_3$ antagonists (e.g., ondansetron)

      v. Cancer chemotherapeutic agents

      vi. Orally administered iron

      vii. Tricyclic antidepressants

   b) Metabolic disturbances

      i. Dehydration

      ii. Hypercalcemia

      iii. Hypokalemia

      iv. Uremia

      v. Hypothyroidism

      vi. Diabetes

   c) Inactivity, weakness, and/or fatigue

   d) Neurologic disorders

      i. Cerebral tumors

      ii. Spinal cord involvement

      iii. Sacral nerve infiltration

      iv. Autonomic dysfunction

   e) Structural abnormalities (e.g., pelvic tumor mass)

   f) Anorexia and/or low-fiber diet

   g) Gastrointestinal motility disorders

   h) Uncontrolled pain associated with defecation (e.g., anorectal pain)

   i) Environmental/cultural—lack of privacy, comfort, or assistance with toileting

4. Assessment

   a) History

      i. Ask time of last bowel movement

      ii. Characteristics of stools—color, texture, quantity, bloody, mucus

      iii. Ask about normal movement pattern

      iv. Explore if any pain or other symptoms associated with bowel movements

      v. Ask about prior history of reliance on bowel preparations

      vi. Current bowel regimen (e.g., laxatives, suppositories)

       vii.   Be aware that definition of constipation varies significantly from patient to patient and the goal is to establish what is normal for each patient

   b)   Physical examination

       i.   Abdominal examination—abdominal distention and/or tenderness; may report feeling of fullness or bloating; bowel sounds may be normal or hypoactive; percussion reveals dullness in otherwise tympanic areas; may be able to palpate stool in colon

       ii.   Rectal examination—presence of hemorrhoids, anal fissures; digital examination may reveal hard, impacted stool

       iii.   Abdominal x-ray may be necessary to rule out obstruction

   c)   Food and fluid intake

   d)   Medication and side effect profile

   e)   Mobility potential

   f)   Change in flatus or nausea/vomiting

5.   Interventions

   a)   Prevention is the goal

   b)   Nonpharmacological

       i.   Increase fluid and fiber intake, if possible and appropriate

          (a)   High fiber foods may include whole grain bread, bran cereal, fruits, and vegetables

       ii.   If ability to consume increased fluids is limited, increase foods containing larger amounts of water (e.g., soups, fruits, gelatin desserts, yogurt, mousse, sauces, supplements)

       iii.   Increase mobility and range of motion, if possible and appropriate

       iv.   Optimize toileting

          (a)   Encourage adequate time after breakfast since most powerful gastrocolic reflex occurs in the morning

          (b)   Provide for privacy

          (c)   Avoid bedpans if possible as they limit intra-abdominal pressure to pass stool

          (d)   Correct positioning—provide footstool if needed or toilet seat with arms

   c)   Pharmacological

       i.   Laxatives

          (a)   Bulk laxatives—provide bulk to intestines to increase mass (e.g., fiber, psyllium, carboxymethylcellulose, methylcellulose); helpful for mild constipation; work best with increased fluid intake so may not be appropriate for end-stage patients

             (i)   Psyllium 2–4 teaspoons daily; action may take 2–3 days

(b) Lubricant laxatives—lubricates stool surface and softens the stool by penetration

   (i) Mineral oil 10–30 mL/day, action may take 1–3 days

(c) Surfactant/detergent laxatives—reduce surface tension, which increases absorption of water and fats into dry stools leading to a softening effect

   (i) Docusate starting at 300 mg daily, action may take 1–2 days

(d) Osmotic laxatives—nonabsorbable sugars that exert an osmotic effect in both small and large intestines; lower ammonia levels, which can improve confusion in hepatic failure patients (lactulose); can cause severe cramping and discomfort

   (i) Lactulose or sorbitol 30–60 mL for severe constipation every 4 hours until bowel movement occurs; 30 mL daily maintenance dose

   (ii) Magnesium hydroxide 30 mL to initiate bowel movement; 15 mL for maintenance dose daily or every other day

   (iii) Magnesium citrate 10 oz. bottle for severe constipation

   (iv) Polyethylene glycol 1 tablespoon, may take 2–4 days

(e) Bowel stimulants—work on colon to increase motility

   (i) Bisacodyl 10–20 mg twice a day, takes 6–12 hours; can cause severe cramping

   (ii) Senna 2 tabs daily, max—4 tabs twice daily

(f) Suppository medications

   (i) Bisacodyl 10 mg per rectum, onset of action 15–60 minutes

   (ii) Saline or oil enemas—should not be used as part of standing bowel regimen; onset of action can be 30 minutes

ii. If patient at risk for constipation or taking medication such as an opioid, start prophylactic stool softener and stimulant (e.g., docusate sodium with senna)

iii. Titrate bowel medications as needed for minimum goal of a bowel movement every 72 hours, regardless of intake

iv. Titrate bowel regimen if opioid dosing increased

v. If no bowel movement in 3 days, suppositories and/or enemas should be considered

vi. Opioid-induced constipation

(a) Methylnaltrexone—inhibits opioid-induced decreased gastrointestinal motility and delay in gastrointestinal transit time; given subcutaneously and dosed according to weight

vii. Rectal pain—hemorrhoid preparations and sitz baths

6. Patient/family education

    a) Explain cause of constipation and instruct in ways to manage

        i. Nonpharmacological interventions—increased food/fluid intake, increased activity

        ii. Pharmacological interventions

        iii. Continually reinforce necessity of bowel regimen, even if patient is not constipated

        iv. Explain medication effects and possible side effects

        v. Reinforce that bowel movement should occur at least every 3 days and further action should be taken if no bowel movement after this time

B. Diarrhea

1. Definitions

    a) Frequent passage of loose, unformed, liquid stool

    b) Associated symptoms can include abdominal cramps, anxiety, lethargy, weakness, dehydration, dizziness, loss of electrolytes, skin breakdown, pain, dry mouth, or weight loss[58]

2. Etiologies

    a) Infection—*Candida* or *Clostridium difficile*

    b) Laxative therapy overuse or dietary fiber

    c) Gastrointestinal-related problems—malabsorption disorders, motility disturbances, partial bowel obstruction, enterocolic fistula, inflammatory bowel disease, pancreatic insufficiency, diverticulitis, ulcerative colitis, Crohn's disease

    d) Tumors—gastrointestinal and carcinoid tumors, pancreatic islet cell tumors, small cell lung tumors

    e) Surgical procedures—gastrectomy, ileal resection, colectomy

    f) Radiation and chemotherapy (pelvic radiation has been shown to cause diarrhea in up to 70% of patients receiving it)[58]

    g) Adverse effects from drugs (e.g., NSAIDs, antibiotics)

    h) Food intolerances or tube feedings

    i) Fecal impaction

    j) Other chronic disorders such as diabetes and hyperthyroidism

3. Assessment

    a) History

        i. Frequency of stools

        ii. Characteristics of stool—quantity, color, bloody

        iii. Explore if any pain or other symptoms associated with bowel movements

        iv. Determine if currently on bowel regimen and review carefully

         v.   Medication review

         vi.   Review diet and intake

         vii. Recent radiation or chemotherapy

         viii. Recent gastrointestinal surgery

  b) Physical assessment

      i.   Abdominal examination—bowel sounds may be hyperactive or hypoactive; may report cramping or pain; palpable masses in abdomen may indicate partial obstruction

      ii.   Signs of dehydration and skin integrity

  c) Stool samples if appropriate, to assess for

      i.   Blood, fat, ova, or parasites

      ii.   Infection (e.g., *Clostridium difficile* toxin, *Giardia lamblia*)

4. Interventions

  a) Treat any reversible cause

  b) Nonpharmacological

      i.   Increase fluid intake, oral fluids recommended over IV fluids

      ii.   Diet teaching—avoid spicy food, high-fat or fried foods, gas causing food, alcohol and caffeine, foods high in sorbitol (e.g., fruit juice), and milk/dairy products

  c) Pharmacological

      i.   Loperamide—start with 4 mg followed by 2 mg after each loose stool, not to exceed 16 mg per day[58]

      ii.   Diphenoxylate and atropine—5 mg 4 times/day until control achieved, then reduce dose; maximum 20 mg per day[58]

      iii. Methylcellulose may help provide bulk to increase consistency of stools

      iv. Scopolamine can reduce gastric secretions and decrease peristalsis

      v.   Octreotide deceases gastrointestinal secretions especially in carcinoid tumors, late-stage human immunodeficiency virus (HIV), or post-gastrointestinal resection

      vi. Corticosteroids (e.g., dexamethasone) can decrease inflammation in partial bowel obstruction and ulcerative colitis

5. Patient and family education

  a) Explain etiology of diarrhea and appropriate interventions relative to etiology

  b) Explain effects of medication and potential side effects

  c) Demonstrate correct hygiene and skin care techniques to prevent skin breakdown

  d) Explain signs, symptoms, and treatment of dehydration

C. Bowel Incontinence[59]

1. Definition—the involuntary passage of solid or liquid stool

2. Prevalence

    a) Although not widely discussed, is common

    b) Most recent epidemiological studies suggest that 1% of adults in the community are affected

    c) Residential settings have not been reliably determined, but one historical study suggests that up to 10% are affected

    d) Nursing home residents are up to 50% affected

3. Etiologies

    a) Can result from any disorder that affects

        i. Neurologic control of defecation at any level, including cognition

        ii. Muscle control of defecation

        iii. Fecal urgency with loose stool

        iv. The sphincter mechanism itself

        v. Gastrointestinal absorption (e.g., Crohn's disease, ulcerative colitis, inflammatory bowel disease)

    b) Risk factors

        i. Frailty

        ii. Loose stool or diarrhea from any cause, including impaction with overflow

        iii. Neurologic or spinal disease or injury, including spina bifida, stroke, multiple sclerosis, and spinal cord injury

        iv. Severe cognitive impairment

        v. Urinary incontinence

        vi. Pelvic organ prolapse and/or rectal prolapse

        vii. Colonic resection or anal surgery

        viii. Pelvic radiotherapy

        ix. Perianal soreness, itching, or pain

        x. Learning disability

        xi. Childbirth, especially after third- and fourth-degree obstetric injury (third-degree tears involve the anal sphincter, fourth-degree tears involve the anal sphincter and the rectal mucosa)

4. Assessment

    a) Goal is to identify reversible causes and contributing factors, also to ascertain the severity of the symptoms and their impact on quality of life

b) All patients should undergo baseline medical assessment

    i. Conduct thorough history of the incontinence

        (a) Current medications

        (b) Previous medical, surgical, and obstetric issues

        (c) General physical examination

        (d) Anorectal examination to exclude impaction

        (e) Cognitive assessment (if appropriate)

        (f) Personal concerns and goals—continence diaries can be helpful

        (g) Red flag symptoms—can be suggestive of serious underlying organic pathology and should usually prompt referral for investigation depending on goals of care

            (i) Unexplained change in bowel habit

            (ii) Rectal bleeding

            (iii) Weight loss

            (iv) Nocturnal abdominal pain or diarrhea

            (v) Fever

            (vi) Anemia

5. Interventions—limited evidence base exists

    a) Address treatable conditions, if known

    b) Nonpharmacologic

        i. Psychological support

        ii. Lifestyle modifications (may take several months to take effect)

            (a) Adequate fluid intake and balanced diet with stool-bulking soluble and insoluble fiber

            (b) Avoidance of gastric stimulants (e.g., caffeine, alcohol, spicy foods)

        iii. Toileting

            (a) Adopt a correct toileting position—lowering of toilet seat and use of a foot stool

            (b) Regular toileting

            (c) Privacy and dignity preservation if patient is not able to be home

        iv. Pelvic floor exercises and biofeedback

        v. Further specialist strategies

            (a) Sacral and tibial nerve stimulation

                (i) Electrical nerve stimulation (ENS) may offer a less invasive alternative to surgery and has a developing evidence base

a.   Stimulation of the sacral nerve helps to improve muscle and sphincter control

b.   Stimulation of the tibial nerve—fairly new with mechanism of action unclear

(b)   Rectal irrigation systems

(i)   Requires a degree of manual dexterity and carries a risk of bowel perforation of 1 per 50 000 irritants

(ii)   Anecdotally, younger patients with spinal cord compression are most likely to find these effective

(c)   Rectal plugs

(d)   Surgical intervention—depending on goals of care

(i)   Colostomy formation and other interventions designed to form an anal sphincter

vi.   Continence pads and absorbent briefs if appropriate

vii.   Skin barrier products

c)   Pharmacologic

i.   Loperamide 2 mg orally per dose after each loose stool

ii.   Codeine 30–60 mg orally divided once to twice a day

iii.   Bulk-forming agents (i.e., psyllium) as directed if patient is able to take in adequate fluids

6.   Patient and family education

a)   Education about diet, toileting techniques, and lifestyle—see above for specifics

D.   Ascites

1.   Definitions

a)   Ascites—the accumulation of excessive fluid in the peritoneal cavity

b)   Malignant ascites—the accumulation of abdominal fluid due to direct effects of cancer[60]

2.   Etiologies

a)   Portal hypertension—obstruction of portal vessels causing leakage into the abdominal cavity. Some causes include

i.   Cirrhosis

(a)   Most common cause of ascites accounting for 75% of all cases in Western Europe or in the United States[61]

ii.   Congestive heart failure

iii.   Portal venous thrombosis

b) Malignancy

  i. Contributing mechanisms

    (a) Tumor-related obstruction of lymphatic drainage

    (b) Increased vascular permeability

    (c) Over activation of the renin-angiotensin-aldosterone system

    (d) Neoplastic fluid production

    (e) Production of metalloproteinases that degrade the extracellular matrix

  ii. Most common cancers associated with ascites

    (a) Ovarian

    (b) Colon

    (c) Gastric

    (d) Pancreatic

    (e) Breast

    (f) Liver/cholangiocarcinoma

  iii. Poor prognostic sign with average life expectancy of 20 weeks from time of diagnosis[62]

c) Decreased osmotic oncotic pressure—decrease in plasma albumin levels, causing fluid to leave plasma and accumulate in abdomen. Some causes include

  i. Cirrhosis

  ii. Nephrotic syndrome

  iii. Malnutrition

d) Other causes can include

  i. Pancreatitis

  ii. Tuberculosis

  iii. Bowel perforation

  iv. Infectious process of the peritoneum

3. Assessment

a) Weight gain

b) Increase in belt size; need for clothing with a larger waist

c) Associated symptoms—distention, pain, early satiety, dyspnea, nausea, decreased appetite, lower extremity edema, reduced mobility, alterations in body image

d) Physical examination

  i. Inspect abdomen for distention and caput medusae; measure abdominal girth

  ii. Fluid wave test

  iii. Shifting dullness test

  iv. Tachycardia, dyspnea, orthopnea

e) Diagnostic tests

    i.   Abdominal x-rays show a hazy appearance

    ii.   Abdominal ultrasound

    iii.   Computed tomography (CT) scan can confirm the presence and demonstrate if the fluid is loculated in discrete areas of the abdomen

f) Laboratory tests

    i.   Serum albumin and protein level

    ii.   Diagnostic paracentesis—checks ascitic fluid white blood cell count, albumin, protein, and cytology

4. Interventions

a) Nonpharmacological

    i.   Diet—reduce daily sodium intake to 2000 mg or less

    ii.   Fluid restriction if moderate to severe hyponatremia

    iii.   Paracentesis

        (a)   Usually a maximum of 5 L of fluid is removed

        (b)   Complications include pain, perforation, hypotension, and secondary peritonitis

        (c)   Usually requires repeated treatments, which may lead to frequent hospital visits; depletes the patient of protein and electrolytes

        (d)   Based on goals of care and quality of life

    iv.   Paracentesis catheters/drainage catheters

        (a)   PleurX® catheter[63]

            (i)   Tunneled catheter with one-way valve to prevent leaks between draining sessions

            (ii)   Used in patients with life expectancy of at least 1 month

            (iii)   Risk of peritonitis, cellulitis, and catheter occlusion

        (b)   Pigtail catheter—simple catheter prone to complications (e.g., peritonitis, accidental removal, leakage, occlusion)

    v.   Vascular shunts

        (a)   Peritoneovenous shunts (PVS) (Denver or LeVeen shunt)

            (i)   Used primarily in nonmalignant ascites but relatively contraindication for advanced heart failure or renal failure due to volume overload

            (ii)   Removes fluid from abdomen and shunts up into the internal jugular vein

            (iii)   High rate of failure related to occlusion and associated with pulmonary edema, thrombosis of major veins, seroma formation, leaks, and disseminated intravascular coagulation (DIC)[64]

(b)   Transjugular intrahepatic portosystemic shunt (TIPS)[63]

(i)   Shunt between the portal vein and hepatic vein with purpose to reduce portal hypertension and improve sodium balance

(ii)   Increased risk of encephalopathy seen

b)   Pharmacological

i.   Diuretics

(a)   Potassium-sparing diuretic—spironolactone 100–400 mg/day

(b)   Loop diuretic—furosemide 40–80 mg/day

5.   Patient and family education

a)   Educate the patient and caregiver on rationale behind fluid and sodium restrictions if diet adjustment appropriate, depending on disease trajectory

b)   Teach about medications and potential side effects

c)   Explain skin problems with ascites and demonstrate proper measures for maintaining skin integrity

d)   Discuss signs and symptoms of infection if paracentesis or catheters are part of treatment plan

e)   Discuss/review patient's goals for overall quality of life; ongoing assessment regarding when risks and inconvenience of paracentesis outweigh benefits

E.   Hiccoughs (also called Hiccups)

1.   Definitions

a)   Involuntary, synchronous, clonic spasms of the intercostal muscles and diaphragm, which produce a sudden inspiration continued by an abrupt glottis closure that results in a characteristic sound[65]

b)   Three categories of hiccoughs

i.   Benign—self-limiting, lasting several minutes to 2 days

ii.   Persistent—chronic, continuing for more than 48 hours but less than 1 month

iii.   Intractable—persist longer than 1 month[12]

2.   Prevalence—1% to 9% of advanced cancer patients[65]

3.   Etiologies

a)   Peripheral nervous system—affecting or irritating the peripheral branches of the phrenic and vagus nerves

i.   Gastric distention—impaired gastric motility, excessive gas

ii.   Abdominal or mediastinal tumors

iii.   Hepatomegaly

iv.   Ascites

v.   Temperature changes—heat, cold

b) Central nervous system—stroke, brain tumor, multiple sclerosis, meningitis, and encephalitis

c) Infectious and toxic disorders—sepsis, pneumonia, uremia, alcohol

d) Inflammatory disorders—pericarditis, pleuritis, esophagitis, gastritis, pancreatitis, hepatitis

e) Metabolic disorders—hyponatremia, hypokalemia, and hypocalcemia

f) Myocardial infarction

g) Medications—steroids, chemotherapy, dopamine antagonists, opioids, muscle relaxants

h) Psychogenic—stress, excitement, personality disorders, anorexia nervosa, conversion/grief reaction

4. Assessment

a) Subjective review level of distress the hiccoughs cause

b) History and duration

c) Assess if interfering with rest, eating, daily routines

d) Identify potential triggers (e.g., eating, drinking, positioning)

e) Review medications

f) Physical examination

    i. General appearance and inspection for signs of a toxic or septic process

    ii. Oral cavity—assess for signs of swelling or obstruction

    iii. Abdominal area—assess for distention, bowel sounds

5. Interventions

a) Treat underlying cause if known

b) Nonpharmacological

    i. Respiratory maneuvers—breath holding, rebreathing in a paper bag, diaphragm compression, drinking ice water slowly, induction of sneeze or cough with spices or inhalants

    ii. Vagal simulation—carotid massage, Valsalva maneuver, digital rectal massage, ocular compression

    iii. Nasal and pharyngeal stimulation—nose pressure, lifting uvula with a spoon or cotton-tip applicator, gargling with water, biting a lemon, swallowing sugar

    iv. Gastric distention relief—nasogastric tube, lavage, induction of vomiting

    v. Psychiatric—distraction, behavioral techniques

    vi. Acupuncture

    vii. Peppermint water to relax lower esophagus

    c)   Pharmacological

       i.   Agents to decrease gastric distention

          (a) Simethicone for gas relief—40–360 mg after meals and at bedtime as needed

          (b) Metoclopramide to promote gastric emptying—10–20 mg oral/IV every 4–6 hours

       ii. Muscle relaxant

          (a) Baclofen 10–20 mg 2–3 times per day

             (i) Monitor for sedation, insomnia, dizziness, ataxia, and mental confusion

      iii. Antiepileptic

          (a) Gabapentin 300 mg orally daily, increasing to 1200 mg daily as needed in divided doses

      iv. Antipsychotics—dopamine agonists

          (a) Chlorpromazine 25–50 mg oral/IV/subcutaneous 3 to 4 times/day

          (b) Haloperidol 1–5 mg orally/IV/subcutaneous every 4–12 hours

          (c) Monitor for sedation and extrapyramidal effects

       v. Calcium channel blockers

          (a) Induces vasodilatation

          (b) Nifedipine 10 mg orally twice a day with gradual increase up to 20 mg 3 times/day if needed

6.   Patient and family education

    a) Promote discussion on severity of symptom and level of distress

    b) Explain etiology if known, and discuss ways to treat

    c) Explain appropriate, safe nonpharmacological techniques that are realistic for individual and patient

    d) Teach about medications and side effects

F. Nausea and Vomiting

1.   Definitions

    a) Nausea—subjective symptom involving an unpleasant sensation experienced in the back of the throat and the epigastrium, which may or may not result in vomiting[66]

       i. Can be accompanied by increased salivation, dizziness, light-headedness, difficulty swallowing, and tachycardia

       ii. Can be acute, anticipatory, or delayed

    b) Vomiting—expulsion of gastric contents through the mouth, caused by forceful contraction of the abdominal muscles[66]

2.   Prevalence

    a)   Nausea occurs in up to 70% of terminally ill patients[67]

    b)   Nausea and/or vomiting occurs in over 50% of patients with advanced cancer[66]

3.   Etiologies

    a)   Gastrointestinal stimulating vagal and sympathetic pathways

        i.   Gastric irritation, distention, stasis, or obstruction

        ii.   Constipation

        iii.   Cancer

        iv.   Intractable cough

        v.   Esophagitis

        vi.   Pancreatitis

        vii.   Hepatitis

        viii.   Radiation

    b)   Metabolic stimulating the chemoreceptor zone within the brain

        i.   Hypercalcemia

        ii.   Hyponatremia

        iii.   Fluid and electrolyte imbalance

        iv.   Adrenocorticoid insufficiency

        v.   Liver failure

        vi.   Renal failure

    c)   Central nervous system

        i.   Raised intracranial pressure

            (a)   Cerebral edema

            (b)   Intracranial tumor

            (c)   Intracranial bleeding

            (d)   Brain metastases

        ii.   Pain

        iii.   Vestibular—nausea aggravated by movement[68]

    d)   Psychological stimulating emetic receptors in brain

        i.   Fear and anxiety

    e)   Drugs

        i.   Chemotherapy

        ii.   Opioids

        iii.   Digoxin

        iv.   Antibiotics

        v.   Antiepileptic

        vi.   Aspirin and NSAIDs

4. Assessment

   a) History—duration, frequency, patterns, or identification of activities that may precipitate or alleviate (e.g., occurring after meals or certain medications)

   b) Assess consistency, frequency, color, and volume of emesis, which may assist in determining cause

      i.   Blood—active gastric bleeding

      ii.   Coffee ground emesis—lower intestinal or older bleeding

      iii.   Fecal matter—partial bowel obstruction

   c) Bowel history

   d) Pain assessment and other distressing symptoms such as anxiety

   e) Medication history

   f) Physical examination

      i.   Oral cavity—assess for thrush or mucositis

      ii.   Abdomen—bowel sounds, distention

      iii.   Rectum—fecal impaction

      iv.   Neurologic signs of intracranial pressure

   g) Laboratory tests—renal and liver function tests, electrolytes, calcium, and serum drug levels

   h) Radiologic tests—abdominal x-rays, head CT, head magnetic resonance angiography (MRA)

5. Interventions

   a) Treat underlying cause if known

   b) Nonpharmacological

      i.   Serve meals at room temperature and avoid strong smells

      ii.   Avoid sweet, salty, fatty, and spicy foods

      iii.   Encourage small meals, slow eating, and correct positioning (to avoid aspiration)

      iv.   Encourage, provide, and/or instruct on good oral care

      v.   Invasive therapies

         (a)   Nasogastric tube to relieve pressure if obstructed

(b)   Draining gastrostomy tube if unresectable obstruction and appropriate based on goals and prognosis

(c)   Surgery to correct obstruction depending on goals, condition, and life expectancy

vi.   Behavioral interventions—distraction, relaxation, biofeedback, self-hypnosis, guided imagery, and systematic desensitization

vii.   Acupuncture, acupressure, and music therapy

c)   Pharmacological (see Table 5-3)

Table 5-3. Pharmacological Treatment of Nausea and Vomiting[66–68]

Class and Drugs	Indication	Dosage, Route, and Schedule	Side Effects	Comments
Anticholinergics hyoscine hydrobromide (scopolamine)	• Intestinal obstruction • Motion sickness • Peritoneal irritation • Increased ICP • Excess secretions	SL: 200–400 mcg every 4–8 hours SC: 200–400 mcg every 8 hours TD: 1.5 mg patch every 72 hours (up to 3 patches)	• Dry mouth, ileus • Urinary retention • Blurred vision • Agitation • Confusion • Sedation • Anticholinergic effects, especially in the elderly	• Useful if nausea and vomiting coexist with colic
Antihistamines diphenhydramine cyclizine	• Intestinal obstruction • Increased ICP • Peritoneal irritation • Vestibular causes	PO: 25–50 mg every 6–8 hours IV: 25–50 mg every 6–8 hours PO: 25–50 mg every 8 hours	• Dry mouth • Blurred vision • Sedation	• Cyclizine is less sedating • Diphenhydramine should be avoided in the elderly
Prokinetic agents Metoclopramide	• Gastric stasis • Ileus	PO: 10–20 mg every 8 hours IV: 1–3 mg/kg every 2–4 hours	• Dystonias • Akathisia • Esophageal spasm • Colic if gastrointestinal obstruction • Headache • Fatigue • Abdominal cramps • Diarrhea	• Can use diphenhydramine to decrease extrapyramidal symptoms
Corticosteroids dexamethasone	• Increased ICP from cerebral metastases • Hypercalcemia from malignancy • Malignant pyloric stenosis	PO/IV: 2–4 mg every 6 hours	• Insomnia • Anxiety • Euphoria • Perirectal burning	• Most effective in combination with other agents

(continued)

Table 5-3. Pharmacological Treatment of Nausea and Vomiting[66–68]
(continued)

Class and Drugs	Indication	Dosage, Route, and Schedule	Side Effects	Comments
Dopamine antagonists haloperidol prochlorperazine	• Opioid-induced nausea • Chemoreceptor zone	PO: 0.5–5 mg every 4–6 hours IV/SC: 0.5–2 mg every 3–4 hours PO: 5–25 mg every 3–4 hours PR: 25 mg every 6–8 hours IV: 20–40 mg every 3–4 hours	• Dyskinesia • Akathisia • Dystonic reaction • Extrapyramidal reactions • Sedation	• Effective when anxiety and anticipatory symptoms aggravate the intensity of nausea and vomiting
5-HT$_3$ receptor antagonists ondansetron	• Postoperative nausea and vomiting • Chemotherapy related emesis	PO: 8 mg 2 times/day IV: 8 mg or 0.15 mg/kg	• Headache • Constipation • Diarrhea • Minimal sedation	• Ideal for elderly or pediatric
Benzodiazepines lorazepam	• Nausea and vomiting exacerbated by anxiety	PO: 1–2 mg every 2–3 hours IV: 2–4 every 4–8 hours	• Sedation • Amnesia • Pleasant hallucinations	• Use with caution in hepatic or renal dysfunction and debilitated patients
Cannabinoids dronabinol	• Second-line agent	PO: 2–10 mg every 4–6 hours	• CNS sedation • Dizziness • Disorientation • Impaired concentration • Dysphoria • Hypotension • Dry mouth • Tachycardia	• Helpful in younger adults
Miscellaneous octreotide acetate	• Nausea and vomiting associated with intestinal obstruction	SC: 100–600 mcg 2–4 doses/day	• Diarrhea • Loose stools • Anorexia • Headache • Dizziness • Seizures	• Monitor liver enzymes, may affect glucose regulation

Key: SC = subcutaneous; CNS = central nervous system; ICP = intracranial pressure; PO = orally; SL = sublingual; TD = transdermal

6. Patient/family education

a) Explain etiology and treatment plan

b) Instruct on nonpharmacological measure to relieve symptoms

c) Explain effects of medications and possible side effects

G. Bowel Obstruction

1. Definitions

   a) Bowel obstruction—blockage of the forward flow of gastric and intestinal contents through the gastrointestinal tract caused by ineffective motility or by an occlusion of the lumen of the bowel[58]

   b) Malignant bowel obstruction—"evidence of bowel obstruction; obstruction beyond the ligament of Treitz in setting of intra-abdominal primary cancer with incurable disease, or non-intra-abdominal primary cancer with clear intraperitoneal disease"[69]

2. Prevalence

   a) Can occur in 5% to 43% of patients with advanced disease[58]

   b) Can occur 5.5% to 42% in ovarian cancer and from 10% to 28% in colorectal cancer[70]

3. Etiologies

   a) Nonmalignant causes

      i. Adhesions from previous surgery

      ii. Hernia

      iii. Inflammatory bowel disease

      iv. Fecal impaction

      v. Bowel ischemia

   b) Malignant causes

      i. Growth of primary tumor in abdominal and pelvic cancers

      ii. Metastatic disease from primary lung, breast, and esophageal tumors

      iii. Post-radiation fibrosis

4. Assessment

   a) History of bowel activity, passing of flatus, and medication usage

      i. Constipation and inability to pass flatus seen in complete obstruction

   b) Assess for associated symptoms—nausea, vomiting, abdominal pain (colicky and/or continuous), constipation, or diarrhea

   c) Physical examination

      i. Abdominal assessment—bowel sounds, palpation for masses or distention

      ii. Rectal exam for presence of stool or distended empty rectum

      iii. Elevated temperature could indicate bowel ischemia and infection

   d) Radiological tests—abdominal x-ray, CT scan, magnetic resonance imaging

5. Interventions

   a) Prevent obstruction whenever possible with an appropriate bowel regimen and patient education

b) Treatment is guided by goals and must take into consideration prognosis and disease state; if recurrent or advanced disease, nonoperative treatments may be most appropriate

c) Nonpharmacological

   i. Bowel rest

   ii. IV fluid replacement

   iii. Nasogastric tube to decompress and drain stomach

   iv. Venting gastrostomy tube (G-tube) or jejunostomy to decompress and if resolves can be means to provide nutrition

   v. Endoscopic stenting improves luminal patency and allows oral intake without surgery

      (a) Complications include misdeployment, malpositioning, perforation, bleeding, stent migration, tumor growth extending through the stent into the lumen

      (b) Advantages to surgery—less invasive, faster resumption of oral intake, and shorter hospital stay and recovery

   vi. Surgery to alleviate obstruction and reestablish continuity and function of bowel

      (a) Increased risk of morbidity and mortality if poor performance status, advanced age, poor nutritional status, previous radiation therapy to the abdomen or pelvis, massive ascites, and/or history of multiple episodes of small bowel obstruction

d) Pharmacological

   i. Octreotide used early may prevent partial obstructions from becoming complete

      (a) Dosing

         (i) Subcutaneous—100–300 mcg 2–3 times/day

         (ii) Continuous IV/subcutaneous—10–40 mcg/hour

         (iii) Intramuscular depot injection—20 mg intragluteally every 4 weeks once stabilized on IV/subcutaneous for at least 2 weeks

      (b) Can be cost-prohibitive

   ii. Hyoscine hydrobromide (scopolamine) reduces gastrointestinal secretions and motility

      (a) Dosing

         (i) IV/subcutaneous infusion 10 mg/hour

         (ii) Transdermally 10 mcg/hour

      (b) Side effects—tachycardia, hypotension, dry mouth, sedation, delirium

   iii. Opioid medications for abdominal pain

   iv. Antiemetics—5-HT$_3$ (e.g., ondansetron), metoclopramide only with incomplete bowel obstruction, dopamine antagonists (e.g., haloperidol)

v.   Steroids to reduce bowel wall inflammation and edema

vi.   Antispasmodic—hyoscine hydrobromide (scopolamine), atropine

vii.   Stool softening agents if obstruction in colon or rectum; avoid stimulant laxatives

6.   Patient and family education

a)   Explain etiology and treatment course of bowel obstruction

b)   Explain medication effects and possible side effects

c)   Demonstrate postoperative care of incisions/gastrostomy tube if appropriate

d)   Explain importance of bowel regimen and assist in initiating a regimen

e)   Support patient and family in review of goals and decision-making, being aware of disease progression

VI.   Genitourinary

A.   Urinary—Incontinence, Retention, Hematuria, and Bladder Spasms

1.   Definitions

a)   Urinary incontinence—the involuntary loss of urine, further specified as functional or urge/stress incontinence[71]

i.   Functional incontinence—loss of urine due to the inability of a patient to reach the toilet and/or coordinate the movements necessary to use the toilet; most common cause of incontinence

ii.   Urge/stress incontinence—loss of urine due to irritability of the detrusor muscle, or uninhibited muscle contractions[72]

b)   Urinary retention—sudden inability to pass urine and is often associated with severe abdominal pain[73]

c)   Hematuria—presence of blood in the urine[74]

d)   Bladder spasm—painful contraction of the bladder described as stabbing, cramping, or colicky[74]

2.   Prevalence

a)   Incontinence—common in patients with life-limiting disease, particularly those with dementia

3.   Etiologies

a)   Incontinence

i.   Functional decline and disease progression

ii.   Irritation caused by atrophic vaginitis, tumor, infection, radiation, or chemotherapy

iii.   Neurologic disorders—dementia, stroke, Parkinson's disease

iv.   Sedative or analgesic medications may reduce awareness of bladder fullness

b) Retention

    i. Bladder outlet obstruction

        (a) Malignant tumors of prostate, urethra, or bladder

        (b) Lesions in central nervous system

        (c) Inflammation of the prostate

    ii. Deficient detrusor contraction strength

        (a) Denervation from large abdominopelvic surgeries (e.g., abdominoperineal resection)

        (b) Radiation or medications

        (c) Neurologic lesions affecting the acral spine or spinal column, multiple sclerosis lesions, and tertiary syphilis

c) Hematuria

    i. Tumor (may be initial complaint or finding with discovery of underlying malignancy)

    ii. Pelvic radiation or chemotherapy causing cystitis

    iii. Infection, nephrolithiasis or trauma

    iv. Coagulation disorder

    v. Benign prostatic hypertrophy

d) Bladder spasm

    i. Tumor and/or blockage of bladder outlet

    ii. Indwelling catheter or ureteral stents secondary to irritative effect on urinary mucosa; catheter occlusion

    iii. Urinary tract infections

    iv. Bladder or lower ureteral calculus

    v. Recent bladder surgery, caustic substances into the bladder, radiation therapy, and chemotherapeutic agents

4. Assessment

    a) History, including nature and duration of symptoms; and urine characteristics—amount, flow, color, if bloody, or cloudy

    b) Continuously assess severity if bleeding, and urinary tract patency—obstruction is considered an end-of-life emergency

    c) Review medications and any recent treatments for cancer if appropriate

    d) Physical examination

        i. Assess bladder for distention and perineum for swelling

        ii. Assess for fecal impaction

        iii. Neurologic examination—cognitive level, sensation, and sensorimotor deficits

        iv. Functional assessment—mobility, ability to perform ADLs

        v.   Skin assessment

        vi.   Signs of uremia—nausea, vomiting, and hypertension

        vii.   Signs of pyelonephritis—fever and chills

e)   Laboratory tests—urinalysis, urine culture and sensitivity testing, other tests as appropriate (e.g., serum urea nitrogen [BUN], creatinine, potassium, complete blood cell count [CBC] if bleeding)

f)   Imaging studies if appropriate (e.g., ultrasonography, cystoscopy, CT scan)

g)   Depression screening

5.   Interventions

a)   Incontinence—functional and urge/stress

        i.   Provide appropriate assistive devices for impaired mobility (e.g., walker, bedside commode)

        ii.   Rearrange furniture if necessary, to easier assist mobility and distance from toilet

        iii.   Schedule voiding times (e.g., every 2 hours) for bladder training

        iv.   Pelvic floor exercises (Kegel exercises)

        v.   Instruct to decrease amount of fluids consumed in evening before bed and limit intake of food/fluids containing caffeine or alcohol

        vi.   Encourage use of absorbent undergarments and/or pads

        vii.   If patient taking diuretics, administer/schedule early in day

        viii. Medications if nonpharmacological therapies not successful

           (a)   Anticholinergic agents that cause retention (e.g., oxybutynin, tricyclic antidepressants)

               (i)   Can be poorly tolerated in palliative population due to other burdensome side effects—constipation, delirium, dry mouth

           (b)   Calcium channel blockers for smooth muscle relaxation

           (c)   Antibiotics for infection if appropriate, with goals

        ix.   Indwelling catheter for terminally ill and dying patient may protect skin from repeated moisture exposure and reduce burden of too frequent hygiene care

        x.   If fecal impaction is present, disimpact and initiate bowel regimen

b)   Retention

        i.   Identify signs of acute renal failure

        ii.   Prompt placement of indwelling urinary catheter

           (a)   Close monitoring of output after insertion to avoid too rapid diuresis causing hemodynamic instability; if output reaches 500 mL, clamp catheter for about 5 minutes before further urine evacuation

           (b)   Intermittent or continuous catheterization may be needed for chronic urinary retention

          iii.   Ureteral stent via cystoscopy for obstruction of the upper urinary tract

          iv.   Percutaneous nephrostomy tube if placement of ureteral stent not feasible

          v.   Medications—belladonna and opium (B&O) suppositories; 1 suppository administered 3–4 times daily

             (a)   Side effects—dry mouth, constipation, drowsiness, and central nervous system depression

    c)   Hematuria

          i.   Prevent ureteral obstruction from clots

             (a)   Encourage increase in fluids

             (b)   Bladder irrigation if clots identified—intermittent versus continuous

          ii.   Replace blood and volume loss if appropriate (e.g., blood transfusions, iron supplementation, intravenous fluids)

          iii.   May be appropriate to hold certain medications—aspirin, NSAIDs, anticoagulation, and antiplatelet therapies

          iv.   Medications include trial of B&O suppositories or oxybutynin if needed for visceral pain

    d)   Bladder spasm

          i.   Treat any reversible cause

          ii.   Indwelling urinary catheter care—change of indwelling catheter as appropriate (every 4 weeks), smaller French size unless patient experiencing buildup of sediment causing catheter blockage, correct positioning of catheter and drainage bag

          iii.   Anticholinergic medications—oxybutynin

6.   Patient and family education

    a)   Educate family members and caregivers that all patients with serious or life-limiting disease, especially those with dementia, will eventually develop incontinence as they decline

    b)   Teach patient and family hygiene and skin care measures

    c)   Teach catheter care if appropriate, and signs of catheter malfunction

    d)   Explain signs and symptoms of urinary tract infection

VII. Skin and Mucous Membrane

A. Xerostomia and Oral Pain

1.   Definitions

    a)   Mucositis—inflammation of mucous membranes in any part of the mouth and upper esophagus; pain can impair eating and drinking[75]

    b)   Xerostomia—dry mouth[12]

2.   Prevalence

    a)   Xerostomia—reported by 30% to 55% of palliative care patients[12]

3.   Etiologies

    a)   Oral pain

        i.   Mucositis—some chemotherapy agents, radiation in head and neck cancer patients

        ii.   Candidiasis—more common in immunosuppressed patients

        iii.   Ulcerations—single ulcerations (e.g., canker sores)

    b)   Xerostomia

        i.   Common symptom—dehydration, medications, stress, and anxiety

4.   Assessment

    a)   Look for reversible etiologies—medication review, oral intake, oral hygiene practices

    b)   Oral exam

        i.   Dry mucous membranes

        ii.   White thick patches—presence of *Candida*

        iii.   Ulcerations

        iv.   Dentition and denture fit

5.   Interventions

    a)   Good oral hygiene with soft toothbrush and gentle flossing to remove food

        i.   Remove dentures at night

    b)   Oral rinses with dilute saline and baking soda solution

        i.   ½ tsp salt + ½ tsp baking soda in 1 cup warm water[76]

    c)   Dry mouth

        i.   Saliva substitute

        ii.   Hard candy, gum, mints—stimulate salivation

        iii.   Avoid products containing lemon or vitamin C

        iv.   Frequent sips of fluid or swabs with water

        v.   Pilocarpine 5–10 mg orally 3 times/day—cholinergic side effects

        vi.   Acupuncture

        vii.   Transcutaneous nerve stimulation (TENS)-like unit[77]

    d)   Treat candidiasis—oral thrush

        i.   Nystatin 4–6 mL orally 4 times/day—hold in mouth for several minutes before swallowing or spitting; continue 48 hours after symptoms resolve

       ii.   Fluconazole 100–200 mg orally daily

       iii.   Clotrimazole 10 mg troche—must be dissolved orally

    e)   Pain relief measures

       i.   Soft moist foods preferred over spicy, acidic, dry, salty foods

       ii.   Topical pain relievers

           (a)   Topical gels and pastes over the counter

           (b)   Medicated mouthwashes using combinations of lidocaine, morphine, doxepin, milk of magnesia, diphenhydramine may provide local relief

               (i)   Lidocaine can compromise the gag reflex and thus impair swallowing

           (c)   Opioids can be added to mouthwashes. Swish and hold for several minutes[78]

           (d)   Systemic pain relievers including opioids should be considered if pain not controlled

    f)   Prevention of chemotherapy induced mucositis

       i.   Ice chips minutes before cytotoxic drug and 30 minutes after completion[76]

6.   Patient and family education

    a)   Use of swabs and need for oral care

    b)   A dry mouth is uncomfortable for patients and thirst from dehydration is not felt by most patients who are actively dying[79]

    c)   Review risks and benefits of IV fluids in addressing expected decline in oral intake with the dying process

    d)   Review dehydration as an expected part of the dying process that may improve comfort status

B. Pruritus

1.   Etiologies[80]

    a)   Mediated by histamine, serotonin, prostaglandins, kinins, proteases, and physical stimuli

    b)   Dermatologic—dryness, maceration, irritation, eczema, psoriasis

    c)   Metabolic—liver and/or kidney failure, hypothyroidism

    d)   Drugs—opioids, aspirin, allergic reactions

       i.   Opioid-related pruritus is not indicative of an allergy

    e)   Infectious—scabies, lice, *Candida*

    f)   Allergy—urticaria (swelling/raised welts, contact dermatitis)

    g)   Psychogenic—associated with psychiatric disorders

2. Prevalence—occurs in 10% to 52% of patients[81]

3. Assessment

    a) Ask about allergies, soaps, new medications, pain with pruritus

    b) Look for signs of dryness and infestations

    c) Describe—diffuse, localized, raised/flat, linear

    d) Note presence of end stage renal disease or liver disease

4. Interventions

    a) Moisturizers—should be first line treatment given dry skin as most common etiology or exacerbating factor[80]

        i. Apply over damp skin after bathing—do not use scent based lotions; petroleum jelly over damp skin and covered with cotton clothing preferred

        ii. Moisturizers containing menthol or calamine may help with itching

    b) Soaps—gentle bathing with tepid water—oil added to bath water for bed baths

        i. Aveeno® oatmeal bath

        ii. Avoid skin irritants—alcohol-based lotions; harsh soaps; hot water baths; tight, heavy clothing

        iii. Attention to trimming nails to avoid scratches

        iv. Use powders for areas between skin folds that are moist

    c) Pharmacological

        i. Antiepileptic—gabapentin in patients with renal failure

        ii. Topical steroids—triamcinolone topical

        iii. Topical anesthetics—lidocaine, prilocaine

        iv. Bile acid sequestrants—cholestyramine in patients with liver disease; may cause nausea, bloating, and constipation

        v. Antidepressants

            (a) Sertraline—in patients with renal failure and liver failure[82]

            (b) Mirtazapine

            (c) Paroxetine

        vi. Ondansetron—for opioid-induced pruritus

        vii. Naltrexone—opioid antagonist; may not be appropriate for patients taking opioids for pain[83,84] as it reverses analgesia

5. Patient and family education

    a) Use of medications and comfort measures to treat and prevent symptoms[82,84,85]

C. **Pressure Ulcers and Wounds**

1. Definition—pressure ulcers are defined by the National Pressure Ulcer Advisory Panel (NPUAP) as "localized injury to the skin and/or underlying tissue usually over a bony prominence as a result of pressure or pressure in combination with shear and/or friction."[86]

2. Prevalence

   a) Pressure ulcers reported in 10% to 28% in hospice patients[87]

3. Etiologies

   a) Pressure ulcers—immobility, loss of sensation, moisture, inactivity in bed, nutrition/weight change, skin condition, friction/shear

   b) Malignant wounds—are not likely to heal

   c) Nonhealing surgical wounds

   d) Venous stasis ulcers/arterial insufficiency ulcers

4. Assessment

   a) Risk factors for pressure ulcers

      i. Advanced age associated with drier skin, fragility, loss of collagen

      ii. Protein–calorie malnutrition associated with cachexia, weakness, debilitation, weight loss, and muscle atrophy

      iii. Cytokines released from injured tissues associated with anorexia, malaise, decreased albumin synthesis, and nitrogen retention

      iv. Immobility—increases with advanced illnesses and exacerbated by fear of pain with movement

      v. Friction and shear—can occur with movement on bed linens, shearing force occurs with sliding down in bed

      vi. Moisture—excess perspiration, wound exudates, urine, and/or feces; sweat between skin folds creates environment for bacteria and yeast

      vii. Soaps—can alter skin pH and increase vulnerability to infection[88]

5. Existing wounds

   a) Measure circumference and depth with dressing changes

   b) Pain with movement, dressing changes

   c) Ability to reposition

   d) Evaluate treatment effectiveness

   e) Infection—erythema, swelling, pain, malodor, fever, elevated white count, serous exudate, delayed healing, change in color of wound bed

   f) Nutritional and hydration status—reversible factors

6. Stage wounds—for pressure ulcers only[86]

   a) Stage I—nonblanchable erythema of intact skin, the heralding lesion of skin ulceration. May be difficult to detect in darkly pigmented individuals

    b)   Stage II—partial thickness loss of dermis. Shallow ulcer with red pink wound bed, without slough or blister

    c)   Stage III—full thickness skin loss. Subcutaneous fat or slough visible but bone, tendon, and muscle are *not* exposed. May include undermining or tunneling

    d)   Stage IV—full thickness tissue loss. Exposed bone, tendon, or muscle present with slough or eschar. Often includes tunneling or undermining

7. Malignant wounds—associated with esthetic distress and pain[89]

    a)   Bleeding risk, pain, odor

    b)   Note patient and family distress, isolation, embarrassment

8. Lower extremity ulcers

    a)   Venous insufficiency

    b)   Arterial insufficiency

    c)   Diabetic foot ulcerations

    d)   Identify factors that may indicate low likelihood of healing[90]

        i.   Wound is more than 3 months old

        ii.   Immobility—spending more than 20 hours in dependent position

        iii.   Incontinent of urine and/or feces

        iv.   Wound associated with diabetes, and/or peripheral vascular disease

        v.   End stage major organ disease state

        vi.   Full thickness wound with tunneling

        vii.   Lab values indicate low protein/albumin stores and diminished immune response

        viii.   Patient is minimally responsive

        ix.   Loss of > 5% of weight or 10 pounds in past 90 days

9. Interventions

    a)   Risk reduction strategies

        i.   Elevate lower extremities to reduce leg edema in venous insufficiency

            (a)   Ulcers caused by arterial insufficiency may cause pain with elevation due to decreased perfusion and blood flow

        ii.   Turning and repositioning every 2 hours as tolerated

        iii.   Keep head of bed elevation less than 30 degrees if tolerated to minimize shearing and friction

        iv.   Consider mattress overlays or sheepskin

        v.   Elevate heels off of bed or use heel protectors and protect other bony prominences

        vi.   Use chair cushion that redistributes pressure

        vii.   Maximize nutrition and hydration support as tolerated[91]

        (a) Feeding tubes are not effective for prevention or improved healing in patients with advanced dementia

        (b) Feeding tubes are associated with increased risk for pressure ulcers when used in long-term care facilities

    viii. Minimize excess moisture from wound exudates, incontinence, or perspiration[88]

b) Provide treatment for pain

    i. Systemic opioids and/or nonsteroidal anti-inflammatory drugs 30 minutes before dressing changes, turning, and procedures

    ii. Topical pain relievers with lidocaine-prilocaine[87] and morphine

    iii. Consider extended-wear dressings to reduce pain associated with dressing changes[88]

c) Wound management

    i. Protect intact skin around wound site from exudates with barrier cream

    ii. Cleanse with saline or warm water

        (a) Minimize damage to wound bed if granulation tissue present

        (b) Irrigation with syringe to remove debris, purulent exudate, or eschar

    iii. Dressings—consult with wound care specialist as needed[87,88]

        (a) Semipermeable film—for shallow small wounds to provide barrier from bacteria, shear and pain relief

        (b) Hydrocolloid—maintains moist environment for low exudate wounds. Provides protective environment for healing and autolytic debridement

        (c) Alginates—for heavy exudative wounds to control secretions and contamination by absorption and formation of hydrophilic gel

        (d) Hydrogels/xerogels—for debridement in the presence of slough and eschar

    iv. Compression bandages if appropriate, for leg edema

    v. Bleeding wounds should be covered with nonadherent layer over absorptive dressing to minimize pain and trauma

        (a) Absorptive dressings—alginate, hydrocolloid

        (b) Compressive dressings for hemostasis of minimally bleeding wounds

        (c) Thromboplastin—clotting agent in powder form

d) Debridement

    i. Surgical or mechanical—uses hydrotherapy or wound irrigation

    ii. Autolytic—hydrocolloids and hydrogels. When healing is not a primary goal. Makes use of the body's natural enzymatic process

    iii. Enzymatic preparations

    iv. Biological—larval or maggot therapy[86,92]

    e)   Vacuum assisted closure (VAC) therapy—promotes healing by extracting infectious materials and other fluids out of the wound

    f)   Wound odor and exudates

        i.   Address distress, social isolation, and embarrassment

        ii.   Topical metronidazole as gel or tablets crushed and applied to wound bed

        iii.   Activated charcoal dressings

        iv.   Room deodorizing methods—cat litter under the bed, jar of vinegar or coffee beans, aromatherapy packs[87,88]

    g)   Treating infections

        i.   Oral antibiotics

        ii.   Topical silver-sulfadiazine and silver impregnated dressings

10.   Patient and family education

    a)   Wound care and management

        i.   Demonstrate correct positioning and turning, wound management

        ii.   Prepare for possible bleeding wounds with dark linens and containment plan

        iii.   Educate family members on role of nutrition and hydration

        iv.   Role of nutrition in wound healing as appropriate

VIII. Psychosocial, Emotional, and Spiritual

A. Sleep Disturbances

1.   Definitions

    a)   Insomnia—"subjective complaint by the patient of sleep disturbance despite adequate opportunity to sleep"[93, p. 1060]

        i.   May be transient, short-term, or chronic

    b)   Primary insomnia—sleep problems not directly associated with any other health condition or problem[93]

    c)   Secondary insomnia—sleep problems because of something else, such as a health condition, medication, or substance[93]

    d)   Sleep–wake cycle disturbances—"perceived or actual alterations in night sleep with resultant daytime impairment"[94]

2.   Prevalence

    a)   In general population

        i.   10% to 15%[95]

        ii.   Up to 33% of Americans are at risk for primary sleep disorders[96]

        iii.   In cancer, insomnia is the most prevalent sleep disturbance in the oncology population; reported in 33% to 55% of people with cancer[95]

3.   Etiologies

a)   Acute insomnia

i.   Significant life stress

ii.   Illness

iii.   Emotional or physical discomfort

iv.   Environmental factors like noise, light, or extreme temperatures that interfere with sleep

v.   Medications—analgesics, antihistamines, antihypertensives, antidepressants, antiemetics, anxiolytics, bronchodilators, corticosteroids[93]

vi.   Interference in normal sleep schedule

b)   Chronic insomnia

i.   Depression and/or anxiety

ii.   Chronic stress

iii.   Pain or discomfort at night

4.   Assessment

a)   Sleep–wake assessment parameters[97]

i.   Total sleep time

ii.   Sleep latency

iii.   Awakenings

iv.   Wake time after sleep onset

v.   Napping during the day

vi.   Excessive daytime sleepiness

vii.   Quality of perceived sleep

viii.   Stability of circadian rhythms

ix.   Sleep efficiency

b)   Sleep assessment includes

i.   Patient's sleep history and patterns—previous sleep disturbance, exercise, caffeine, alcohol, tobacco use, rituals that promote sleep (sleep hygiene)[17]

ii.   Current risk factors related to diagnosis—treatment modality and adverse effects, pain, anxiety, fear

iii.   Assess for unmet emotional or spiritual needs

iv.   Does the patient have signs/symptoms of sleep apnea?

v.   Environmental factors—noise, light, interruptions

vi.   Screening tools

(a)   The Pittsburgh Sleep Quality Index

(b)   The Insomnia Severity Index

(c)   Have patient keep a daily diary of sleep-wake patterns for 2 weeks

vii. Other studies—done in specialized sleep clinics[95]

(a) Polysomnography (sleep study)—includes an overnight recording of the patient's sleep

(b) Wrist actigraphy—noninvasive tool used to measure 24-hour sleep activity cycle by assessing wrist movement

5. Interventions

a) Requires multimodal treatment, including pharmacological and nonpharmacological interventions

b) Cognitive Behavioral Therapy for Insomnia (CBT-I) considered standard treatment based on high level of empirical support[95,98]

i. Cognitive therapy targets negative perceptions from prior experiences

ii. Behavioral therapy uses positive and negative reinforcement to modify behaviors in the present

iii. Goal is to lessen high-risk behaviors and patterns

iv. Specific CBT-I interventions include stimulus control therapy; sleep restriction therapy; relaxation therapies; and sleep hygiene education[99]

c) Pharmacological interventions[93]

i. Used in conjunction with nonpharmacological interventions

ii. Benefits of using these medications must be balanced against the risk of interaction among other medications

iii. Consider both short- and long-acting sleep aids

iv. Nonbenzodiazepines are generally better tolerated and more effective than benzodiazepine medications. There is reduced dependency, reduced rebound insomnia, and a reduced tendency for drowsiness upon awakening[17]

(a) Zolpidem—5–10 mg

(b) Ramelteon—8 mg

(c) Melatonin as directed

v. Benzodiazepines—can be used to aid in anxiety; not effective with continuous use[100]

(a) Lorazepam 2–4 mg (may start with a lower dose in the elderly population)

vi. Antihistamines—used for seasonal allergies, but have the effect of making someone sleepy

(a) Diphenhydramine 25–50 mg, not recommended for the elderly

vii. Antidepressants—may have some added benefit of improving sleep[100]

(a) Trazodone 25–50 mg

6. Patient/family education

a) Educate patient/family on treatment options, medications, and anticipated side effects

      b) Provide education to patient/family in promoting healthy sleep practices

         i. Interventions to help relax before sleep—calming music, meditation

         ii. Warm milk, scent of lavender

         iii. Limit time spent in bed only for sex and to the period of the night set aside for sleeping

         iv. Avoid daytime napping; promote daytime activities[17]

         v. Avoid consuming alcohol or coffee in the 3 hours before bedtime

         vi. Maintain comfortable environment in the bedroom

         vii. Maintaining a sleep–wake diary

         viii. If unable to fall asleep within 10 minutes, get out of bed and do something else until sleepy again[17]

IX. Nutrition and Metabolic

A. Anorexia, Cachexia, and Dehydration

1. Definitions

  a) Anorexia—loss of a desire to eat and is a symptom that accompanies many common illnesses[101]

  b) Cachexia—complex metabolic syndrome associated with underlying illness and characterized by loss of muscle with or without loss of fat mass; frequently associated with anorexia[102]

  c) Anorexia/cachexia syndrome (ACS)—debilitating condition characterizing the clinical journey of patients suffering from chronic diseases and cancer that negatively impacts patients' morbidity, mortality, and quality of life[103]

  d) Dehydration—loss of normal body water[104]

2. Prevalence

  a) Anorexia—common in elderly, chronic diseases, and advanced cancer

  b) Cachexia—may occur in up to 80% of patients with advanced cancer[105] and highly prevalent in patients with advanced congestive heart failure, chronic obstructive pulmonary disease, HIV, and renal disease

  c) Dehydration—very common at the end of life, though assessment varies among practitioners[104] making prevalence difficult to determine

3. Etiologies

  a) Pain

  b) Primary or metastatic disease sites with cancers having direct effects on organs of digestion (i.e., gastric, pancreatic)[101]

  c) Alteration in taste or smells in food

  d) Alteration in mucous membranes—candidiasis, xerostomia, mucositis

  e) Gastrointestinal alterations—gastroparesis, constipation, nausea/vomiting

f) Chronic fatigue or depression

g) Altered mental status—depression, dementia, confusion, anxiety

h) Medications—antibiotics, antihistamines, amphetamines, antiretroviral therapy, anticholinergics

i) Aging—food intake diminishes secondary to decreased energy needs due to reduced physical activity and decreased energy expenditure; changes in taste and smell can lead to decreased desire to eat

j) Radiation or chemotherapy

k) Alcoholism or other substance dependence

l) Reversible Causes of Anorexia-Cachexia[106]

   i. Aches and pains

   ii. Nausea and gastrointestinal dysfunction

   iii. Oral candidiasis

   iv. Reactive (or organic) depression

   v. Evacuation problems (constipation, retention)

   vi. Xerostomia

   vii. Iatrogenic (radiation, hemotherapy, drugs)

   viii. Acid-related problems (gastritis, peptic ulcers)

m) Anorexia/cachexia syndrome

   i. Increased nutritional losses related to etiologies associated with anorexia and cachexia

   ii. Alternations of brain neurochemistry leading to anorexia and reduced food intake

   iii. Endogenous metabolic abnormalities

     (a) Abnormal protein metabolism leading to increased basal metabolic rate and decreased albumin

     (b) Abnormal carbohydrate metabolism due to inefficient energy metabolism (i.e., decreasing anabolism, increasing catabolism) leading to insulin resistance, muscle wasting, and fatigue

     (c) Abnormal lipid metabolism leading to overall depletion of body fat

     (d) Change in fluid and electrolyte balance (increase in extracellular fluid and total body sodium and decrease in intracellular fluid and total body potassium)[103]

4. Assessment

a) Appetite—history and changes transformed into a numerical assessment scale if possible

   i. Edmonton Symptom Assessment Scale

   ii. Memorial Symptom Scale

    b)   Nutritional intake—measured retrospectively by diet recall or prospectively by calorie count

    c)   Inspection/observation—muscle wasting, loss of strength and decreased fat, mucous membranes and skin dryness

    d)   Complete bowel assessment

    e)   Assessment of oral cavity

        i.   Check mouth/oral mucosa for dryness, sores, candidiasis, or other signs of infection

        ii.   Properly fitting dentures and/or dental pain

    f)   Other diagnostics to assess nutritional status

        i.   Subjective Global Assessment for Nutrition (SGA)[107]

        ii.   Anthropometric testing

            (a)   Weight—typically decreases but can increase secondary to fluid accumulation or heart failure

            (b)   Body mass index (BMI)

            (c)   Mid-arm muscle circumference

            (d)   Triceps skinfold thickness

        iii.   Laboratory testing—serum albumin (late marker as half-life about 20 days), electrolytes (i.e., dehydration is indicated by hyperchloremia, hyperkalemia)[108]

        iv.   Medication review

        v.   Patient food preferences—likes and dislikes

        vi.   Psychosocial—meaning of food or eating to patient and family; changes in self-image; cultural influences and beliefs

        vii.   Patient and family goals—stage of illness and goals of care should be clearly determined before detailed assessment and intervention are planned or initiated[101]

5.   Interventions

    a)   Pain and symptom management

    b)   Good basic oral hygiene

    c)   Oral nutritional support

        i.   Improved nutritional quality of foods (increased protein and calories)

        ii.   Eliminate dietary restrictions and encourage patient's favorite foods

        iii.   Small, frequent meals on the patient's schedule

        iv.   Smaller portions at mealtime with pleasing appearance

    v.   Room temperature and less spicy foods may be preferable

    vi.   Limit fluids without nutritional value (e.g., carbonated soda) and spacing intake of foods and fluids to limit early satiety

    vii.   Preserve cultural or social traditions around mealtime, if possible; share mealtime and continue habits such as glass of wine with meals, if medically appropriate[101]

    viii.   Encourage nutritional supplements if tolerated

d)   Consultation with a nutritionist or dietitian as appropriate

e)   Enteral feeding and nutrition

    i.   Via nasoenteral tube, gastrostomy, or jejunostomy

    ii.   Appropriate in small subset of terminally ill patients such as head and neck cancer with dysphagia secondary to radiation, or in a defined trial in chronically ill patients

f)   Parenteral feeding, nutrition, and hydration

    i.   Total parenteral nutrition (TPN) or peripheral parenteral nutrition (PPN)

        (a)   Assessed on individual basis but rarely indicated in terminally ill patients, can be commonly seen in chronically ill patients

        (b)   Systematic review evaluating use in cancer patients found very limited benefit;[109] worsening of peripheral edema, ascites, and bronchial secretions were noted[110]

        (c)   Greater chance of complications and difficult to implement and continue in home environment

    ii.   Hypodermoclysis (subcutaneous hydration)—when oral and intravenous routes are not available and hydration is desired. Can be administered in the home setting. A variety of insertion sites can be used (e.g., upper chest, upper arm, abdomen, outer thigh, upper back, scapula). Infusion amount is limited to 1500 mL per 24 hours. Common complications are edema, inflammation, and infection at insertion site. Not recommended for those with severe dehydration, heart failure, pulmonary edema, renal failure on dialysis, thrombocytopenia, and/or coagulopathy[111]

g)   Pharmacological interventions (see Table 5-4)

Table 5-4. Medications Commonly Used for Anorexia-Cachexia[79,112,113]

Class of Drug	Medication and Common Dosing	Indications	Side Effects and Considerations
Progestational agents	Megestrol acetate 160–800 mg/day	• Improves appetite to assist with weight gain • No significant impact on quality of life	• Venous thrombosis, edema • Nausea • Adrenal suppression • Hypertension • Menstrual irregularities • Impotence • 20% to 30% advanced cancer patients have weight gain > 5% • Median time to response 6–8 weeks
Corticosteroids	Dexamethasone 4–8 mg/day	• Improves appetite without typically increase in body mass • Beneficial effects on pain, asthenia, and mood	• Hyperglycemia • Immunosuppression • Masks infection • Hypertension • Myopathy • Gastrointestinal disturbances • Dermal atrophy • Increased intracranial pressure (ICP) • Electrolyte imbalances • Delirium • Avoid abrupt cessation
Cannabinoids	Dronabinol 5–20 mg/day; start 2.5 mg twice daily	• Increases appetite and decreases anxiety	• Hypotension with reflex tachycardia • Somnolence • Confusion • Dysphoria • Side effects worse in elderly • Costly
Gastrokinetic agents	Metoclopramide 10 mg before meals	• Improves gastric emptying • Decreases early satiety • Improves appetite	• Diarrhea • Restlessness • Fatigue • Drowsiness • Extrapyramidal side effects

6.   Patient and family education

   a)   Encourage patient to eat as often as desired, but assure patient it is acceptable not to eat if it is uncomfortable

   b)   Explain dying process to patient and family, especially that anorexia is normal in last days of life

   c)   Encourage open communication regarding nutrition

B. Fatigue

1. Definitions

    a) Fatigue—a subjective feeling of tiredness, weakness, or lack of energy[114]

    b) Cancer-related fatigue—a distressing persistent, subjective sense of physical, emotional, and/or cognitive tiredness or exhaustion related to cancer or cancer treatment that is not proportional to recent activity and interferes with usual functioning[115]

2. Prevalence

    a) Estimates are between 60% and 90% in cancer and other chronic diseases, including cardiac, COPD, renal, HIV, and multiple sclerosis[116]

3. Etiologies

    a) Disease-related

        i.   Stage and extent of disease

        ii. Comorbidities

        iii. Common causes

            (a) Anemia (severe anemia hemoglobin [Hgb] ≤ 8 g/dL and possibly moderate anemia Hgb ≤ 11 g/dL)

            (b) Electrolyte imbalances

                (i) Hyponatremia, hypokalemia, hypomagnesemia

                (ii) Hypercalcemia

            (c) Nutritional imbalance/impairment

            (d) Infection/fever

            (e) Hyperglycemia

            (f) Uncontrolled pain

            (g) Organ failure (e.g., heart, lungs, kidneys, liver)

            (h) Adverse environment (heat or cold extremes)

            (i) CNS injury—disrupts the electrical pathway within the nervous system

            (j) Hypoxia

            (k) Thyroid disorders

            (l) Sleep disturbance

    b) Psychosocial factors

        i.   Mental and emotional state—depression, fear, anxiety, psychological or spiritual distress, family distress

        ii. Impaired mobility/activity intolerance/immobility resulting from disease process or treatment can lead to impaired ability to participate in activities of daily living, causing sense of loss or loss of role,[117] and can lead to progressive deconditioning[118]

        iii. Environmental—multiple sensory stimuli (e.g., noise, lights, odors)

c)   Treatment-related

    i.   Cancer treatment (surgery, chemotherapy or radiation) can cause distressing symptoms such as skin reaction, pain, dyspnea, constipation, diarrhea, sleep disruption, depression, anxiety

    ii. Medication issues—side effects, polypharmacy, taste changes, use of over-the-counter medications

4.   Assessment

a)   History—onset, history of change in functional status

b)   Subjective data

    i.   Description of fatigue

    ii.   Verbal rating scale—0 (no fatigue) to 10 (extreme fatigue) and ask the patient to rate level of fatigue in past 24 hours

    iii. Exacerbating and alleviating factors

    iv.   Duration, patterns, and temporal characteristics

    v.   Ability to complete ADLs

    vi.   Assess if a specific part of the body is most fatigued

    vii. Investigate if medications improve or worsen

    viii. Assess if underlying anxiety and/or depression

    ix.   Discern if patient is experiencing difficulty concentrating

    x.   Assess the functional impact on daily living

c)   Assess adequacy of pain control and other distressing symptoms (e.g., nausea, vomiting, dyspnea, anxiety, depression)

d)   Objective data

    i.   Vital signs to assess for fever, abnormal heart rate or respiratory rate

    ii.   Evaluate hydration status

    iii. Test muscle strength, symmetry, and endurance of upper and lower extremities to determine if neurologic changes are present

    iv.   Inability to complete ADLs (e.g., odor from not bathing, not changing clothing) and not keeping up with house work

    v.   Evidence of immobility (e.g., decubitus ulcers)

e)   Laboratory data

    i.   Oxygenation status—assess for sign of hypoxia

    ii.   CBC—assess for infection or anemia

    iii. Thyroid function

5.   Interventions

    a)   Should be directed toward correcting identifiable causes (e.g., elimination of sedating drugs, correction of anemia or electrolyte imbalance, improving mobility)

    b)   Nonpharmacologic

        i.   Assess and control symptoms contributing to or coexisting with fatigue—pain, insomnia, depression, nausea, diarrhea, constipation, electrolyte imbalances, dyspnea, dehydration, infection

        ii.   Recommend blood transfusions if appropriate, with goals and directed toward improving quality of life

        iii.   Encourage frequent rest periods, adjust method/pace of care

        iv.   Prioritize and save energy for important events

        v.   Use energy conservation techniques or assist devices (e.g., bedside commode, wheelchair, shower chair)

        vi.   Obtain physical therapy consult if appropriate

            (a)   May help joint flexibility and prevent pain

            (b)   May offer valuable input regarding potential interventions

        vii.   Participating in exercise program may decrease the severity of fatigue[118]

        viii.   If appropriate, consider nutritional consultation or provide diet education (e.g., high protein, nutrient dense food)

        ix.   Encourage activities to restore energy—meditating, gardening, praying, hobbies

        x.   Encourage spending time with family/friends engaging in passive activities such as riding in a car or watching meal preparation

        xi.   Provide assistance and services (e.g., home health, hospice) that helps the person to maintain independence and functional abilities for as long as possible

    c)   Pharmacological (see Table 5-5)

Table 5-5. Medications for Fatigue[116,119]

Class of Drug	Medication and Common Adult Dosing	Actions and Indications	Side Effects and Considerations
Psychostimulants	Methylphenidate: 5–10 mg at breakfast and 5 mg at lunch daily Modafinil: 100–400 mg daily in the morning; start with 50 mg every morning and titrate as necessary	• CNS stimulant • Improve QOL, reduce fatigue, and along with exercise, increase functional capacity • Methylphenidate may counteract opioid somnolence	• HTN • Angina • Anxiety • Insomnia • Use with caution if concomitant CV and psychiatric disorder • Elderly may require downward dose adjustment • Abuse potential with methylphenidate • Avoid methylphenidate in patients with valvular heart disease
Antidepressants	Bupropion: 100 mg daily for 3 days, then can increase to 100–150 mg 3 times daily at least 6 hours apart	• Norepinephrine dopamine reuptake inhibitor that may act as stimulant • Shows some improvement, especially if concurrent depression	• CV effects (e.g., HTN, tachycardia) • Anxiety • Insomnia • Weight loss
Cholinesterase inhibitors	Donepezil: 5 mg daily at bedtime; can titrate to 10 mg at bedtime after 4–6 weeks	• Reversible acetylcholinesterase inhibitor that enhances cholinergic function and may act as stimulant	• Studies show some improvement but efficacy still being researched • CV effects (e.g., HTN, angina) • Insomnia • Gastrointestinal effects
Corticosteroids	Prednisone: 7.5–10 mg daily Dexamethasone: 1–2 mg daily	• Mimic effects of cortisol • Shows improvement for short term use (1–2 weeks)	• Significant toxicity and side effects • Insomnia • Fluid retention • Anxiety/agitation • Hyperglycemia
Hematopoietic growth factors	Erythropoietin alpha: doses vary:[120] 10 000 U SC 3 times weekly to 40 000 U weekly	• Increase hemoglobin levels for some cancer patients	• Possible thromboembolic events

Key: CNS = central nervous system; CV = cardiovascular; HTN = hypertension; QOL = quality of life; SC = subcutaneous; U = units

6. Patient and family education

    a) Educate about fatigue to normalize symptom

    b) Promote adaptation/adjustment through setting realistic goals

    c) Instruct regarding balancing activities and rest

    d) Discuss expected medication effects and potential side effects, especially as they may contribute to fatigue or sedation

        i. Consider tapering or discontinuing medicine if appropriate

            (a) If opioid induced, fatigue may resolve when patient develops tolerance, usually 48–72 hours after start or dose increase

    e) Educate family in terminal phase regarding end stage disease process and encourage setting realistic goals

X. Immune/Lymphatic System

A. Hematologic and Immune

1. Definitions

    a) Hemorrhage—excessive bleeding

    b) Clotting—systemic response to disease or medication that initiates coagulation cascade causing clotting

    c) Cytopenias—reductions in bone marrow blood cell components which can precipitate a systemic response

        i. Neutropenia—reduction in white blood cells; decreases ability to respond to infections

        ii. Thrombocytopenia—reduction in platelets; increases potential for frank, uncontrolled bleeding

        iii. Anemia—reductions in production or maturation of red blood cells; low hemoglobin; decreased oxygen carrying capacity that may cause increased dyspnea, fatigue

        iv. Pancytopenia—reduction in all blood cells

    d) Fever—body temperature greater than 38°C/100.4°F, rechecked every hour for 3 hours or 1 reading greater than 38.5°C/101.3°F

2. Etiologies

    a) Hemorrhage may be caused by tumor erosion into blood vessels or disruption of clotting factors

        i. Hepatic failure—inability to synthesize clotting factors[121]

        ii. Advanced hematologic malignancies failure of bone marrow production[122]

    b) Venous thromboembolism (VTE)—deep vein thrombosis (DVT) and pulmonary embolism (PE) can be caused by activation of clotting system, venous stasis, and endothelial injury/vessel wall injury

        i. Cancer patients at significantly greater risk for VTE

        ii. Surgery, trauma, sepsis, heart failure, and chemotherapy

        iii. Hepatic failure—inability to remove activated clotting factors[121]

    c) Cytopenias—treatment or disease related

        i. HIV—CD4 T-cell counts of less than 200 cells/mm^3 indicate impaired immune status and increased susceptibility to infections[123]

        ii. Treatments—chemotherapy, radiation, antibiotics

        iii. Hematologic malignancies—leukemia, myelomas, lymphomas

        iv. Anemia—chronic versus acute

        v. Renal failure reduces erythropoietin production predisposing patients to anemia

    d) Fevers—inflammation (including malignancy), infection, immunologic disorders, and hypermetabolic states

3. Assessment

    a) Recent history and physical exam

        i. Orthostatic blood pressures if appropriate

    b) Bleeding location to determine strategies

        i. Identify underlying etiologies if possible

        ii. External bleeding from wound or cancer erosion

        iii. Hemoptysis

        iv. Hematemesis

        v. Easy bruising, bleeding with oral care

    c) Symptoms of DVT

        i. Unilateral swelling in an extremity, pain, and erythema

    d) Symptoms of pulmonary embolism (PE)

        i. Shortness of breath, pleuritic chest pain, hemoptysis, unexplained fever

    e) Fever

        i. Identify possible source of infection—skin, wound, bladder, respiratory, viral, gastrointestinal

        ii. History of cancer and recent treatments

        iii. Level of discomfort, diaphoresis, timing of fevers

4. Interventions

    a) Emergent interventions for bleeding, dependent on goals

        i. Activating emergency response system in the setting of life-prolonging goals

        ii. Dark towels for external bleeding with local pressure

        iii. Opioids for pain and dyspnea

        iv. Emotional support

    b) Cytopenias

        i. Transfusion of blood products—as per goals of care (e.g., life expectancy, expected improvement), comorbid heart failure increases the risk of fluid overload. End stage diseases may be associated with declining symptomatic response to transfusions[124]

        ii. Neutropenia—utilize universal precautions (e.g., decrease contact with those with active infection, diligent hand washing)

        iii. Thrombocytopenia—utilize injury protection measures (e.g., electric razors, soft toothbrushes, fall precautions)

        iv. Anemia

            (a) See section on bleeding for acute blood loss

            (b) Depending on goals of care, continue or start treatment according to cause (e.g., monthly vitamin B_{12} for pernicious anemia, daily folate preparations for folate deficiency anemia)[125]

    c) Treatment for DVT and PE—dependent on goals of care

        i. Warfarin difficult to manage in debilitated patients who have poor intake; may require frequent venipuncture

        ii. Rivaroxaban—oral factor Xa inhibitor with no anecdote in the event of supratherapeutic international normalized ratio (INR)

        iii. Injectable agent that does not require blood draws and, if at home, requires someone who is able to give the injection

            (a) Enoxaparin—often used short-term as a bridge until INR on warfarin is therapeutic

        iv. Oxygen and opioids for dyspnea

        v. Compression stockings for DVT prevention

    d) Treatment for fever dependent on etiology and goals of care

        i. Antipyretics—acetaminophen, aspirin, ibuprofen

        ii. Steroids—may reduce fever but have immunosuppressive effects

        iii. Cool cloths to forehead, ice packs to axillary and femoral areas, bathing in tepid water

        iv. Meticulous oral hygiene and skin care

            v.   Intravenous/subcutaneous fluids

            vi.   Antibiotic therapy

    5.   Patient and family education

       a)   Review rationale of disease processes and related cytopenias

       b)   Review plan for bleeding crisis with patient and family

       c)   Review risks and benefits with patients and families for continuing/initiating/discontinuing anticoagulation therapy

XI.　Mental Status Changes

A.　Altered Mental Status (Confusion, Delirium, Agitation, Terminal Agitation)

    1.   Definitions

       a)   Confusion

          i.   Can range from delirium, dementia, psychosis, obtundation, etc.[126]

          ii.   Changes in cognition/impaired cognitive function, impaired perceptions, and/or emotional disturbances

       b)   Delirium

          i.   Hallmark is an acute change in level of arousal or cognitive function

          ii.   Features include altered sleep/wake cycles, mumbling speech, disturbance of memory and attention, and perceptual disturbances with delusions or hallucinations[127]

          iii. Disturbance develops over a short period of time (hours-to-days) and tends to fluctuate over the course of the day[127]

          iv. Interferes with recognition and control of other physical and psychological symptoms

          v.   Negatively impacts both quantity and quality of life

          vi.   Affects ability to participate in medical decision-making

          vii. Categories of delirium[128]

              (a) Hyperactive delirium—symptoms include constant movement. Common symptoms include hyperarousal; hyperalertness; hallucinations; delusions; disorientation; trying to get out of bed; removing clothing, IV lines, or catheters; may be misdiagnosed as anxiety

              (b) Hypoactive delirium—reduced awareness of an interaction with surroundings. Common symptoms include hypoarousal, hypoalert, lethargy, sedation, decreased psychomotor activity, impaired ability to sustain attention

              (c) Mixed delirium—alternating characteristics of hyperactive and hypoactive delirium (see Table 5-6)

Table 5-6. Comparison of Delirium, Depression, and Dementia

	Delirium	Depression	Dementia
Onset	Sudden/over hours to days	Slow onset	Gradual/months-to-years
Disturbance of arousal	Hypoaroused; hyperalert; drowsy	Normal level of arousal	Normal level of arousal
Cognitive changes	Short-term memory loss; decreased attention and concentration	Mild cognitive deficits may be present	Short-term memory loss; decreased attention and concentration
Sleep–wake cycle	Severely disordered	May be impaired	May be normal
Level of consciousness	Impaired/fluctuates	Normal	Normal
Hallucinations	Frequent/often vivid; present in up to 75% of patients[129]	Rarely present[129]	Rare
Level of activity	Abnormally reduced or increased	Usually hypoactive or withdrawn	Normal

c) Agitation

   i.   A group of symptoms that may include physically and/or verbally aggressive behaviors (e.g., hiding or hoarding behaviors) and/or nonaggressive behaviors (e.g., pacing, inappropriate dressing, repetitive actions)

   ii.   Can occur at any time during a disease process and is an objective result of confusion or delirium

   iii.   Terminal agitation—seen in the imminently dying phases

      (a)   Excessive restlessness, increased mental and physical activity

      (b)   Commonly seen features are frequent, nonpurposeful motor activity, inability to concentrate or relax, disturbances in sleep or rest patterns, potential for progression to agitation

2.   Prevalence

   a)   Most common neuropsychiatric complication experienced by patients with advanced illness, occurring in up to 85% of the patients in the last week of life[129–132]

   b)   Some studies show 13% to 46% of patients experience agitation/hyperactive delirium[129]

   c)   Some studies show up to 80% of patients near the end of life develop hypoactive delirium[129]

   d)   Although hyperactive delirium is more readily identified, prevalence of delirium is thought to be much higher than recognized because symptoms of hypoactive delirium are common and frequently go undiagnosed[133–135]

3. Etiologies

    a) Often multifactorial[136]

    b) Direct CNS pathology—brain tumor or metastases, stroke

    c) Medications—anticholinergics; sedative/hypnotics; opioids

    d) Opioid or benzodiazepine withdrawal

    e) Nicotine or alcohol withdrawal

    f) Treatment side effects—chemotherapy or radiation therapy

    g) Metabolic disturbance—hypocalcemia, uremia, fluctuations in glucose, increased ammonia, anemia, hypoxemia

    h) Infection/sepsis

    i) Extreme, uncontrolled anxiety, sleep disturbance

    j) Nutritional deficiencies, dehydration

4. Assessment

    a) Thorough assessment to distinguish between confusion, delirium, depression, dementia[137]

    b) History and physical examination

        i. Basic needs—hot/cold, hungry/thirsty, full bladder, constipation, use of glasses/hearing aid(s)

        ii. Onset of symptom history

        iii. Personality and/or emotional coping abilities

        iv. Alcohol abuse and/or recent nicotine use

        v. Signs of infection—febrile, hypotensive, tachycardia, tachypnea, diaphoresis

        vi. Basic laboratory data—CBC, basic metabolic panel (BMP), renal and liver function

        vii. Brain imaging, if appropriate

    c) Delirium assessment scales

        i. Memorial Delirium Assessment Scale (MDAS)

        ii. Delirium Rating Scale (DRS)

        iii. Confusion Assessment Method (CAM)

        iv. Mini-Mental Status Examination (MMSE)

    d) Medication review—review current medications for compliance, effects, and iatrogenic effects that may contribute to altered mental status

    e) Pain assessment—unrelieved pain may alter ability to identify and/or express symptoms

5. Interventions

    a) Etiology of altered mental status and goals of care will determine intervention plan

    b) Discontinue or reduce medications thought to be contributing

    c) Correct metabolic imbalance

    d) Support withdrawal from alcohol, drugs, and/or nicotine as indicated

    e) Treat infection as appropriate

    f) For impaction—disimpact; establish aggressive bowel regimen

    g) For urinary retention, straight or retention catheter

    h) Provide for safety—follow agency policy regarding use of restraints

    i) Avoid sedation if possible

    j) Pharmacological interventions

        i. Although psychotropic drugs do not reverse altered mental status they may calm distressing agitation, paranoia, or hallucinations

        ii. Dosing guideline, no matter which drug is chosen, is to start low and increase the dose slowly

        iii. Neuroleptics—first-line treatment (e.g., haloperidol, chlorpromazine)[138,139]

        iv. New atypical neuroleptics—little evidence supporting these drugs; not to be considered as first-line treatment (e.g., olanzapine, quetiapine, risperidone)[138,140]

        v. Avoid benzodiazepines; potential for paradoxical worsening of symptoms (except in cases of suspected alcohol withdrawal)[140]

    k) Nonpharmacological interventions

        i. Should always be utilized

        ii. Environmental modifications

            (a) Reduce or increase the sensory stimulation

            (b) Avoid restraints or catheters if possible

            (c) Normalize sleep cycle; facilitate sleep hygiene

            (d) Have familiar people and/or objects nearby

            (e) Use soft voice tones and physical contact

            (f) Limit number of visits/visitors at bedside at one time

            (g) Avoid distressing extreme sensory experiences (heat, cold, lights)

            (h) Avoid changing the position of the bed

        iii. Other interventions

            (a) Pastoral and psychological support for patient and family

            (b) Relaxation techniques—visualization, distraction, massage, music, pet therapy

6. Patient and family education

   a) Communicate the delirium experience for family members—definition, characteristics of delirium, relationship to disease, role of therapies, and fluctuation of cognition

      i. Fluctuation in mental status are to be expected and may be worse at night[11]

   b) Communicate the role of opioids; families may feel that opioid is to blame and may withhold the drug *or* they might increase the dose if they think the delirium can be alleviated by additional doses

   c) Clarify goals of care

   d) Identify and explore family/caregiver expectations for behaviors; educate to adjust expectation if necessary

   e) Discuss therapeutic response to intervention(s), including potential sedating effects

   f) Discuss safety needs of patient during periods of altered mental status

   g) Instruct patient and family regarding sleep health/habits

   h) If terminal agitation, prepare family for patient's death

CITED REFERENCES

1. National Consensus Project for Quality Palliative Care. *Clinical Practice Guidelines for Quality Palliative Care.* Pittsburgh, PA: National Consensus Project; 2013. www.nationalconsensusproject.org/Guidelines_Download2.aspx. Accessed May 23, 2014.

2. Centers for Medicare & Medicaid Services (CMS). *Title 42: Public Health; Part 418—Hospice Care.* 2014. www.ecfr.gov/cgi-bin/text-idx?c=ecfr&sid=818258235647b14d2961ad30fa3e68e6&rgn=div5&view=text&node=42:3.0.1.1.5&idno=42#42:3.0.1.1.5.3.4.12. Accessed September 30, 2014.

3. American Nurses Association. *The Nursing Process.* 2014. www.nursingworld.org/EspeciallyForYou/What-is-Nursing/Tools-You-Need/Thenursingprocess.html. Accessed August 18, 2014.

4. Howden CW. Management of acid-related disorders in patients with dysphagia. *Am J Med.* 2004;117(5A Suppl):44S-48S.

5. American Speech-Language-Hearing Association (ASHA). 2014. www.asha.org. Accessed February 1, 2014.

6. Mann G, Hankey GJ. Initial clinical and demographic predictors of swallowing impairment following acute stroke. *Dysphagia.* 2001;16(3):208-215.

7. Crisan D, Shaban A, Boehme A, et al. Predictors of recovery of functional swallow after gastrostomy tube placement for dysphagia in stroke patients after inpatient rehabilitation: a pilot study. *Ann Rehabil Med.* 2014;38(4):467-475. doi: 10.5535/arm.2014.38.4.467. Epub August 28, 2014.

8. Nguyen NP, Frank C, Moltz CC, et al. Aspiration rate following chemoradiation for head and neck cancer: an underreported occurrence. *Radiother Oncol.* 2006;80(3):302-306. Epub August 4, 2006.

9. Nguyen NP, Moltz CC, Frank C, et al. Long-term aspiration following treatment for head and neck cancer. *Oncology.* 2008;74(1-2):25-30. doi: 10.1159/000138976. Epub June 10, 2008.

10. Aslam M, Vaezi MF. Dysphagia in the elderly. *Gastroenterol Hepatol (N Y).* 2013;9(12):784-795.

11. Quill T, Holloway RG, Stevens MS, Caprio TV, Olden AM, Storey CP. *Primer of Palliative Care.* 5th ed. Chicago, IL: American Academy of Hospice and Palliative Medicine; 2010.

12. Dahlin C, Cohen AK, Goldsmith, T. Dysphagia, xerostomia, and hiccups. In: Ferrell BR, Coyle N, eds. *Oxford Textbook of Palliative Nursing.* New York, NY: Oxford University Press; 2010:239-267.

13. Blush III RR, Larsen PD. Gastrointestinal symptoms. In: Matzo M, Sherman DW, eds. *Palliative Care Nursing: Quality Care to the End of Life.* 4th ed. New York, NY: Springer Publishing Company, LLC; 2015:560-588.

14. Pasero C, Quinn TE, Portenoy RK, McCaffery M, Rizos A. Opioid analgesics. In: Pasero C, McCaffery M, eds. *Pain Assessment and Pharmacological Management.* St. Louis, MO: Mosby Inc.; 2011: 277-622.

15. Wilson RK, Weissman DE. Neuroexcitatory effects of opioids: treatment. 2nd ed. *Fast Facts and Concepts.* 2006; 58. www.eperc.mcw.edu/EPERC/FastFactsIndex/ff_058.htm. Accessed October 3, 2014.

16. DeMonaco N, Arnold R. Myoclonus. *Fast Facts and Concepts.* 2009; 114. www.eperc.mcw.edu/EPERC/FastFactsIndex/ff_114.htm. Accessed October 3, 2014.

17. Wrede-Seaman L. *Symptom Management Algorithms: A Handbook for Palliative Care.* 3rd ed. Yakima, WA: Intellicard, Inc.; 2009.

18. Connelly J, Weissman DE. Seizure management in the dying patient. *Fast Facts and Concepts.* 2010; 229. www.eperc.mcw.edu/EPERC/FastFactsIndex/ff_229.htm. Accessed October 3, 2014.

19. Krouwer HGJ, Pallagi JL, Graves NM. Management of seizures in brain tumor patients at the end of life. *J Palliat Med.* 2000;3(4):465-475.

20. Top T. Seizures at the end of life. *J Palliat Med.* 2009;12(7):661-662.

21. Hospice and Palliative Nurses Association (HPNA). TIPS for Seizures. 2010. hpna.advancingexpert care.org/education/tips-sheets/. Accessed October 20, 2014.

22. Tenback DE, van Harten PN. Epidemiology and risk factors for (tardive) dyskinesia. In: Borthie J, Berzard E, Jenner P, eds. *Pathophysiology, Pharmacology, and Biochemistry of Dyskinesia, Volume 98 (International Review of Neurology).* New York, NY: Elsevier, Inc.; 2011:212.

23. Gopal S, Liu Y, Alphs L, Savitz A, Nuamah I, Hough D. Incidence and time course of extrapyramidal symptoms with oral and long-acting injectable paliperidone: a posthoc pooled analysis of seven randomized controlled studies. *Neuropsychiatr Dis Treat.* 2013:9:1381-1392. doi: 10.2147/NDT. S49944. Epub September 20, 2013.

24. Sterns RH; Wolters Kluwer Health. Pathophysiology and etiology of edema in adults. *UpToDate.* 2013. www.uptodate.com/contents/pathophysiology-and-etiology-of-edema-in-adults. Accessed August 25, 2014.

25. Simoff MJ, Lally B, Slade MG, et al. Symptom management in patients with lung cancer: diagnosis and management of lung cancer, 3rd ed: American College of Chest Physicians evidence-based clinical practice guidelines. *Chest.* 2013;143(5 Suppl):e455S-e497S. doi: 10.1378/chest.12-2366.

26. Drews RE, Rabkin DJ; Wolters Kluwer Health. Malignancy-related superior vena cava syndrome. *UpToDate.* 2013. www.uptodate.com/contents/malignancy-related-superior-vena-cava-syndrome?source=search_result&search=Malignancy-related+superior+vena+cava+syndrome& selectedTitle=1%7E150. Accessed October 6, 2014.

27. Sterns RH. General principles of the treatment of edema in adults. *UpToDate.* 2013. www.uptodate. com/contents/general-principles-of-the-treatment-of-edema-in-adults?source=search_result&search= General+principles+of+the+treatment+of+edema+in+adults&selectedTitle=1%7E150. Accessed October 6, 2014.

28. Go AS, Mozaffarian D, Roger VL, et al. Heart disease and stroke statistics—2014 update: a report from the American Heart Association. *Circulation.* 2014;129(3):e28-e292. doi: 10.1161/01. cir.0000441139.02102.80. circ.ahajournals.org/content/129/3/e28.full. Accessed September 5, 2014.

29. Tierney P, McKenna N. Management of angina in the older adult. *Nurs Residential Care.* 2014;16(2): 78-82.

30. Murphy SL, Xu J, Kochanek KD. U.S. Department of Health and Human Services (HHS). Deaths: final data for 2010. *National Vital Statistics Reports.* 2013;61(4):1-17. www.cdc.gov/nchs/data/nvsr/ nvsr61/nvsr61_04.pdf. Accessed July 29, 2014.

31. National Heart, Lung, and Blood Institute (NHLBI). *What is Angina?* 2011. www.nhlbi.nih.gov/ health/health-topics/topics/angina/. Accessed September 26, 2014.

32. Jessup M, Abraham WT, Casey DE, et al. 2009 focused update: ACCF/AHA guidelines for the diagnosis and management of heart failure in adults: a report of the American College of Cardiology Foundation/American Heart Association Task Force on practice guidelines: developed in collaboration with the International Society for Heart and Lung Transplantation. *Circulation.* 2009;119(14):1977–2016. doi: 10.1161/CIRCULATIONAHA.109.192064. Epub March 26, 2009.

33. Wee B, Browning J, Adams A, et al. Management of chronic cough in patients receiving palliative care: review of evidence and recommendations by a task group of the Association for Palliative Medicine of Great Britain and Ireland. *Palliat Med.* 2012; 26(6);780-787. doi: 10.1177/02692163114 23793. Epub October 12, 2011.

34. Janssen DJA, Spruit MA, Uszko-Lencer NH, Schols JMGA, Wouters EFM. Symptoms, comorbidities, and health care in advanced chronic obstructive pulmonary disease or chronic heart failure. *J Palliat Med.* 2011;14(6):735-743.

35. Bausewein C, Booth S, Gysels M, Kühnbach R, Haberland B, Higginson IJ. Understanding breathlessness: cross-sectional comparison of symptom burden and palliative care needs in chronic obstructive pulmonary disease and cancer. *J Palliat Med.* 2010;13(9):1109-1118.

36. Truesdale K, Jurdi A. Nebulized lidocaine in the treatment of intractable cough. *Am J Hosp Palliat Med.* 2013;30(6):587-589. doi: 10.1177/1049909112458577. Epub September 9, 2012.

37. Ryan NM, Birring SS, Gibson PG. Gabapentin for refractory chronic cough: a randomised, double-blind, placebo-controlled trial. *Lancet.* 2012;380(9853):1583-1589. doi: 10.1016/S0140-6736(12)60776-4. Epub August 28, 2012.

38. Parshall MB, Schwartzstein RM, Adams L, et al. An official American Thoracic Society statement: update on the mechanisms, assessment, and management of dyspnea. *Am J Respir Crit Care Med.* 2012;185(4):435-452. doi: 10.1164/rccm.201111-2042ST.

39. Kamal AH, Maguire JM, Wheeler JL, Currow DC, Abernethy AP. Dyspnea review for the palliative care professional: treatment goals and therapeutic options. *J Palliat Med.* 2012;15(1):106-114.

40. Kamal AH, Maguire JM, Wheeler JL, Currow DC, Abernethy AP. Dyspnea review for the palliative care professional: assessment, burdens, and etiologies. *J Palliat Med.* 2011;14(10):1167-1172.

41. Hui D, Morgado M, Vidai M, et al. Dyspnea in hospitalized advanced cancer patients: subjective and physiologic correlates. *J Palliat Med.* 2013;16(3):274-280.

42. Yancy CW, Jessup M, Bozkurt B, et al. 2013 ACCF/AHA guideline for the management of heart failure: a report of the American College of Cardiology Foundation/American Heart Association Task Force on practice guidelines. *Circulation.* 2013;128(16):e240-327. doi: 10.1161/CIR.0b013e31829e8776. Epub June 5, 2013.

43. Campbell ML, Templin T, Walch J. A respiratory distress observation scale for patients unable to self-report dyspnea. *J Palliat Med.* 2010;13(3):285-290.

44. Norweg A, Collins EG. Evidence for cognitive-behavioral strategies improving dyspnea and related distress in CPOD. *Int J Chron Obstruct Pulmon Dis.* 2013;8:439-451. doi: 10.2147/COPD.S30145. Epub September 25, 2013.

45. Campbell M, Yarandi H. Death rattle is not associated with patient respiratory distress: is pharmacologic treatment indicated? *J Palliat Med.* 2013;16(10):1255-1259.

46. Shimizu Y, Miyashita M, Morita T, Sato K, Tsuneto S, Shima Y. Care strategy for death rattle in terminally ill cancer patients and their family members: recommendations from a cross-sectional nationwide survey of bereaved family members' perceptions. *J Pain Symptom Manage.* 2014;48(1):2-12. doi: 10.1016/j.jpainsymman.2013.07.010. Epub October 23, 2013.

47. Abernethy AP, McDonald CF, Frith PA, et al. Effect of palliative oxygen versus room air in relief of breathlessness in patients with refractory dyspnea: a double-blind, randomised controlled trial. *Lancet.* 2010;376(9743):784-793. doi: 10.1016/S0140-6736(10)61115-4.

48. Clemens KE, Faust M, Bruera E. Update on combined modalities for the management of breathlessness. *Curr Opin Support Palliat Care.* 2012;6(2):163-167. doi: 10.1097/SPC.0b013e3283530fee.

49. Smight TJ, Ritter JK, Poklis JL, et al. ABH gel is not absorbed from the skin of normal volunteers. *J Pain Symptom Manage.* 2012;43(5):961-966. doi: 10.1016/j.jpainsymman.2011.05.017.

50. Farless LB, Steil N, Williams BR, Bailey FA. Intermittent subcutaneous furosemide: parental diuretic rescue for hospice patients with congestive heart failure resistant to oral diuretic. *Am J Hosp Palliat Care*. 2013;30(8):791-792. doi: 10.1177/1049909112465795. Epub November 6, 2012.

51. Galbraith S, Fagan P, Perkins P, Lynch A, Booth S. Does the use of a handheld fan improve chronic dyspnea? A randomized, controlled, crossover trial. *J Pain Symptom Manage*. 2010;39(5):831-838.

52. Mularski RA, Munjas BA, Lorenz KA, et al. Randomized controlled trial of mindfulness-based therapy for dyspnea in chronic obstructive lung disease. *J Altern Complement Med*. 2009;15(10): 1083-1090. doi: 10.1089/acm.2009.0037.

53. Campion J, Snyder L. Palliative care of dyspnea in patients with advanced COPD. *Elder Care*. 2011. aging.arizona.edu/sites/default/files/palliative_care_of_dyspnea_in_pts_with_copd.pdf. Accessed October 6, 2014.

54. Bobb BT. Urgent syndromes at the end of life. In: Ferrell BR, Coyne N, eds. *Oxford Textbook of Palliative Nursing*. 3rd ed. New York, NY: Oxford University Press; 2010:501-523.

55. Myatt R. Diagnosis and management of patients with pleural effusions. *Nurs Stand*. 2014;28(41): 51-58. doi: 10.7748/ns.28.41.51.e8849.

56. Larkin PJ, Sykes NP, Centeno C, et al. The management of constipation in palliative care: clinical practice recommendations. *Palliat Med*. 2008;22(7):796-807. doi: 10.1177/0269216308096908.

57. Sykes, N. Constipation and diarrhea. In: Hanks G, Cherney NI, Christakis NA, Fallon M, Kaasa S, Portenoy, RK, eds. *Oxford Textbook of Palliative Medicine*. 4th ed. New York, NY: Oxford University Press; 2011:833-849.

58. Economou DC. Bowel management: constipation, diarrhea, obstruction, and ascites. In: Ferrell BR, Coyle N, eds. *Oxford Textbook of Palliative Nursing*. 3rd ed. New York, NY: Oxford University Press; 2010:269-289.

59. Price RO, Bradley R. Assessing and treating faecal incontinence. *Nurs Older People*. 2013;25(7): 16-23. doi: 10.7748/nop2013.09.25.7.16.e484.

60. LeBlanc K, Arnold RA. Evaluation of malignant ascites. *Fast Facts and Concepts*. 2009; 176. www. eperc.mcw.edu/EPERC/FastFactsIndex/ff_176.htm. Accessed October 10, 2011.

61. European Association for the Study of the Liver. EASL clinical practice guidelines on the management of ascites, spontaneous bacterial peritonitis, and hepatorenal syndrome in cirrhosis. *J Hepatol*. 2010; 53(3):397-417. doi: 10.1016/j.jhep.2010.05.004. Epub June 1, 2010.

62. Sangisetty SL, Miner TJ. Malignant ascites: a review of prognostic factors, pathophysiology, and therapeutic measures. *World J Gastrointest Surg*. 2012;4(4):87-95. doi: 10.4240/wjgs.v4.i4.87.

63. Keen J. Jaundice, ascites, and encephalopathy. In: Hanks G, Cherney NI, Christakis NA, Fallon M, Kaasa S, Portenoy RK, eds. *Oxford Textbook of Palliative Medicine*. 4th ed. New York, NY: Oxford University Press; 2010:863-887.

64. Rosenburg S. Palliation of malignant ascites. *Gastroenterol Clin North Am*. 2006;35:189-199.

65. Calsina-Berna A, Garcia-Gomez G, Gonzalez-Barboteo J, Porta-Sales J. Treatment of chronic hiccups in cancer patients: a systematic review. *J Palliat Med*. 2012;15(10):1142-1150. doi: 10.1089/jpm. 2012.0087. Epub August 14, 2012.

66. King C, Tarcatu D. Nausea and vomiting. In: Ferrell BR, Coyle N, eds. *Oxford Textbook of Palliative Nursing*. 3rd ed. New York, NY: Oxford University Press; 2010:221-238.

67. Mannix KA. Palliative of nausea and vomiting. In: Hanks G, Cherney NI, Christakis NA, Fallon M, Kaasa S, Portenoy, RK, eds. *Oxford Textbook of Palliative Medicine.* 4th ed. Oxford, UK: Oxford University Press; 2010:801-812.

68. Glare P, Miller J, Nikolova T, Tickoo R. Treating nausea and vomiting in palliative care: a review. *Clin Interv Aging.* 2011;6:243-259. doi: 10.2147/CIA.S13109. Epub September 12, 2011.

69. Anthony T, Baron T, Mercadante S, et al. Report of the clinical protocol committee: development of randomized trials for malignant bowel obstruction. *J Pain Symptom Manage.* 2007;34(1 Suppl): S49-S59.

70. Ripamonti C, De Conno F, Ventafridda V, Rossi B, Baines MJ. Management of bowel obstruction in advanced and terminal cancer patients. *Ann Oncol.* 1993;4(1):15-21.

71. Kapo J, Morrison LJ, Liao S. Palliative care in the older adult. *J Palliat Med.* 2007;10(1):185-209.

72. Abrams P, Cardozo L, Fall M, et al. The standardisation of terminology of lower urinary tract function: report from the Standardisation Sub-Committee of the International Continence Society. *Neurourol Urodyn.* 2002;21(2):167-178.

73. Thomas K, Oades G, Taylor-Hay C, Kirby RS. Acute urinary retention: what is the impact on patient's quality of life? *BJU Int.* 2005;95(1):72-76. doi: 10.1111/j.1464-410X.2004.05254.x

74. Gray M, Sims T. Urinary tract disorders. In: Ferrell BR, Coyle N, eds. *Oxford Text of Palliative Nursing.* 3rd ed. New York, NY: Oxford University Press; 2010:321-340.

75. McIllmurray M. The medical treatment of cancer in palliative care. In: Hanks G, Cherney NI, Christakis NA, Fallon M, Kaasa S, Portenoy RK, eds. *Oxford Textbook of Palliative Medicine.* 4th ed. New York, NY: Oxford University Press; 2010:513-525.

76. von Gunten CF, Gafford E. Treatment of non-pain-related symptoms. *Cancer J.* 2013;19(5):397-404. doi: 10.1097/PPO.0b013e3182a65ecf.

77. Wong RK, James JL, Sagar S, et al. Phase 2 results from Radiation Therapy Oncology Group Study 0537: a phase 2/3 study comparing acupuncture-like transcutaneous electrical nerve stimulation versus pilocarpine in treating early radiation-induced xerostomia. *Cancer.* 2012;118(17):4244-4252. doi: 10.1002/cncr.27382. Epub January 17, 2012.

78. Jacobsen J. Topical opioids for pain. *Fast Facts and Concepts.* 2010; 185. www.eperc.mcw.edu/ EPERC/FastFactsIndex/ff_185.htm. Accessed October 6, 2014.

79. Del Ferraro C, Grant M, Koczywas M, Dorr-Uyemura LA. Management of anorexia-cachexia in late-stage lung cancer patients. *J Hosp Palliat Nurs.* 2012;14(6):397–402.

80. von Gunten CF, Ferris F. Pruritus. 2nd ed. *Fast Facts and Concepts.* 2005; 37. www.eperc.mcw.edu/ EPERC/FastFactsIndex/ff_037.htm. Accessed October 6, 2014.

81. Sun V. Management of treatment-induced dermatologic toxicities in palliative care. *J Hosp Palliat Nurs.* 2012;14(1):80-85. doi: 10.1097/NJH.0b013e31823e2159.

82. Chan KY, Li CW, Wong H, et al. Use of sertraline for antihistamine-refractory uremic pruritus in renal palliative care patients. *J Pallliat Med.* 2013;16(8):966-970. doi: 10.1089/jpm.2012.0504. Epub June 18, 2013.

83. Seccareccia D, Gebara N. Pruritus in palliative care. *Can Fam Physician.* 2011;57(9):1010-1014.

84. Berger TG, Steinhoff M. Pruritus and renal failure. *Semin Cutan Med Surg.* 2011;30(2):99-100. doi: 10.1016/j.sder.2011.04.005.

85. Levy C. Management of pruritus in patients with cholestatic liver disease. *Gastroenterol Hepatol (NY).* 2011;7(9):615-617.

86. National Pressure Ulcer Advisory Panel, European Pressure Ulcer Advisory Panel, Pan Pacific Pressure Injury Alliance; Haesler E, ed. *Prevention and Treatment of Pressure Ulcers: Quick Reference Guide*. Perth, AU: Cambridge Media; 2014. www.npuap.org/wp-content/uploads/2014/08/Quick-Reference-Guide-DIGITAL-NPUAP-EPUAP-PPPIA.pdf. Accessed October 6, 2014.

87. Burt T. Palliative care of pressure ulcers in long-term care. *Annuals Long-Term Care*. 2013;21(3): 20-28.

88. Lengemo DK, Black J; Panel, National Pressure Ulcer Advisory. Pressure ulcers in individuals receiving palliative care: a national pressure ulcer advisory panel white paper. *Adv Skin Wound Care*. 2010;23(2):59-72. doi: 10.1097/01.ASW.0000363502.84737.c8.

89. Maida V, Ennis M, Kuziemsky C, Trozzolo L. Symptoms associated with malignant wounds: a prospective case series. *J Pain Symptom Manage*. 2009;37(2):206-211. doi: 10.1016/j.jpainsymman.2008.01.009. Epub July 10, 2008.

90. Graves ML, Sun V. Providing quality wound care at the end of life. *J Hosp Palliat Nurs*. 2013;15(2): 68-73.

91. Teno JM, Gozalo P, Mitchell SL, Kuo S, Fulton AT, Mor V. Feeding tubes and the prevention or healing of pressure ulcers. *Arch Intern Med*. 2012;172:697-701.

92. Ramundo JM. Wound debridement. In: Bryant RA, Nix DP, eds. *Acute & Chronic Wounds: Current Management Concepts*. 4th ed. St. Louis, MO: Elsevier Mosby; 2012:279-284.

93. Sateia MJ, Byock IR. Sleep in palliative care. In: Hanks G, Cherny NI, Christakis NA, Fallon M, Kaasa S, Portenoy RK. *Oxtford Textbook of Palliative Medicine*. 4th ed. New York, NY: Oxford University Press; 2010:1059-1083.

94. Page MS, Berger AM; Oncology Nursing Society (ONS). Oncology Nursing Society: PEP Topics: *Sleep-Wake Disturbances*. 2009. www.ons.org/practice-resources/pep/sleep-wake-disturbances. Accessed October 7, 2014.

95. Dambrosio NM, Mazanec P. "Nurse, I can't sleep!": approaches to management of insomnia in oncology patients. *J Hosp Palliat Nurs*. 2013;15(5):267-275.

96. National Sleep Foundation (NSF). *Insomnia*. 2014. sleepfoundation.org/sleep-disorders-problems/insomnia. Accessed October 10, 2014.

97. Berger AM, Parker KP, Young-McCaughan S, et al. Sleep wake disturbances in people with cancer and their caregivers: state of the science. *Oncol Nurs Forum*. 2005;32(6):E98-E126.

98. Siebem AT, Manber R. Insomnia and its effective non-pharmacologic treatment. *Med Clin North Am*. 2010;94(3):581-591. doi: 10.1016/j.mcna.2010.02.005.

99. Woodward S. Cognitive-behavioral therapy for insomnia in patients with cancer. *Clin J Oncol Nurs*. 2011;15(4):E43-E51. doi: 10.1188/11.CJON.E42-E52.

100. Kendall AR. Finding a good night's sleep: understanding insomnia. *J Palliat Med*. 2008;11(5): 805-806.

101. Wholihan D, Kemp C. Anorexia and cachexia. In: Ferrell BR, Coyne N, eds. *Oxford Textbook of Palliative Nursing*. 3rd ed. New York, NY: Oxford University Press; 2010:211-219.

102. Evans WJ, Morley JE, Argiles J, et al. Cachexia: a new definition. *Clin Nutr*. 2008;27(6):793-799.

103. Laviano A, Inui A, Marks DL, et al. Neural control of the anorexia-cachexia syndrome. *Am J Physiol Endocrinol Metab*. 2008;295(5):E1000-E1008. doi: 10.1152/ajpendo.90252.2008. Epub August 19, 2008.

104. Gabriel MS, Kedziera, Coyle N. Hydration, thirst, and nutrition. In: Ferrell BR, Coyle N, eds. *Oxford Textbook of Palliative Nursing*. 3rd ed. New York, NY: Oxford University Press; 2010:291-302.

105. Jatoi A. Pharmacologic therapy for the cancer anorexia/weight loss syndrome: a data-driven, practical approach. *J Support Oncol*. 2006;4(10):499-502.

106. Policzer J, Sobel J; Storey CP, Levine S, Shega, JW, eds. *Management of Selected Nonpain Symptoms of Life-Limiting Illness*. 3rd ed. Glenview, IL: American Academy of Hospice and Palliative Medicine; 2008.

107. Subjective Global Assessment. *A Highly Reliable Nutritional Assessment Tool*. 2012. subjectiveglobal assessment.com/. Accessed August 25, 2014.

108. Pagana KD, Pagana TJ. *Mosby's Diagnostic and Laboratory Test Reference*. 11th ed. St. Louis, MO: Elsevier Mosby; 2013.

109. Bruera E, Hui D, Dalal S, et al. Parenteral hydration in patients with advanced cancer: a multicenter, double-blind, placebo-controlled, randomized trial. *J Clin Oncol*. 2012;31:111-118.

110. Nakajima N, Hata Y, Kusumuto K. A clinical study on the influence of hydration volume on the signs of terminally ill cancer patients with abdominal malignancies. *J Palliat Med*. 2013;16(2):185-189. doi: 10.1089/jpm.2012.0233.

111. Gabriel J. Subcutaneous fluid administration and the hydration of older people. *Br J Nurs*. 2014; 23(14):S10-S14.

112. Ruiz Garcia V, López-Briz E, Carbonell Sanchis R, Gonzalvez Perales JL, Bort-Marti S. Megestrol acetate for treatment of anorexia-cachexia syndrome. *Cochrane Database Syst Rev*. 2013;28;3: CD004310. doi: 10.1002/14651858.CD004310.pub3.

113. Loprinzi CL, Jatoi A. Pharmacologic management of cancer anorexia/cachexia. *UpToDate*. 2014. www.uptodate.com/contents/pharmacologic-management-of-cancer-anorexia-cachexia?source= search_result&search=anorexia+cachexia&selectedTitle=2%7E150. Accessed August 26, 2014.

114. Radbruch L, Straaser F, Elsner F, et al; Research Steering Committee of the European Association for Palliative Care (EAPC). Fatigue in palliative care patients—an EAPC approach. *Palliat Med*. 2008; 22(1):13-32. doi: 10.1177/0269216307085183.

115. National Clinical Practice Guidelines in Oncology. NCCN Clinical Practice Guidelines in Oncology: Cancer-related Fatigue. *National Comprehensive Cancer Network (NCCN)*. 2012. www.nccn.org/ professionals/physician_gls/pdf/fatigue.pdf. Accessed November 9, 2013.

116. Anderson PR, Dean GE, Piech MA. Fatigue. In: Ferrell BR, Coyle N, eds. *Oxford Textbook of Palliative Nursing*. 3rd ed. New York, NY: Oxford University Press; 2010:187-209.

117. Borneman T. Assessment and management of cancer-related fatigue. *J Hosp Palliat Nurs*. 2013; 15(2):77-86.

118. van den Dungen IA, Verhagen CA, van der Graaf WT, van den Berg JP, Vissers KC, Engels Y. Feasibility and impact of a physical exercise program in patients with advanced cancer: a pilot study. *J Palliat Med*. 2014;17(10):1091-1098. doi: 10.1089/jpm.2013.0638.

119. Borneman T. Assessment and management of cancer-related fatigue. *J Hosp Palliat Nurs*. 2013;15(2): 77-86.

120. Reisfield GM, Wilson GR. Cancer related fatigue. *Fast Facts and Concepts*. 2009; 173. www.eperc. mcw.edu/EPERC/FastFactsIndex/ff_173.htm. Accessed October 10, 2014.

121. Bobb BT; Coyne PJ, ed. *Compendium of Treatment of End Stage Non-Cancer Diagnoses: Hepatic*. 2nd ed. Pittsburgh, PA: Hospice and Palliative Nurses Association; 2012.

122. Schrijvers D, van Fraeyenhove F. Emergencies in palliative care. *Cancer J.* 2010;16(5):514-520. doi: 10.1097/PPO.0b013e3181f28a8d.

123. Whitehead P; Coyne PJ, ed. *Compendium of Treatment of End Stage Non-Cancer Diagnoses: HIV/ AIDS.* 2nd ed. Pittsburgh, PA: Hospice and Palliative Nurses Association; 2013.

124. Torres MEU, Rodríguez JNR, Ramos JLS, Gómez FA. Transfusion in palliative cancer patients: a review of the literature. *J Palliat Med.* 2014;17(1):88-104. doi: 10.1089/jpm.2013.0387.

125. Rote NS, McCance KL. Alterations of erythrocyte function. In: McCance KL, Huether SE, Brashers VL, Rote NS. *Pathophysiology: The Biological Basis for Disease in Adults and Children.* 6th ed. Maryland Heights, MO: Mosby Elsevier; 2010:989-1013.

126. Kaasa S, Loge JH. Quality of life in palliative care—principles and practice. In: Hanks G, Cherny NI, Christakis NA, Fallon M, Kaasa S, Portenoy RK. *Oxford Textbook of Palliative Medicine.* 4th ed. New York, NY: Oxford University Press; 2010:443-461.

127. Dahlin CM, Carr A, Mahler A, Telles J; Coyne PJ, ed. *Compendium of Treatment of End Stage Non-Cancer Diagnoses: Dementia.* 2nd ed. Pittsburgh, PA: Hospice and Palliative Nurses Association; 2014.

128. Breitbart W, Chochinov HM, Passik SD. Psychiatric symptoms in palliative medicine. In: Hanks G, Cherny NI, Christakis NA, Fallon M, Kaasa S, Portenoy RK, eds. *Oxford Textbook of Palliative Medicine.* 4th ed. New York, NY: Oxford University Press; 2010:1453-1482.

129. Breitbart W, Alici Y. Agitation and delirium at the end of life. *JAMA.* 2008;300(24):2898-2910. doi: 10.1001/jama.2008.885.

130. Gangon PR. Treatment of delirium in supportive and palliative care. *Curr Opin Support Palliat Care.* 2008;2(1):60-66.

131. Leonard M, Spiller J, Keen J, MacLullich A, Kamholtz B, Meagher D. Symptoms of depression and delirium assessed serially in palliative-care inpatients. *Psychosomatics.* 2009;50(5):506-514. doi: 10.1176/appi.psy.50.5.506.

132. Voyer P, Richard S, Doucet L, Carmichael PH. Detecting delirium and subsyndromal delirium using different diagnostic criteria among demented long-term care residents. *J Am Med Dir Assoc.* 2009;10(3):181-188. doi: 10.1016/j.jamda.2008.09.006. Epub January 8, 2009.

133. Spiller JA, Keen JC. Hypoactive delirium: assessing the extent of the problem for inpatient specialist palliative care. *Palliat Med.* 2006;20(1):17-23.

134. Wada T, Wada M, Wada M, Onishi H. Characteristics, interventions, and outcomes of misdiagnosed delirium in cancer patients. *Palliat Support Care.* 2010;8(2):125-131. doi: 10.1017/S1478951509990861. Epub March 23, 2010.

135. Hosie A, Davidson PM, Agar M, Sanderson Cr, Phillips J. Delirium prevalence, incidence, and implications for screening in specialist palliative care inpatient settings. *Palliat Med.* 2013;27(6):486-498. doi: 10.1177/0269216312457214. Epub September 17, 2012.

136. Breitbart W, Alici Y. Evidence-based treatment of delirium in patients with cancer. *J Clin Oncol.* 2012;30(11):206-1214. doi: 10.1200/JCO.2011.39.8784. Epub March 12, 2012.

137. Marchington KL, Carrier L, Lawlor PG. Delirium masquerading as depression. *Palliat Support Care.* 2012;10(1):59-62. doi: 10.1017/S1478951511000599.

138. Quijada E, Billings AJ. Pharmacologic management of delirium: update on newer agents, 2nd ed. *Fast Facts and Concepts.* 2009; 60. www.eperc.mcw.edu/EPERC/FastFactsIndex/ff_060.htm. Accessed October 7, 2014.

139. Heidrich DE, English N. Delirium, confusion, agitation, and restlessness. In: Ferrell BR, Coyle N, eds. *Oxford Textbook of Palliative Nursing*. 3rd ed. New York, NY: Oxford University Press; 2010:449-467.

140. Close JF, Long CO. Delirium: opportunity for comfort in palliative care. *J Hosp Palliat Nurs*. 2012; 14(6):386–394. doi: 10.1097/NJH.0b013e31825d2b0a.

PSYCHIATRIC/PSYCHOLOGICAL SYMPTOMS AND DIAGNOSES

Nan Grottanelli, ARNP, AGPCNP-BC, CHPN®
Pamela Shockey Stephenson, PhD, RN, AOCNS, PMHCNS-BC

I. Introduction

A. This section focuses on

1. The care of persons with preexisting, serious, and persistent mental illness (SPMI) who also receive a terminal diagnosis

2. Persons who develop new onset depression and/or anxiety after receiving a terminal diagnosis

B. Individuals with a SPMI are "suffer[ing] from a prolonged or recurrent mental illness, are impaired in activities of daily living and require long-term treatment"[1, p. 725]

C. Changing Priorities

1. Palliative and hospice professionals are responsible for the psychological care of their patients[2]

2. The right for persons with SPMI to access quality end-of-life care has been largely ignored

3. A call for improved end-of-life care for persons with SPMI has been made

4. In its *2015–2018 Research Agenda*, the Hospice and Palliative Nurses Association (HPNA) included research on delivery systems of care for patients with both a psychiatric illness and a life-limiting illness as a potential research topic[3]

5. The Academy of Psychosomatic Medicine[4] has called for the implementation of further clinical research, targeted educational programs, and improved policies to reduce the barriers to excellent end-of-life care for persons with SPMI

6. Patients with serious mental illness have a 2 to 3 times higher mortality rate as compared to the general population[5,6]

7. Patients who have mental illness experience the same fears and symptoms that patients in the general population experience

8. One of the most important facets of palliative care, as well as psychiatric care, is therapeutic communication and establishing a trusting relationship

D. Barriers to Care

1. Patients with SPMI are marginalized and less likely to access healthcare. Many are

    a) Transient, homeless, or live in group homes making access to home care services challenging[7]

    b) Unmarried, estranged from families, and left without anyone to care for them[1,8,9]

    c) Fearful or distrustful of the healthcare system[1,10]

    d) Unable to communicate and be understood by health professionals[1,10]

    e) Deemed incompetent by the courts and, therefore, ineligible to participate in healthcare decisions[10]

    f) Assigned a court-appointed healthcare proxy who may not know the patient or understand their fears or desires[1]

2. Symptoms of existing mental disorders may exacerbate during the stress of a serious or life-threatening illness[11]

3. There is a gap between the nursing skills that medical/surgical and psychiatric nurses are comfortable employing

    a) Nurses who care for medical patients are uncomfortable caring for psychiatric patients and vice versa[7]

        i. Nurses who are uncomfortable or lack confidence may not be able to provide the best care

    b) Some clinicians view psychological symptoms such as depression and anxiety as expected consequences of having a serious illness and thought to be a normal part of the dying process that does not warrant treatment[2]

4. Discussion of advanced directives needs to be done to try to honor patient wishes, but may spur on a competency hearing to determine the course of a patient's treatment

5. Multiple studies have indicated that pain is undertreated in patients with a psychiatric history[12,13]

6. Family involvement may be an issue in caring for someone with a serious mental illness, due to estrangement, or other family dysfunctions. Thus, emotional support for this patient can be a challenge. Involvement of psychiatric personnel who may have a long-standing involvement with this patient should be considered

E. Suggestions for Improving Care

1. An interdisciplinary team approach that includes mental health professionals and a clinical pharmacist is essential for providing palliative care to patients with mental illness

2. Learn about the needs of persons with a SPMI and how to care for them[1]

3. Incorporate detailed psychiatric histories into routine intake assessments[2]

4. Develop creative strategies to reach out to patients with SPMI wherever they live

   a) For many with SPMI "home" may be a group home, homeless shelter, or long-term inpatient mental health facility

   b) "Family" may be the staff members at these facilities[10]

   c) Collaborate with the care facility staff to allow the patient to remain in their "home" environment[1]

5. Consult with a clinical pharmacist to ensure medications for palliative care (e.g., analgesics, antiemetics) do not interact with medications for psychiatric diagnosis(es) (e.g., antidepressants, antipsychotics)

II. Schizophrenia

A. Definition[14]

1. The *Diagnostic Statistical Manual for Mental Illness-5* (DSM-5)[14] defines schizophrenia by the presence of delusions, hallucinations, and/or disorganized speech for a significant portion of time along with at least 1 additional of the previous symptoms or grossly disorganized or abnormal motor behavior and/or negative symptoms[14]

   a) Delusions[14]

      i. A fixed false belief that is not amenable to change, even with evidence to the contrary

      ii. Common types of delusions

         (a) Delusion of persecution—belief of going to be harmed

         (b) Delusion of grandeur—belief that he/she is exceptional

         (c) Delusion of reference—belief that comments, gestures, and so forth are directed toward him/her

         (d) Delusion of control—belief that an outside force is controlling him/her

         (e) Somatic delusion—preoccupation with health or organs

         (f) Nihilistic delusion—conviction that a major catastrophe will occur

         (g) Erotomanic delusion—false belief that another person is in love with him/her

   b) Hallucinations[14,15]

      i. A sensory experience that does not exist outside the patient's mind

      ii. May involve any sense, but auditory is the most common

      iii. Must occur while the patient is awake, not while falling asleep or waking up

   c) Disorganized thinking

      i. Inferred through content and form of speech

      ii. Common types of disorganized thinking

(a) Association looseness—quick movement between topics without logical sequence

(b) Neologisms—making up new words

(c) Concrete thinking—thinking comes from only what one can sense, lacks abstract thinking or the ability to generalize

(d) Clang associations—linking words based on similar sounds, rhyming

(e) Word salad—confused speech that lacks logical sequence, often repetitious

(f) Circumstantiality—included unnecessary word and detail; hard to get to point

(g) Tangentiality—only briefly mentions and moves to new thought

(h) Mutism—unable to speak

(i) Preservation—stuck on an idea, repetition

d) Grossly disorganized or abnormal motor behavior

   i. Varies from childlike silliness and catatonia to unpredictable agitation

   ii. Leads to difficulties in performing activities of daily living

e) Negative symptoms

   i. Diminished verbal and nonverbal expression of emotion

   ii. Avolition—decrease in motivated and self-initiated purposeful activities

   iii. Alogia—diminished speech

   iv. Anhedonia—decreased ability to experience pleasure

2. Individuals have impairments in a range of cognitive domains

3. Psychotic disorders are varied, and symptom severity can predict the degree of cognitive or neurobiological deficits

4. Many patients who are on antipsychotics have the associated medical problem of metabolic syndrome (a cluster of conditions—increased blood pressure, a high blood glucose level, excess body fat around the waist, and abnormal cholesterol levels—that occur together, increasing risk of heart disease, stroke, and diabetes)

5. Severe mania or depression can also prompt psychotic symptoms such as hallucinations or delusions making bipolar disorder easily confused with schizophrenia

B. Treatment

1. Nonpharmacological interventions

   a) Communication

      i. Always speak plainly and clearly in words that cannot be misunderstood

      ii. Focus conversations on reality and remain calm

      iii. Convey acceptance, but the patient must understand that you do not view the delusion or hallucination as real

        iv.   Use reasonable doubt, "I realize that you believe this is true, but I find it hard to accept (or I do not see or hear the hallucination)"

        v.   Maintain an assertive, matter-of-fact yet natural approach with suspicious patients

        vi.   If the patient is having an auditory hallucination, ask, "What are the voices saying to you?" This is important to avoid injury to the patient and others from command hallucinations

        vii.   When referring to hallucinations, refer to them as "the voices," never use the word "they"

        viii.   If the patient is using unusual speech patterns, state, "I don't understand what you mean. Would you please explain to me?"

b)   Milieu

        i.   Remove all dangerous objects from the patient's environment

        ii.   Intervene at the first sign of increased anxiety, agitation, aggression, or hostility

        iii.   Maintain a low level of stimuli in the patient's environment to decrease potential for violence

        iv.   Avoid physical contact when possible, or warn the patient when you are about to perform a procedure

        v.   Avoid laughing, talking, or whispering where the patient cannot hear what is being said

        vi.   Provide a predictable, calm, organized environment of time, place, and staff

        vii.   If restraint is absolutely necessary, make sure you have enough staff for safety

c)   Psychotherapy/group therapy/family therapy

        i.   Consult with the interdisciplinary team for a psychiatrist, psychologist, or psychiatric nurse practitioner who could assist with therapy

        ii.   Extra psychosocial support is best provided by professionals who already have a relationship with the patient

d)   Behavior therapy

        i.   Clearly define goals and how they will be measured

        ii.   Attach positive, negative, and aversive reinforcements to adaptive and maladaptive behavior

        iii.   Use simple, concrete instructions and prompts to elicit the desired behavior

2.   Pharmacological interventions

    a)   One of the biggest challenges is getting people who have schizophrenia to take their medications. Creativity is necessary. There are usually multiple problems due to learning difficulties, organizational skills, side effects they do not like, lack of understanding, need to continue therapy when they feel better, or stigmatization

    b)   First generation antipsychotic agents for positive symptoms[16]

        i.   Haloperidol

        ii.   Chlorpromazine

        iii.   Perphenazine

        iv.   Fluphenazine

    c)   First generation antipsychotic agent side effects[16]

        i.   Rigidity

        ii.   Persistent muscle spasms

        iii.   Tremors

        iv.   Restlessness

        v.   Tardive dyskinesis—involuntary movements, especially of tongue, lips, and mouth

    d)   Second generation antipsychotic agents for negative symptoms[16]

        i.   Risperidone

        ii.   Olanzapine

        iii.   Quetiapine

        iv.   Ziprasidone

        v.   Aripiprazole

        vi.   Paliperidone

        vii.   Clozapine

    e)   Second generation antipsychotic agent side effects[16]

        i.   Weight gain (monitor weight, glucose levels, and lipid levels)

        ii.   Clozapine has been known to cause agranulocytosis. Check white blood cell (WBC) count every week

III. Bipolar and Related Disorders

A. Definition[14]

    1.   According to the DSM-5,[14] bipolar disorders consist of

        a)   Manic episodes

            i.   Extended periods of excessively happy or exuberant moods, often leading to extreme irritability

            ii.   May participate in inappropriate and risky behaviors such as rapid speech, flight of ideas, restlessness, impulsivity, insomnia, and unrealistic beliefs in their abilities

b) Hypomanic episodes

    i.   Similar symptoms to mania but to a lesser degree

    ii.   More apt to maintain productivity in hypomanic state

    iii. Hypomania that is not treated can progress into full mania or depression

c) Depressive episodes

    i.   Prolonged periods of overwhelming sadness or hopelessness with a loss of interest in nearly all previously enjoyed activities

    ii.   Many depressive symptoms overlap with common complaints in serious illness and at the end of life such as extreme fatigue, restlessness, changes in sleeping and eating patterns, and poor concentration and memory

d) Mixed episode

    i.   Manic and depressive symptoms occur simultaneously. Persons experiencing a mixed episode will demonstrate profound sadness and hopelessness while also feeling extremely energetic[14]

2. Chronic and potentially severe mental disorders affecting mood, energy levels, and activity

3. Symptoms usually occur intermittently throughout one's lifetime

4. Can also experience difficulty with relationships, school, and work

5. Patients can continue to have persistent symptoms despite treatment[14,17]

6. Severe mania or depression can also prompt psychotic symptoms such as hallucinations or delusions making bipolar disorder easily confused with schizophrenia

a) Hallucinations are interpretations of a stimulus that is not present. They can be visual (seeing something that is not present), auditory (hearing voices that are not really there), or tactile (feelings things that are not really there)

b) Delusions are thought perceptions that are misinterpreted as something other than what it is. They are "fixed beliefs" in that the delusional patient cannot be convinced that they are misinterpreting the stimulus[14]

7. Individuals in both manic and depressive phases are at an increased **suicide risk**

a) Nearly one-third of persons with bipolar disorder will attempt suicide, making it one of the worst mental health disorders for suicide risk[18]

b) See "When to Call for Help" at the end of this section for suicidal interventions

8. DSM-5 classifications of bipolar disorders[14]

a) Bipolar disorder I includes

    i.   Manic or mixed episode lasting at least 7 days

    ii.   Severe manic symptoms requiring immediate hospitalization

    iii. With or without psychosis and/or major depression

b)   Bipolar disorder II includes

   i.   At least 1 hypomanic episode with at least 1 major depressive episode and without previous manic or mixed episodes

   ii.   Clustering symptoms cannot be better described by another type of mental disorder (e.g., schizoaffective, unspecified schizophrenia, or psychotic disorder)

c)   Cyclothymia includes

   i.   Frequently displayed symptoms of hypomania and depressive episodes over the course of 2 years without the demonstration of a full manic episode or major depression

d)   Substance-/medication-induced bipolar disorder includes

   i.   The demonstration of "maniclike" symptoms (e.g., high excitability, energy, irritability) as a result of substance use, and which cannot be better described by another psychological condition

e)   Bipolar and related disorder due to another medical condition includes

   i.   The demonstration of "maniclike" symptoms (e.g., high excitability, energy, or irritability) in the presence of an underlying medical condition (e.g., conditions requiring steroid use), and which cannot be described by a better psychological condition

f)   Unspecified bipolar disorder includes

   i.   Behaviors are abnormal but they do not meet criteria for any of the previously described bipolar disorders[14]

B.   Treatment

1.   Bipolar disorder is not curable but can be managed

2.   The presence of additional psychological disorders (e.g., alcoholism) or medical conditions complicates the course of treatment[1]

3.   Nonpharmacological intervention

a)   Communication

   i.   Communicating with patients in manic or depressive episodes can be challenging for nurses

b)   During a manic episode, patients may be excessively talkative and energetic. Nurses should

   i.   Remain calm and not be drawn into a chaotic situation

   ii.   Recognize that it may be difficult for patients to sit still. Allowing them to walk freely will help to expend energy

      (a)   Terminal patients who are not ambulatory might expend energy by doing something repetitive with their hands (e.g., folding small towels repeatedly)

   iii.   Set parameters for the hospitalized patients to protect their safety and the privacy of others[7]

c)   Explain your rationale for the restrictions, rather than merely telling the patient what they can and cannot do. This will convey that you care about their safety

d)   Call the patient by first name to convey that you value them as a person

e)   Monitor family dynamics, which can be strained or dysfunctional[19,20]

4.   Pharmacological interventions

a)   Pharmacological treatment options for bipolar disorder can be complex depending on frequent psychiatric and medical comorbidities, incomplete patient histories, substance abuse, and previous suicide attempts[21]

b)   Commonly used agents include

i.   Mood stabilizers to restore chemical balance affecting emotional states

(a)   Lithium

(i)   Monitor for lithium toxicity, hypothyroidism, or kidney dysfunction[22]

ii.   Antiepileptics also act as mood stabilizers for bipolar mania

(a)   Valproic acid

(b)   Lamotrigine

(c)   Gabapentin

(d)   Oxcarbazepine

(e)   Patients taking antiepileptics to treat bipolar disorder should be monitored for suicidal ideation[22,23]

iii.   Atypical antipsychotics may also be used to treat delirium or psychosis[24]

(a)   Olanzapine

(b)   Aripiprazole

(c)   Quetiapine

(d)   Risperidone

(e)   Ziprasidone

(f)   Patients taking atypical antipsychotics should be monitored for tardive dyskinesia (TD), a condition resulting in uncontrollable muscle movement and muscle spasms around the mouth. This can be serious if the medication is not discontinued right away[22]

iv.   Antidepressants can be prescribed to manage depressive symptoms

(a)   Fluoxetine

(b)   Paroxetine

(c)   Sertraline

(d)   Bupropion[22]

v.   Miscellaneous agents include several drugs that may already be familiar to hospice or palliative patients and are in various stages of investigation for the treatment of bipolar symptoms, including

(a)   Tamoxifen—an antiestrogen agent most commonly used to treat women with receptor positive breast cancer

(b)   Memantine—approved for moderate to severe Alzheimer's disease

(c)   Galantamine—approved for the treatment of mild to moderate dementia in patients with Alzheimer's disease

(d)   Allopurinol—approved to reduce uric acid level in the treatment and prevention of gout[25]

C.   When to Call for Help

1.   Patient exhibits signs of mania (e.g., hyperexcitability, rapid speech, participation in risky behaviors)

2.   Patient demonstrates extreme depression or suicide risk

3.   Patients at greatest risk for suicide include those with

   a)   Rapidly progressing disease

   b)   Uncontrolled symptoms such as intractable pain

   c)   Previous history of mental illness or suicide attempts

4.   To assess for suicide risk, the nurse should question if the patient has

   a)   Thoughts about ending their life

   b)   A plan about how they would end their life

   c)   Access to lethal resources (e.g., gun, pills) to carry out the plan

5.   Patients with a plan, the means, and the resources should be evaluated immediately by a trained mental health professional, hospitalized, and placed under constant surveillance[26]

IV.   Depressive Disorders

A.   Definition[14]

1.   Types of severe depression described by the DSM-5[14]

   a)   Major depressive disorder

      i.   Depression that interferes with the quality of life, including productivity (work or school), eating, and participation in activities previously considered to be pleasurable

      ii.   Often described as "not wanting to get out of bed or move"

      iii.   Can occur as a single occurrence or recurrent episodes

   b)   Dysthymia

      i.   Depression lasting for 2 years or longer

      ii.   May be interspersed with major depressive episodes but the depression is always simmering and never completely goes away

        iii.   Individuals may be able to maintain some level of productivity in work or school but with great effort

   c)   Minor depression

        i.   Exhibits depressive symptoms but not significant enough to qualify as major depression

        ii.   Minor depression can lead to major depression disorder if not treated

   d)   Psychotic depression

        i.   Severe depressive symptoms accompanied by psychosis in the form of hallucinations (hearing or seeing things that are not real) or delusions (having false beliefs)

   e)   Seasonal affective disorder

        i.   The onset of depressive symptoms during months with limited natural sunlight

2.   Prevalence in patients with depression who have a chronic (versus terminal) illness

   a)   Depression is commonly seen in

        i.   Cardiovascular disease—14% to 21% (1 in every 5 patients experience depressive symptoms)[27]

        ii.   Chronic obstructive pulmonary disease—7% to 42%[28]

        iii.   Chronic kidney disease—20%[29]

        iv.   Stroke—30% to 50%[30]

        v.   Cancer—10% to 25%[31]

B.   **Data in other non-cancer diagnoses (e.g., central nervous system [CNS], autoimmune, and endocrine disorders) is widely lacking; nonetheless, depression is a common comorbidity[32]**

1.   Patients with a terminal illness can develop depression after a terminal diagnosis or have a history of depression that can exacerbate in the face of a terminal illness

2.   Depression after a terminal diagnosis

   a)   Many dying patients experience sadness, anticipatory grief, anger, and fear[26]

   b)   Symptoms of depression are often overlooked when they mirror common signs of a terminal illness

        i.   Poor appetite

        ii.   Insomnia

        iii.   Withdrawal[26]

   c)   Contributing factors of depression

        i.   Uncontrolled physical symptoms[33]

            (a)   Pain management

            (b)   Constipation

          (c)   Insomnia

          (d)   Loss of appetite

ii.   Medications associated with increased risk for depression[2]

          (a)   Antihypertensives

          (b)   Analgesics

          (c)   Antiparkinsonian agents

          (d)   Steroids

          (e)   Hypoglycemic

          (f)   Chemotherapy

          (g)   Hormones

          (h)   Antimicrobials

          (i)   L-Dopa

          (j)   Benzodiazepines

          (k)   Alcohol

          (l)   Phenothiazines

          (m)   Amphetamines

          (n)   Cimetidine

iii.   Psychological challenges

          (a)   Previous mental health diagnoses

          (b)   Fear of death

          (c)   Loss of independence

          (d)   Loss of control

          (e)   Changes in body image and deterioration

          (f)   Anticipatory loss (financial and social)[2]

iv.   Lack of social support[2]

d)   Assessment

    i.   Depression is influenced by cultural variables in how it is accepted and managed

    ii.   Allow cultural tendencies among racial and ethnic groups to guide patient care but not dictate stereotypical beliefs of what patients will want[34]

    iii.   Assessment should not only investigate the illness but also distinguish the preferences of the patient based on cultural beliefs, keeping in mind that there can be a wide variation within a culture. For example

          (a)   African-American elders described depression as "a crisis of spirit" signifying the need to address spiritual concerns and/or use spiritual interventions to manage depression[35]

(b)   Others view depression as controllable and the inability to control it is a sign of weakness and lack of self-control. More severe depression indicates greater lack of control, which leads to embarrassment, shame, rejection, and denial[36]

(c)   Traditional Mexican beliefs view mental illness as an imbalance of mind, body, and spirit. Treatment is often kept within the cultural community by healers and family members[36]

(d)   Mental illness is strongly stigmatized among Chinese-Americans and for terminally ill patients and their families, the significance of a history of mental illness might have been minimized for many years. Also, a patient with new onset depression stemming from terminal illness may be resistant to accept the diagnosis of depression[37]

iv.   Listen carefully for the way that patients describe a depressed mood and use the same language when talking about depression

(a)   "Sadness," "nerves," "down in the dumps," "out of sorts"

v.   Ask open-ended questions

(a)   Tell me, how has your mood been lately?

(b)   What does the future look like to you?

(c)   Ask questions about specific situational factors affecting mood (e.g., relationships, finances)

vi.   Assess for and manage comorbid symptoms that could contribute to depression (e.g., pain)[2]

vii.   Continue to monitor for progressive symptoms of more severe anxiety or depression warranting more aggressive interventions[26]

3.   Treatment

a)   Combinations of psychotherapy (counseling), medications, and education can be beneficial but some patients who are terminally ill may not have the energy needed to participate in these therapies[26]

b)   Nonpharmacological interventions

i.   Before starting medications[38]

(a)   Assess previous sources of strength and arrange for patient to have access to them (e.g., personal relationships, faith)

(b)   Ensure that distressing symptoms have been optimally managed

(c)   Review current medications for side effects of depressive symptoms and the possibility of interactions with new medications[2,26]

(d)   Consider the side effect profiles, patient's preferences, and previous experience with drugs before starting new[26]

ii.   Consider the cultural influence in how depression is accepted and expressed[34]

iii.   Facilitate autonomy as often as possible (e.g., offer opportunities for decision-making to patient)

        iv.   Provide the patient with opportunities to process their feelings, concerns, and anticipatory grief by talking about their situation[26,38]

        v.   Reminiscing is beneficial to patients trying to make sense of their lives, illness, and dying

        vi.   Consider the need to consult a mental health professional to evaluate for treatment options[2]

    c)   Pharmacological interventions

        i.   Few studies have examined the use of antidepressants with terminal patients. Most information is anecdotal[26]

        ii.   Side effects of antidepressants may be intolerable to terminally ill patients[26]

        iii.   Antidepressants may not be useful to patients with a less than 1 month life expectancy as drugs could take longer to reach a therapeutic level[39]

        iv.   Antidepressants effect neurotransmitters (i.e., serotonin, norepinephrine, dopamine) and include several classes[22,26]

            (a)   Selective serotonin reuptake inhibitors (SSRIs) may be beneficial to terminal patients by demonstrating a therapeutic response within 1 week

                (i)   Fluoxetine

                (ii)   Sertraline

                (iii)   Escitalopram

                (iv)   Paroxetine

                (v)   Citalopram

            (b)   Serotonin and norepinephrine reuptake inhibitors (SNRIs)

                (i)   Venlafaxine

                (ii)   Duloxetine

            (c)   Tricyclic antidepressants

                (i)   Amitriptyline

                (ii)   Nortriptyline

    d)   When to call for help

        i.   When patient exhibits signs of suicide risk

        ii.   For management of suicidal risk, see "When to Call for Help" under Bipolar Disorder

V. Anxiety Disorders

A. Definitions[14]

    1.   According to the DSM-5, anxiety disorders are those that share features of excessive anxiety and fear with related behavioral disturbances

2. These disorders differ from normal fear and anxiety in their being excessive and persisting beyond developmentally appropriate periods, typically lasting 6 months or more

    a) Separation anxiety—anxiety or fear about separation from an attachment figure

    b) Selective mutism—consistent failure to speak in social situations

    c) Social anxiety—fear or anxiety about social interactions or situations

    d) Panic disorder—recurrent panic attacks

    e) Phobias—fear of a specific object or situation

    f) Generalized anxiety disorder—persistent or excessive anxiety and worry about various domains

B. Treatment

1. Nonpharmacological interventions

    a) Establish a trusting relationship

    b) Be aware of any anxiety that you as a nurse may have that may be picked up on

    c) Do not leave a person experiencing an anxiety disorder exacerbation alone

    d) Maintain a calm, nonthreatening, manner-of-fact approach

    e) Keep stimuli minimized

    f) Use simple words and brief messages that are calmly and clearly explained

    g) Discuss the reality of the situation

    h) Include person on decision-making to feel more in control

    i) Encourage exploration of underlying feelings that contribute to irrational fears

    j) Teach and reinforce stress management/relaxation techniques

2. Pharmacological interventions[40,41]

    a) Antianxiety drugs are called anxiolytics

    b) Actions include depressing subcortical levels of the central nervous system (CNS)

    c) Potentiates the neurotransmitter gamma-aminobutyric acid (GABA)

    d) Buspirone is the only anxiolytic that does not depress the CNS

    e) Use caution with the elderly due to decreased hepatic or renal function

    f) Contraindicated in pregnancy, narrow-angle glaucoma, shock, and coma

    g) Decreased effects with smoking and caffeine

    h) Potentiated (increased) with kava root, valerian, alcohol, barbiturates, narcotics, antipsychotics, antidepressants, antihistamines, neuromuscular blocking agents, cimetidine, or disulfiram

    i) Anxiolytics

        i. Antihistamines

            (a) Hydroxyzine

      ii.   Benzodiazepines

          (a)   Alprazolam

          (b)   Chlordiazepoxide

          (c)   Clonazepam

          (d)   Clorazepate

          (e)   Diazepam

          (f)   Lorazepam

          (g)   Oxazepam

      iii. Carbamate derivative

          (a)   Meprobamate

      iv. Azaspirodecanedione

          (a)   Buspirone

j)   Side effects of anxiolytics

      i.   Drowsiness, confusion, lethargy

      ii.   Tolerance

      iii. Orthostatic hypotension

      iv. Dry mouth

      v.   Nausea and vomiting

      vi. Blood dyscrasias

      vii. Delayed onset of effect (10–14 days) with buspirone

k)   Medications for specific disorders

      i.   Panic and generalized anxiety disorder

          (a)   Anxiolytics

          (b)   Antidepressants

          (c)   Antihypertensive agents

              (i)   Beta-blockers

              (ii) Alpha-2 receptor agonists

      ii.   Phobic disorders

          (a)   Anxiolytics

          (b)   Antidepressants

          (c)   Antihypertensive agents

VI. Obsessive-Compulsive Disorders

A. Definition[14]

1. According the DSM-5, obsessive-compulsive disorders differ from preoccupations and rituals by being excessive and beyond the developmentally-appropriate periods[14]

   a) Obsessions are repetitive and persistent thoughts or urges that are not pleasurable or experienced as voluntary and may cause distress or anxiety

   b) Compulsions are performed in response to obsessions, and the aim is to reduce distress or anxiety

2. Disorders in this section include obsessive-compulsive disorder, body dysmorphic disorder, hoarding disorder, trichotillomania, and excoriation

   a) Obsessive-compulsive disorder may vary among individuals, but certain symptoms are common such as cleaning, symmetry (repetitive ordering and counting compulsions), forbidden or taboo (religion or sexual), and harm (fear of harm to oneself or others)

   b) Body dysmorphic disorder is characterized by a preoccupation with perceived defects or flaws in physical appearance and repetitive behavior such as checking mirrors, grooming, skin picking, or seeking reassurance

   c) Hoarding disorder is characterized by a persistent difficulty in parting with possessions to the point of excess

   d) Trichotillomania is characterized by a repetitive pulling out of one's hair, eyebrows, or eyelashes, resulting in hair loss

   e) Excoriation is characterized by a repetitive picking of one's skin resulting in lesions

B. Treatment

1. Nonpharmacological

   a) Establish a trusting relationship

   b) Understand the underlying theme of the obsessive-compulsive behavior (e.g., contamination by germs, having things orderly or symmetrical)

   c) Be aware of your behavior that may create issues in patient and/or family (e.g., washing your hands and using hand sanitizer and asking permission before using or moving any personal items in the home)

   d) Do not leave a person experiencing an exacerbation alone

   e) Maintain a calm, nonthreatening matter-of-fact approach

   f) Keep stimuli minimized

   g) Do not be judgmental or verbalize disapproval of their behavior

   h) Support efforts toward exploration of meaning and purpose of behavior

   i) Assist in identifying types of situations that trigger behavior

   j) Assist with learning of how to interrupt obsessive thoughts or ritualistic behavior

   k) If possible, gradually limit amount of time for ritualistic behavior

2.   Consultation—work with interdisciplinary team about consulting a psychologist, psychiatrist, or psychiatric nurse practitioner for individual psychotherapy, cognitive therapy, or behavior therapy when symptoms cannot be controlled with nonpharmacological or pharmacological methods

3.   Psychopharmacology

    a)   Obsessive-compulsive disorder

        i.   Antidepressants

    b)   Body dysmorphic disorder

        i.   Antidepressants

    c)   Trichotillomania[42,43]

        i.   Chlorpromazine

        ii.   Amitriptyline

        iii.   Lithium carbonate

        iv.   SSRIs

        v.   Olanzapine

    d)   Excoriation[44]

        i.   Fluvoxamine

VII. Trauma and Stressor-Related Disorders

A.   Definition[14]

1.   According to the DSM-5, trauma and stressor-related disorders occur as the direct result of exposure to traumatic or stressful events[14]

2.   Traumatic or stressful events can be the terminal diagnosis itself, or from other life stressors that occurred at various times and in various situations

3.   This section focuses on 2 traumatic events that can complicate the dying process for patients and families, patients with a history of involvement with abusive relationships or events, and patients experiencing posttraumatic stress disorder (PTSD)

B.   Involvement in Abusive Relationships or Events

1.   The incidence of abuse is thought to be under reported and, therefore, unknown. However, scenarios for abuse to occur are numerous, increasing the possibility that nurses will care for patients with these histories

    a)   Chronically- and terminally-ill persons can be affected by histories of abuse as victims, perpetrators, or witnesses to violence

    b)   Incidents of abuse can occur during childhood, adolescence, and/or adulthood

    c)   Individuals can be involved in one type of abuse with one relationship, several types of abuse within one relationship, or multiple abuses within multiple relationships

d) Patients can have abusive encounters as part of their past or currently be involved in an ongoing abusive relationship

e) Remote memories of abuse or neglect can resurface at the end of life, causing distress to the patient searching for meaning and life closure

f) Nurses must be alert for clues that patients are affected by past or present episodes of violence (e.g., recoiling from a touch, reacting out of proportion to an examination or a procedure [catheterization, perineal care], uncomfortable around men/women)

2. Specific types of violence described by the Centers for Disease Control and Prevention include[45]

a) Child abuse defined as, "Any recent act or failure to act on the part of a parent or caretaker which results in death, serious physical or emotional harm, sexual abuse or exploitation"

b) Child neglect defined as "An action or failure to act which presents an imminent risk of serious harm"

c) Elder abuse—"any abuse and neglect of persons age 60 and older by a caregiver or another person in a relationship involving an expectation of trust."[46] Forms of abuse include physical, sexual, psychological, emotional, financial, neglect, or abandonment

d) Intimate partner violence—"describes physical, sexual, or psychological harm by a current or former partner or spouse. This type of violence can occur among heterosexual or same-sex couples and does not require sexual intimacy"[47]

e) "Sexual violence (SV) is any sexual act that is perpetrated against someone's will. SV encompasses a range of offenses, including a completed nonconsensual sex act (i.e., rape), an attempted nonconsensual sex act, abusive sexual contact (i.e., unwanted touching), and non-contact sexual abuse (e.g., threatened sexual violence, exhibitionism, verbal sexual harassment)"[48]

3. For this discussion, "participants of abuse" refers to aggressors, recipients, witnesses, or any combination of participation. Each point of view can be wrought with unique difficulties at the end of life

4. Challenges to end-of-life care[49]

a) Though life reviews are common at the end of life, they should be used cautiously if prior or current abuse is known or suspected as they may open psychic wounds from previous abuse

b) Physical examinations can be considered intrusive for persons with a history of abuse, particularly in histories of sexual abuse

c) Recipients of abuse may experience helplessness from the physical deterioration of advanced disease, which mirrors the helplessness experienced during violent episodes

d) Patients may be fearful if the aggressor is also the primary caregiver

   i. Patients who do not divulge their history of abuse with hospice caregivers cannot be supported or assisted by the healthcare team and will suffer in silence if the hospice team is not observant to their distress

e) Some participants of abuse (whether aggressors, recipients, or witnesses of abuse) may choose to disclose the abuse for the first time as they approach death in an attempt to achieve life closure

f)   Patients who elect to disclose or process abuse may receive resistance from other family members who prefer to deny or minimize the abuse

g)   In general, negative family dynamics can compromise the support needed for persons at the end of life

5.   Assessment

a)   Identifying patients who may have a history of abuse involvement is difficult

b)   Family relationships involving abuse can be complicated as each party may have a different interpretation of the events[49]

c)   Symptoms associated with this type of stressor are similar to other sources of stress (e.g., anxiety, depression, insomnia, withdrawal) that the patient may be experiencing with advanced disease[49]

d)   Nurses who suspect a history of abuse should ask the patient while in a private and safe setting. Do not approach the topic while others are around and assure confidentiality

   i.   Explain to the patient which situations you are required to report to legal authorities depending on the individual state's law

   ii.   For example, most states require reports of abuse, neglect, or homicidal threats

e)   Patients may be reluctant to discuss the abuse with members of the hospice team due to guilt, shame, and self-blame[49]

f)   Respect their decision but be sure to give them permission to talk to you should they change their mind[49]

g)   Explain that they are not alone and many people have had similar situations. Tell them they will not be judged for what has happened

h)   Some patients might not associate what happened to them as "abuse." Listen closely to what they say and the words they use to describe the negative behaviors

   i.   Recipients of abuse are often told that the aggressive behaviors are a symbol of the "love" the aggressor has for them[49]

i)   If the patient describes something that sounds like they might be a recipient of abuse, try to determine if the aggression is ongoing and if they are currently in danger of harm

   i.   If the abuse is ongoing, the nurse must know his/her state's laws for reporting abuse

   ii.   For more information about individual state's requirement see www.childwelfare.gov/systemwide/laws_policies/state/

   iii. Seek assistance from the team social worker and supervisor to assure that the patient is removed from any risk of imminent danger and that legal responsibilities are carried out

6.   Treatment

a)   Nonpharmacological interventions

   i.   Recent research is lacking that explains how having previous experiences with abusive situations affect the dying process

ii. The evidence that currently exists is limited and dated

iii. Communicating with patients who want to discuss the abuse

    (a) Create a safe, nonjudgmental environment for the patient to disclose to the team member

    (b) Validate the importance of the abuse

    (c) Provide reassurance

    (d) Protect the patient's autonomy as this is something that might have been compromised in the past

    (e) Ask the patient for permission to involve the social worker or chaplain. Find out who they would prefer to talk to

    (f) The team may need to support the patient around other family members who deny the significance of the event[49]

iv. Take a team approach

    (a) Meeting several team members allows patients to select with whom they are more comfortable confiding

    (b) The team can also support each other as these family dynamics are often challenging

        (i) Stories of abuse can be difficult for nurses to hear, but nurses must remain nonjudgmental and supportive for the patient and family

    (c) Team members should

        (i) Discuss family dynamics at team meetings to assemble the most comprehensive view of how these stories are revealed, processed, and played out

        (ii) Remain aware of how these situations make them feel and strive to maintain a neutral stance throughout encounters

        (iii) Be diligent not to insinuate a particular point of view or make judgmental statements about other family members involved in the abusive dynamic

        (iv) Be careful not to make positive or negative statements about family members that could be construed as taking sides by the other family members

        (v) Remember that each family member may have a different interpretation of the abusive events and team members must not make judgments about the roles family members play

        (vi) Be realistic with the patient's ability to resolve the stress associated with the abuse. For some, resolving the occurrence and effects can take years, which the patient may not have[49]

    (d) Ongoing aggression

        (i) If the abusive relationship is ongoing, the team must take the appropriate steps to ensure that the patient is safe and protected

    (e) Patients with histories of abuse can suffer anxiety and/or depression

        b)   Pharmacological interventions

            i.   Prescribing appropriate medications to treat these conditions should be initiated as needed

            ii.   See sections on anxiety and depression for additional information about pharmacological interventions

        c)   When to call for help

            i.   With evidence of severe depression or suicide risk

                (a)   For management of suicidal risk, see "When to Call for Help" under Bipolar Disorder

            ii.   With evidence of ongoing physical abuse or neglect or if the patient's safety is in jeopardy

            iii.   With reports of the abuse of a minor or elder and which falls within the reporting requirements for the individual state

C.   Posttraumatic Stress Disorder (PTSD)[14]

1.   A disorder associated with exposure to serious threat of death, injury, or sexual violence in one of several ways

        a)   Experiencing trauma as a single or repeated event (e.g., first responder, combat Veteran)

        b)   Witnessing trauma

        c)   Often occurs with comorbid psychiatric disorders (e.g., anxiety, depression, substance abuse)

        d)   Learning about trauma involving a close friend or family member

2.   Symptomatology of one or more of the following include

        a)   Recurrent, involuntary, and intrusive memories causing distress

        b)   Recurrent dreams that are distressing

        c)   Flashbacks of the traumatic event

        d)   Ongoing psychological distress or guilt

        e)   Avoidance of stressors or reminders associated with the trauma

        f)   Descriptions of feeling "numb"

        g)   Hyperexcitability (e.g., volatile, jumpy, edgy)

3.   The presence of symptoms can greatly influence the quality of life at the end of life

4.   Terminally-ill patients can develop new-onset PTSD from the trauma of their diagnosis or suffer from the exacerbation of symptoms of previous incidents of PTSD

5.   Assessment

        a)   Ask about a prior history of exposure to trauma or PTSD

            i.   Symptoms of PTSD can be exacerbated at the end of life

        b)   Monitor sleep and nutritional patterns[50]

6. Treatment

    a) Nonpharmacological interventions

        i. Treatment can be extremely complex. Refer patients for psychiatric consult with signs of exacerbated or severe symptoms of PTSD

            (a) Individual or group psychotherapy has been successful for the management of PTSD

            (b) Limited life expectancy warrants managing those symptoms most troublesome to the patient

        ii. Family dynamics may be strained[50]

    b) Pharmacological interventions

        i. Antidepressants approved for the treatment of PTSD

            (a) Sertraline

            (b) Paroxetine

        ii. Benzodiazepines for sleep, anxiety, and hyperexcitability symptoms

        iii. Antiepileptics (mood stabilizers) to treat irritability, hyperarousal, and impulsivity

            (a) Valproate

            (b) Carbamazepine

            (c) Gabapentin[50]

    c) When to call for help

        i. With exacerbations of distressful symptoms

        ii. With patient report of suicide risk

        iii. For management of suicidal risk, see "When to Call for Help" under Bipolar Disorder

VIII. Personality Disorders

A. Definition[14]

1. According to the DSM-5, personality disorder is a continuous pattern of inner experience and behavior that deviates from cultural and social norms, and is pervasive and inflexible[14]

2. The onset is usually in adolescence or early adulthood

3. Predictors of aggressive behavior[12]

    a) Impulsivity

    b) Hostility

    c) Family history of abusive or violent behavior

    d) Substance use

    e) Irritability

4.   The disorder manifests in 2 or more of the following areas

    a)   Cognition (i.e., ways of perceiving and interpreting self, other people, and events)

    b)   Affectivity (emotional response)

    c)   Interpersonal functioning

    d)   Impulse control

B.   Personality Disorder

1.   Cluster A—odd or eccentric

    a)   Paranoid—has a pattern of distrust and suspiciousness

    b)   Schizoid—has a pattern of detachment from social relationships with restricted range of emotional expression

    c)   Schizotypal—has a pattern of acute discomfort in close relationships, cognition or perceptual distortions, and eccentric behavior

2.   Cluster B—dramatic, emotional, erratic

    a)   Antisocial—has a pattern of disregard for and violence against the rights of others

    b)   Borderline—has a pattern of instability in relationships, self-image, affect, and marked impulsivity

    c)   Histrionic—has a pattern of excessive emotionality and attention-seeking

    d)   Narcissistic—has a pattern of grandiosity, need for admiration, and lack of empathy

3.   Cluster C—anxious and fearful

    a)   Avoidant—has a pattern of social inhibition, feelings of inadequacy, and hypersensitivity to negative comments/evaluation

    b)   Dependent—has a pattern of submissive and clinging behavior related to an excessive need to be taken care of

    c)   Obsessive-compulsive—has a pattern of preoccupation with orderliness, perfectionism, and control

C.   Nonpharmacological Interventions[12]

1.   Observe behavior and establish a trusting relationship by showing interest and empathy

2.   Focus on monitoring appropriate levels of concern and the boundaries of a therapeutic relationship

3.   Observe in order to prevent harm to self and others

    a)   Persons with borderline disorders are prone to self-mutilation or suicide

    b)   Persons with antisocial disorders are prone to violence against others

4.   Secure verbal or written contracts against violence to self or others

5.   Role model appropriate expression of feelings

6.   Encourage communications about feelings

7. Increase team communication and consistency to prevent splitting (an attempt on the part of one person to make another, third individual, look wrong, bad, guilty)

8. Identify cues or triggers to assist with notification for assistance

9. Remove dangerous objects

10. Redirect unacceptable behaviors into acceptable outlets such as exercise or meditation

11. Provide a structured environment

12. Have sufficient number of staff when needed

13. Explore with the person the true source of emotions

14. Explain the behaviors associated with the normal grieving process

15. Encourage recognition of maladaptive behaviors such as splitting, clinging, distancing, etc.

16. Maintain a low level of stimuli in the environment when possible

17. Explore alternative ways of handling frustrations

18. Remain calm

19. Provide positive feedback for acceptable behavior

20. Whenever conversing, maintain attitude of "it is not you, but your behavior that is unacceptable"

21. Focus on strengths

22. Encourage journal writing

23. Restrain only as a last resort

24. Consult with the interdisciplinary team about resources for psychotherapy, group therapy, cognitive-behavior therapy, or anger management training as needed

D. Pharmacological Interventions

1. Cluster A disorders who show psychotic symptoms may respond to antipsychotics

2. Cluster B disorders may benefit from mood-stabilizing or second generation antipsychotics alone or with antidepressants

3. Cluster C may benefit from serotonergic antidepressants

IX. Substance-Related Disorders

A. Definition[14]

1. According to the DSM-5, any drug class taken in excess that then activates the brain's reward system producing a pleasurable sensation that reinforces behavior and produces memories[14]

2. The drug produces such an intense activation of the reward system that the person neglects normal activities

3. Predisposition factors to substance abuse are lower levels of self-control, genetics, low self-esteem, depression, punitive superego, social learning from peers or family, conditioning, or antisocial personality

4. While abuse, misuse, and diversion must always be considered, it should not generate fear in the palliative care team, which leads to undertreatment of pain

5. Psychiatric diagnoses associated with this disorder

   a) Psychosis

   b) Bipolar

   c) Depression

   d) Anxiety

   e) Obsessive-compulsive disorder (OCD)

   f) Sleep disorders

   g) Sexual disorders

   h) Delirium

   i) Neurocognitive disorders

6. The 10 classes of drugs with the most abuse

   a) Alcohol

   b) Caffeine

   c) Cannabis

   d) Hallucinogens

   e) Inhalants

   f) Opioids

   g) Sedatives

   h) Hypnotics

   i) Anxiolytics

   j) Stimulants

   k) Tobacco

   l) Bath salts

B. Substance Use Disorder (Addiction)[14]

1. Use of the substance interferes with activities of daily living and relationships

2. Craving for the substance consumes an excessive amount of time

3. Use of the substance interferes with judgment and the person continues to use it even knowing this fact

4. Tolerance develops, thus the amount of substance required to achieve the desired effect continues to increase

C.   Substance-Induced Disorder (Intoxication and Withdrawal)[14]

1.   Substance intoxication is the excessive use of a substance followed by a reversible syndrome of symptoms that is substance specific. There is direct effect on the central nervous system with impairment of physical functioning, impaired judgment, maladaptive behavior, and impaired social functioning

2.   Substance withdrawal occurs with abrupt reduction or discontinuance of a substance that has been used regularly for a prolonged time. The syndrome of symptoms is substance specific. There are physical, thinking, feeling, and behavioral changes

3.   See Table 6-1 for a summary of withdrawal and intoxication symptoms

Table 6-1. Summary of Symptoms Associated with the Syndromes of Intoxication and Withdrawal

Class of Drugs	Intoxication	Withdrawal	Comments
Alcohol	Aggressiveness, impaired judgment, impaired attention, irritability, euphoria, depression, emotional lability, slurred speech, incoordination, unsteady gait, nystagmus, flushed face	Tremors, nausea/vomiting, malaise, weakness, tachycardia, sweating, elevated blood pressure, anxiety, depressed mood, irritability, hallucinations, headache, insomnia, seizures	Alcohol withdrawal begins within 4–6 hours after last drink. May progress to delirium tremens on 2nd or 3rd day. Use of chlordiazepoxide or oxazepam is common for substitution therapy
Amphetamines and related substances	Fighting, grandiosity, hypervigilance, psychomotor agitation, impaired judgment, tachycardia, pupillary dilation, elevated blood pressure, perspiration or chills, nausea, and vomiting	Anxiety, depressed mood, irritability, craving for the substance, fatigue, insomnia or hypersomnia, psychomotor agitation, paranoid, and suicidal ideation	Withdrawal symptoms usually peak within 2–4 days, although depression and irritability may persist for months. Antidepressants may be used
Caffeine	Restlessness, nervousness, excitement, insomnia, flushed face, diuresis, gastrointestinal complaints, muscle twitching, rambling flow of thought and speech, cardiac arrhythmia, periods of inexhaustibility, psychomotor agitation	Headache	Caffeine is contained in coffee, tea, colas, cocoa, chocolate, energy drinks, some over-the-counter analgesics, "cold" preparations, and stimulants
Cannabis	Euphoria, anxiety, suspiciousness, sensation of slowed time, impaired judgment, social withdrawal, tachycardia, conjunctival redness, increased appetite, hallucinations	Restlessness, irritability, insomnia, loss of appetite, depressed mood, tremors, fever, chills, headache, stomach pain	Intoxication occurs immediately and lasts 3 hours. Oral ingestion is more slowly absorbed and has longer lasting effects

(continued)

Table 6-1. Summary of Symptoms Associated with the Syndromes of Intoxication and Withdrawal *(continued)*

Class of Drugs	Intoxication	Withdrawal	Comments
Cocaine	Euphoria, fighting, grandiosity, hypervigilance, psychomotor agitation, impaired judgment, tachycardia, elevated blood pressure, pupillary dilation, perspiration or chills, nausea/vomiting, hallucinations, delirium	Depression, anxiety, irritability, fatigue, insomnia or hypersomnia, psychomotor agitation, paranoid or suicidal ideation, apathy, social withdrawal	Large doses of the drug can result in convulsions or death from cardiac arrhythmias or respiratory paralysis
Inhalants	Belligerence, assaultive, apathy, impaired judgment, dizziness, nystagmus, slurred speech, unsteady gait, lethargy, depressed reflexes, tremor, blurred vision, stupor or coma, euphoria, irritation around eyes, throat, and nose		Intoxication occurs within 5 minutes of inhalation. Symptoms last 60–90 minutes. Large doses can result in death from CNS depression or cardiac arrhythmia
Nicotine		Craving for the drug, irritability, anger, frustration, anxiety, difficulty concentrating, restlessness, decreased heart rate, increased appetite, weight gain, tremor, headaches, insomnia	Symptoms of withdrawal begin within 24 hours of last drug use and decrease in intensity over days, weeks, or sometimes longer
Opioids	Euphoria, lethargy, somnolence, apathy, dysphoria, impaired judgment, pupillary constriction, drowsiness, slurred speech, constipation, nausea, decreased respiratory rate and blood pressure	Craving for the drug, nausea/vomiting, muscle aches, lacrimation or rhinorrhea, pupillary dilation, piloerection or sweating, diarrhea, yawning, fever, insomnia	Withdrawal symptoms appear within 6–8 hours after last dose, reach a peak in the 2nd or 3rd day, and subside in 5–10 days. Times are shorter with meperidine and longer with methadone
Phencyclidine and related substances	Belligerence, assaultive, impulsiveness, psychomotor agitation, impaired judgment, nystagmus, increased heart rate and blood pressure, diminished pain response, ataxia, dysarthria, muscle rigidity, seizures, hyperacusis, delirium		Delirium can occur within 24 hours after use of phencyclidine, or may occur up to a week following recovery from an overdose of the drug

Table 6-1. Summary of Symptoms Associated with the Syndromes of Intoxication and Withdrawal *(continued)*

Class of Drugs	Intoxication	Withdrawal	Comments
Sedatives, hypnotics, and anxiolytics	Disinhibition of sexual or aggressive impulses, mood lability, impaired judgment, slurred speech, incoordination, unsteady gait, impairment in attention or memory disorientation, confusion	Nausea/vomiting, malaise, weakness, tachycardia, sweating, anxiety, irritability, orthostatic hypotension, tremor, insomnia seizures	Withdrawal may progress to delirium, usually within 1 week of last use. Long-acting barbiturates or benzodiazepines may be used in withdrawal substitution therapy

D.   Treatment

1.   Nonpharmacological

a)   Multidisciplinary approach—employs the expertise of the entire team, in addition to consultants, in management of not just a patient problem, but also a family problem. Maintain communication lines to prevent splitting of the team by the patient and/or family. Be careful of countertransference reactions to the patient/family by the team (objectivity is impaired; the care providers are emotionally entangled with the patient and/or family). Assess and address the patient and/or family's behavior with medications, and do not be afraid to address addiction[13]

b)   Assess substance use. Utilizing the principles of therapeutic communication find out what substance or substances have been used, how long, how much, how long since the last use. Explain in nonjudgmental terms that this is knowledge that is necessary so that their pain can be adequately treated. Find out how the substance(s) have been helpful to the patient. Find out how the patient handles stress, sleep problems, and anger. Do not forget to ask about caffeine and nicotine, which also impact care. Find out if the patient has been through rehabilitation, who the professionals were that worked with the patient, and what treatments have helped in the past[51]

c)   Assess psychiatric history. Find out if patient is taking medications for illness, any episodes of violence to self or others, name of mental agency or professionals that have been working with the patient, and length of time since last appointment. Find out what treatments have helped in the past

d)   Recognize and document specific drug abuse behaviors and communicate with the team

e)   Use a written agreement to control drug usage and treat pain. The agreement should contain expectations of patient behavior, roles of the different team members, risks and benefits of the proposed medications, consequences of behavior, use of only 1 pharmacy for obtaining medications, routine pill counts, consequences of lost or stolen medications, random urine testing for drugs, rationale for these procedures and policies, and signed consent for this agreement[13,41,51]

f)   Assess using standardized risk assessment tools such as the CAGE questionnaire for alcohol use and the TADD or TADD-5 for alcohol or drug use. Sensitive to the situation

i.   There are many other risk assessment tools available

ii. Risk assessment tools are used as part of an assessment continuum that begins with a concern about use and/or abuse, then screening assessment, and then formal assessment and a plan for intervention. This should always be done as part of interdisciplinary and collaborative team care

iii. When using these risk assessment tools, be mindful of the goals of care and the patient's place on the disease trajectory

iv. Also be mindful that these tools are for clinical decision-making and are not diagnostic tools

v. If using a risk assessment tool, assure the patient and family that no answers will negatively influence effective pain and symptom management[13]

g) Use adjuvants such as relaxation therapy, distraction, biofeedback, and journals when possible

h) Use the 12-step approach and participation in a program, if possible

i) Frequent family meetings to keep everyone on board with goals of treatment and troubleshoot problems before they become issues. Use meetings to identify family members who may be alcohol or drug users or enablers to the patient

j) If opioid medications are necessary, utilize lock boxes, or daily delivery of medications in small amounts

k) Random urine toxicology screens

l) Set realistic goals in plan of care

m) Consult with psychiatric personnel for issues that cannot be controlled

2. Pharmacological treatments[13]

a) Choose an around-the-clock dosing opioid that is long acting. If given in sufficient amounts, they can minimize break-through use, lessen cravings, and decrease the risk of abuse

b) Provide only limited amounts of break-through medication that is counted at each visit

c) Use nonopioid adjuvants when possible, and then monitor compliance

d) If continue to have issues, consult with psychiatric personnel who can assist with additional substance abuse issues

e) Assess aberrant drug-seeking behaviors that may be indicative of unrelieved pain

f) If using methadone, be aware that it impedes withdrawal for longer periods than it relieves pain

g) Methylphenidate is being studied as a method to improve self-control and manage cravings in cocaine addiction[52]

h) Tiagabine or carbamazepine can be used to treat alcohol withdrawal, anxiety, and cocaine craving

CITED REFERENCES

1. Woods A, Willison K, Kington C, Gavin A. Palliative care for people with severe persistent mental illness: a review of the literature. *Can J Psychiatry*. 2008;53(11):725-736.

2. Hultman T, Reder EA, Dahlin CM. Improving psychological and psychiatric aspects of palliative care: the National Consensus Project and the National Quality Forum Preferred Practices for Palliative and Hospice Care. *Omega (Westport)*. 2008;57(4):323-339.

3. Hospice and Palliative Nurses Association. *Hospice and Palliative Nurses Association 2015–2018 Research Agenda*. Pittsburgh, PA: HPNA; 2015. hpna.advancingexpertcare.org/wp-content/uploads/2014/11/2015-2018-HPNA-Research-Agenda.pdf. Accessed January 5, 2015.

4. Academy of Psychosomatic Medicine (APM). *Psychiatric Aspects of Excellent End-of-Life Care* [Position Statement] 2014. www.apm.org/papers/eol-care.shtml. Accessed September 23, 2014.

5. Laursen TM. Life expectancy among persons with schizophrenia or bipolar affective disorder. *Schizophr Res*. 2011;131(1-3):101-104. doi: 10.1016/j.schres.2011.06.008. Epub July 7, 2011.

6. Sweers K, Dierckx de Casterlé B, Detraux J, De Hert M. End-of-life (care) perspectives and expectations of patients with schizophrenia. *Arch Psychiatr Nurs*. 2013;27(5):246-252. doi: 10.1016/j.apnu.2013.05.003. Epub June 10, 2013.

7. McCasland LA. Providing hospice and palliative care to the seriously and persistently mentally ill. *J Hosp Palliat Nurs*. 2007;9(6):305-313. doi: 10.1097/01.NJH.0000299313.99514.0c.

8. Melamed Y, Kimchi R, Barak Y. Guardianship for the severely mentally ill. *Med Law*. 2000;19(2):321-326.

9. Piatt E, Munetz MR, Ritter C. An examination of premature mortality among decedents with serious mental illness and those in the general population. *Psychiatr Serv*. 2010;61(7):663-668. doi: 10.1176/appi.ps.61.7.663.

10. Foti ME, Okun SN, Wogrin C, Corbeil YJ. *End-of-Life Care for Persons with Serious Mental Illness: The Curriculum for Mental Health Providers. Promoting Excellence in End-of-Life Care*. September 2003. www.promotingexcellence.org/downloads/mass/Curriculum_%20for_%20Mental_Health_Providers.pdf. Accessed October 13, 2014.

11. Billings JA, Block SD. Integrating psychiatry and palliative medicine: the challenges and opportunities. In: Chochinov HM, Breitbart W, eds. *Handbook of Psychiatry in Palliative Medicine*. 2nd ed. New York, NY: Oxford University Press; 2009:13-19.

12. Morgan B. End-of-life care for patients with mental illness and personality disorders. In: Ferrell BR, Coyle N, eds. *Oxford Textbook of Palliative Nursing*. 3rd ed. New York, NY: Oxford University Press; 2010:757-766.

13. Kirsh K, Compton P, Passik SD. Caring for the drug-addicted patient at the end of life. In: Ferrell BR, Coyle N, eds. *Oxford Textbook of Palliative Nursing*. 3rd ed. New York, NY: Oxford University Press; 2010:817-828.

14. American Psychological Association. *Diagnostic and Statistical Manual of Mental Disorders*. 5th ed. Washington, DC: American Psychiatric Publishing; 2013.

15. Goghari VM, Harrow M, Grossman LS, Rosen C. A 20-year multi-follow-up of hallucinations in schizophrenia, other psychotic, and mood disorders. *Psychol Med*. 2013;43(6):1151-1160. doi: 10.1017/S0033291712002206.

16. U.S. Department of Health and Human Services. Agency for Healthcare Research and Quality. *First-Generation Versus Second-Generation Antipsychotics in Adults: Comparative Effectiveness*. Agency for Healthcare Research and Quality; Comparative Effectiveness Review; No. 63.2013. www.ncbi.nlm.nih.gov/pubmedhealth/PMH0049182/pdf/TOC.pdf. Accessed September 22, 2014.

17. National Institutes of Mental Health (NIMH). *Bipolar Disorder*. 2013. www.nimh.nih.gov/health/topics/bipolar-disorder/index.shtml. Accessed October 13, 2014.

18. Cassidy F. Risk factors of attempted suicide in bipolar disorder. *Suicide Life Threat Behav*. 2011;41(1):6-11. doi: 10.1111/j.1943-278X.2010.00007.x. Epub January 24, 2011.

19. Proudfoot J, Doran J, Manicavasaqar V, Parker G. The precipitants of manic/hypomanic episodes in the context of bipolar disorder: a review. *J Affect Disord*. 2011;133(3):381–387. doi: 10.1016/j.jad.2010.10.051. Epub November 23, 2010.

20. Fusar-Poli P, Howes O, Bechdolf A, Borqwardt S. Mapping vulnerability to bipolar disorder: a systematic review and meta-analysis of neuroimaging studies. *J Psychiatry Neurosci*. 2012;37(3): 170-184. doi: 10.1503/jpn.110061.

21. Musetti L, Del Grande C, Marazziti D, Dell'Osso L. Treatment of bipolar depression. *CNS Spectr*. 2013;18(4):177-187. doi: 10.1017/S1092852912001009. Epub February 8, 2013.

22. Skidmore-Roth L. *Mosby's Drug Guide for Nursing Students*. 10th ed. St. Louis, MO: Elsevier; 2013.

23. Vieta E. Valenti M. Pharmacological management of bipolar depression: acute treatment, maintenance, and prophylaxis. *CNS Drugs*. 2013;27(7):515-529. doi: 10.1007/s40263-013-0073-y.

24. Breitbart W, Lawlor P, Friedlander M. Delirium in the Terminally Ill. In: Chochinov HM, Breitbart W, eds. *Handbook of Psychiatry in Palliative Medicine*. 2nd ed. New York, NY: Oxford University Press; 2009: 81-100.

25. Mathews DC, Henter ID, Zarate CA, Jr. New drug developments for bipolar mania. *Psychiatric Times*. December 12, 2012. www.psychiatrictimes.com/bipolar-disorder/new-drug-developments-bipolar-mania/page/0/1?GUID=516DDE24-2C81-40D5-A546-F0B3930EA5BF&rememberme=1&ts=31052013. Accessed October 13, 2014.

26. Ward J, Smith J. Management of mood disorders in patients with advanced illness. *Br J Hosp Med (Lond)*. 2009;70(4):204-207.

27. Chung ML, Lennie TA, Mudd-Martin G, Dubar SB, Pressler SJ, Moser DK. Depressive symptoms in patients with heart failure negatively affect family caregiver outcomes and quality of life. *Eur J Cardiovasc Nur*. May 14, 2014. doi: 10.1177/1474515114535329.

28. Hegerl U, Mergl R. Depression and suicidality in COPD: understandable reaction or independent disorders? *Eur Respir J*. 2014;44(3):734-743. Epub May 29, 2014.

29. Bautovich A, Katz I, Smith M, Loo CK, Harvey SB. Depression and chronic kidney disease: a review for clinicians. *Aust N Z J Psychiatry*. 2014;48(6):530-541.

30. Feng C, Fang M, Liu XY. The neurobiological pathogenesis of poststroke depression. *Scientific World Journal*. 2014:521349. doi: 10.1155/2014/521349. eCollection 2014.

31. Breitbart W, Chochinov HM, Passik SD. Psychiatric symptoms in palliative medicine. In: Hanks G, Cherny NI, Christakis NA, Fallon M, Kaasa S, Portenoy RK, eds. *Oxford Textbook of Palliative Medicine*. 4th ed. New York, NY: Oxford University Press; 2010:1453-1482.

32. Pasacreta JV, Minarik PA, Nield-Anderson L. Anxiety and depression. In: Ferrell BR, Coyle N, eds. *Oxford Textbook of Palliative Nursing*. 3rd ed. New York, NY: Oxford University Press; 2010:425-448.

33. National Cancer Institute (NCI). *Depression (PDQ®)*. 2014. www.cancer.gov/cancertopics/pdq/supportivecare/depression/healthprofessional. Accessed July 10, 2014.

34. Spector RE. *Cultural Diversity in Health and Illness*. 7th ed. Upper Saddle River, NJ: Pearson; 2009.

35. Black HK, Gitlin L, Burke J. Context and culture: African-American elders' experiences of depression. *Mental Health Religion Culture*. 2011;14(7):643-657. doi:10.1080/13674676.2010.505233.

36. Clark L, Colbert A, Flaskerud JH, et al. Culturally based healing and care modalities. *J Transcult Nurs*. 2010;21(1 Suppl):236S-306S.

37. Yang LH, Purdie-Vaughns V, Kotabe H, et al. Culture, threat, and mental illness stigma: identifying culture-specific threat among Chinese-American groups. *Soc Sci Med*. 2013;88:56-67.

38. Kravits K, Berenson S. Complementary and alternative therapies in palliative care. In: Ferrell BR, Coyle N, eds. *Oxford Textbook of Palliative Nursing*. 3rd ed. New York, NY: Oxford University Press; 2010:545-565.

39. Shimizu K, Akechi T, Shimamoto M, et al. Can psychiatric intervention improve major depression in very near end-of-life cancer patients? *Palliat Support Care*. 2007;5(1):3-9.

40. Roth AJ, Massie MJ. Anxiety in palliative care. In: Chochinov HM, Breitbart W, eds. *Handbook of Psychiatry in Palliative Medicine*. 2nd ed. New York, NY: Oxford University Press; 2012:69-80.

41. Townsend MC. *Essentials of Psychiatric Mental Health Nursing: Concepts of Care in Evidence-Based Practice*. Philadelphia, PA: F.A. Davis Co.; 2014.

42. Golomb R, Franklin M, Grant JE, et al. *Expert Consensus: Treatment Guidelines for Trichotillomania, Skin Picking, and Other Body-Focused Repetitive Behaviors*. Trichotillomania Learning Center. 2011. www.trich.org/dnld/ExpertGuidelines_000.pdf. Accessed September 23, 2014.

43. Van Ameringen M, Mancini C, Patterson B, Bennett M, Oakman J. A randomized, double-blind, placebo-controlled trial of olanzapine in the treatment of trichotillomania. *J Clin Psychiatry*. 2010;71(10):1336-1343. doi: 10.4088/JCP.09m05114gre. Epub April 20, 2010.

44. Arnold L, Mutasim DF, Dwight MM, Lamerson CL, Morris EM, McElroy SL. An open clinical trial of fluvoxamine treatment of psychogenic excoriation. *J Clin Psychopharmacol*. 1999;19(1):15-18.

45. Centers for Disease Control and Prevention (CDC). *Injury Prevention & Control: Division of Violence Prevention. Violence Prevention at CDC*. 2014. www.cdc.gov/violenceprevention/overview/index.html. Accessed October 7, 2014.

46. Centers for Disease Control and Prevention (CDC). *Injury Prevention & Control: Division of Violence Prevention. Elder Abuse: Definitions*. 2014. www.cdc.gov/violenceprevention/elderabuse/definitions.html. Accessed October 7, 2014.

47. Centers for Disease Control and Prevention (CDC). *Injury Prevention & Control: Division of Violence Prevention. Intimate Partner Violence: Definitions*. 2014. www.cdc.gov/violenceprevention/intimatepartnerviolence/definitions.html. Accessed October 7, 2014.

48. Centers for Disease Control and Prevention (CDC). *Injury Prevention & Control: Division of Violence Prevention. Sexual Violence: Definitions*. 2014. www.cdc.gov/ViolencePrevention/sexualviolence/definitions.html. Accessed October 7, 2014.

49. Wygant C, Hui D, Bruera E. Childhood sexual abuse in advanced cancer patients in the palliative care setting. *J Pain Symptom Manage*. 2011;42(2):290-295. doi: 10.1016/j.jpainsymman.2010.11.011. Epub March 27, 2011.

50.   Woods AB. The terror of the night: posttraumatic stress disorder at the end of life. *J Hosp Palliat Care*. 2003;5(4):196-204.

51.   Starr TD, Rogak LJ, Casper DJ, Kirsh KL, Passik SD. Palliative care for patients with substance abuse and patients with personality disorders. In: Chochinov HM, Breitbart W, eds. *Handbook of Psychiatry in Palliative Medicine*. New York, NY: Oxford University Press; 2009:122-138.

52.   Konova AB, Moeller SJ, Tomasi D, Volkow ND, Goldstein RZ. Effects of methylphenidate on resting-state functional connectivity of the mesocorticolimbic dopamine pathways in cocaine addiction. *JAMA Psychiatry*. 2013;70(8):857-868. doi: 10.1001/jamapsychiatry.2013.1129.

CHAPTER VII

CARE OF THE FAMILY

Katherine P. Supiano, PhD, LCSW, FT, F-GSA
Judith C. Lentz, RN, MSN, FPCN®
Bridget Sumser, LMSW

I. **Introduction**

    A. **Palliative care, which includes hospice, provides**

        1.   A holistic approach that focuses on the patient and family as the unit of care

        2.   Care that incorporates the expertise of several disciplines who collaborate to meet the needs of patient, family, and caregiver, and who, in addition to their own expertise, have knowledge about physical, psychosocial, spiritual, and bereavement issues that enhance their ability to recognize the need for referral to team specialists

        3.   Care that is based in recognition that assessment, planning, and intervention are the ongoing responsibility of all team members and reflect attention to all dimensions of the patient and family situation[1]

        4.   Care that respects the reality that patients and families form unique relationships with both past medical providers and with team members, and that the perspectives and expertise of these individual clinicians can be invaluable in the identification of needs, in solving problems, clarifying conflicts, and facilitating resolutions

        5.   Care that recognizes that the needs and perspectives of patients, family, and caregivers are unique to them as individuals and unique to their relationships with the patient and that each views the illness trajectory through their own experiences, feelings, and fears

II. **Definitions**

    A. **Family can be defined as blood relatives, relationships established through an emotional commitment, or a group of individuals with whom a person feels most connected**

        1.   The family as a system—one way to consider families and how they function

            a)   A complex entity comprised of interrelated and interacting individuals functioning within a socioeconomic, political environment, as well as a healthcare setting who have some degree of emotional or social ties to each other

b)   The primary objective of the system is to maintain equilibrium in environment, which facilitates individual and family development

c)   System seeks to maintain equilibrium or balance through dynamic process of homeostasis

B.   Caregiver refers to anyone who provides and/or arranges for assistance to someone else who requires it.[2,3] *Informal caregiver* is a term used to refer to an unpaid individual such as family members and friends who provide care. Formal caregivers are volunteers or paid providers associated with a service system

C.   Goals of Care

1.   Establishing patient-driven goals of care is a core competency of palliative care practitioners

2.   Criteria for best practice are written in the *Clinical Practice Guidelines for Quality Palliative Care, 3rd edition*.[4] See Chapter XIII, *National Guidelines and RN Practice* for more on the guidelines

3.   Goals of care are the outcome of advance care planning (ACP) with patient/family

   a)   ACP is a process of multiple conversations[5]

   b)   Patient and family is the unit of care

   c)   Based on holistic patient assessments

   d)   Patient-centered decision-making

   e)   Establishes wishes and preferences of patient and family as a written document to be honored and respected by healthcare providers

   f)   Promote autonomy to empower patient and family

   g)   Grounded in legal doctrine of consent[6] and ethical principle of autonomy

   h)   Requires iterative conversation on multiple occasions

   i)   Allows for ethical justification of decision making[7]

   j)   Significant increase on ACP research has occurred over the past decade

   k)   Target times for conversations are early in disease course, when delivering bad news, discussing prognosis, considering withholding or withdrawing treatments, discussing hospice options, determining code status, and other preferences for care (e.g., medical directives such as POLST/MOLST [physician/provider/medical order for life-sustaining therapy], out of institution resuscitation orders)

   l)   Documentation and revisions of goals of care should occur following each conversation, which includes executing an advance directive or amending an existing one; this varies state-by-state

      i.   Differentiating between an advance directive and POLST/MOLST[8]

         (a)   POLST/MOLST forms

            (i)   Provide medical orders for current treatment

            (ii)   For persons with a serious illness at any age

     (iii) Guides actions by emergency medical personnel

     (iv) Guides inpatient treatment decisions when made available

   (b) Advance directive

     (i) Provides instructions for future treatment

     (ii) For persons 18 years and older

     (iii) Does not guide emergency medical personnel

     (iv) Appoints a healthcare representative

     (v) Guides inpatient treatment decisions when made available

  m) Record conversations for benefit of patient and family if necessary

4. Several models or guides for goals of care conversations exist. One example is a 6-step process[9] sometimes referred to as SPIKES (**S**et up, **P**erception, **I**nvitation, **K**nowledge, **E**motions, Summary/Strategy)[2, p. 172]

  a) Prepare and plan

  b) Ask what patient/family wants to know

  c) Discuss medical information, clarify what they already know

  d) Respond empathetically

  e) Identify and resolve conflicts

  f) Set patient driven goals, summarize

5. Other models guide principles of therapeutic behaviors during advance care planning or a goals of care conversation—VALUE mnemonic[2,10]

  a) **V**alue family statements

  b) **A**cknowledge family emotions

  c) **L**isten to the family

  d) **U**nderstand patient as a person

  e) **E**licit family questions

6. Communication styles are critical

  a) Build trust, recognizing that this may take time

  b) Offer benefits and burdens for options presented

  c) Acknowledge expressed emotions

  d) Acknowledge normalcy of reactions

  e) Explore what is behind emotions

  f) Empathize

  g) Explore coping strategies

h)   Use silence effectively (e.g., pause to allow the patient, family, and those present to think, formulate questions, reflect); silence communicates respect and acknowledges that the patient, family, and close others are in control

i)   Present "bad news" softly

j)   Do periodic rechecks

k)   Use "dying" word cautiously (i.e., pick up or mirror the words the patient and family use and answer questions honestly while validating that the message is clear)

l)   Provide empathic responses such as, "I wish the outcome was better" or "I'm sorry that the treatment was not successful"

m)   Build opportunities to experience control

n)   Preserve dignity

o)   Respect boundaries

p)   Honor decisions

7.   Assure truthful and complete disclosure of all information for maximum decision-making

a)   Prevent and advocate against a "conspiracy of silence"[11,12] (a tacit agreement not to talk about some situation or event)

b)   Be a patient/family advocate

8.   Barriers to effective advance care planning and determination of goals of care

a)   Fear

b)   Anxiety

c)   Belief that all diseases can be cured

d)   Belief in or counting on spiritual healing

e)   Denial—note what seems like denial is often something else (e.g., lack of information, lack of clarity about the goals of care, fragmented care)

f)   Misunderstanding purpose of advance care planning (e.g., limiting care rather than assuring that the patient receives the care they desire should he/she not be able to speak for themselves)

9.   Favorable outcomes to advance care planning and clarifying the goals of care[13]

a)   Improves patient and family satisfaction

b)   Reduces stress, anxiety, and depression in family members

c)   Improves provider communication

d)   Develops readiness to talk about wishes/empowerment

e)   Clarifies understanding of illness and treatment options

f)   Provides context for patient and family to express their values and beliefs

g)   Good death[14]

i.   Which could be considered as a death on one's own terms

ii.   Symptoms managed

        iii.   Decision-making is clear

        iv.   Prepared for death to the extent possible

        v.   Completion of pre-death wishes—life review, faith issues, resolving conflicts, saying goodbye

        vi.   Not being alone, if that is what the patient desires

III. Psychosocial Aspects of Care

A. Assessment—an ongoing, shared responsibility of the interdisciplinary team (IDT)[15]

1. Requires active listening

2. Requires reassessment along the continuum of illness progression, patient, and family/caregiver adaptation and as the situation changes. Plans must continually be reassessed and altered

3. Involves understanding the individual as well as the family as a unit; their history, current functioning, expectations, and vision for the future

4. Is shared and enhanced by observations, input, and clinical expertise of IDT members as well as those who provided care earlier in the illness trajectory

5. Presupposes that the patient, family, and caregiver perspectives and coping may differ; that they impact each other; and that clinicians need to inquire, respect, and intervene according to these unique views

6. Involves observation and interpretation of verbal and nonverbal behaviors and observations from patient, family, caregivers, and interdisciplinary colleagues

7. Is based on verbal, nonverbal, and symbolic communication impacted by

   a) Literacy/numeracy levels

   b) Language/cultural differences

      i.   Adopt an attitude of cultural respect, humility, and inquiry

      ii.   Acquire knowledge about the predominant cultures in your community

      iii.   Avoid using family as translators; use professional interpreters, colleagues, LanguageLine Solutions®[16]

      iv.   Provide educational materials in the language of choice

   c) Communication challenges

      i.   Physical symptoms—dyspnea, pain, tracheostomy, mouth sores, cognitive impairments, visual/hearing impairment, fatigue; important to address symptoms if at all possible before psychosocial assessment and intervention

      ii.   Environmental—noise, interruption, lack of privacy

      iii.   Psychological—depression, anxiety, distress, guilt

      iv.   Accommodate assessment tools, environment, and questions—when necessary, minimize need for patient to speak (i.e., ask questions that can be answered in few words or in nonverbal response)

8. Involves specific areas of assessment that apply to patient, family, and caregiver[17]

    a) Past and present patient and family (including children and adolescents)/caregiver functioning (i.e., physical, psychological, social, cultural, spiritual)

    b) Developmental tasks, sexual orientation/preference, gender identity, where the family is in their life cycle

    c) Risk factors such as psychiatric illness, addiction, physical, and/or sexual abuse

    d) Understanding of medical situation, history, and impact of illness on roles, relationships, values, and hopes

    e) Individual and family coping styles and strengths

        i. Individual attitudes and beliefs about information and the need to know; how much, how little, specifics or generalities, who is to know, and who is to tell

        ii. Learning styles and decision-making process of individuals to assist in customizing interventions

        iii. Need for control; range of ability to delegate and maintain sense of self as valued and life as meaningful in the setting of progressing illness and the consequent emotional, social, and physical impacts

        iv. History of and experience in coping with the unknown, with healthcare systems, with change, and with losses (e.g., physical, psychological, social, cultural, spiritual)

        v. Values, attitudes, and beliefs that infuse individual and family coping, and may be expressed by phrases reflecting a trust in God, desire to keep fighting, trying new treatments, never giving up

    f) Patient's, family's, and caregiver's individual needs, distress, and perspectives related to pain, symptoms, illness progression, caregiver tasks, prognosis, advance care planning, caregiver fatigue, unresolved issues, place of death

    g) Needs of extended or geographically distant family

    h) Needs of emotionally distant/estranged family members

    i) Ongoing evaluation of impact of illness to inform an evolving IDT care plan that might include respite care, alternate care settings, and enhanced supports such as continuous home care, volunteer services, and agency referrals

    j) Community supports and resources including friends, neighbors, clergy and church, or other communities

    k) Emotional and cognitive functioning of patient, family, and caregivers. The following symptoms or behaviors can be very distressing to patients, family, caregivers, and staff; and require vigilant assessment and intervention

        i. Anger and hostility

            (a) Possible etiologies—feelings of isolation, loneliness, infantilization, helplessness, frustration, actual or perceived loss of control or autonomy, perceived threats to feelings of competence, fears of abandonment, disease progression, uncontrolled or new symptoms

            (b) Anxiety—see Chapter VI, *Psychiatric/Psychological Symptoms and Diagnoses*

ii.   Confusion, delirium, agitation, terminal restlessness—see Chapter V, *Symptom Management*

iii. Denial

   (a)   Definition—an unconscious process designed to protect against an overwhelming reality as distinguished from avoidance, which is a conscious process that protects the individual from bringing distressing aspects of their reality to the forefront. As an "unconscious" process, any decision to challenge denial requires a thorough clinical evaluation

   (b)   Possible etiologies—disbelief, fear, needing more time and experience with distressing reality, uncertainty about ability to cope; and in some situations what looks like denial is actually a reflection of the fact that appropriate, understandable, and timely information has never been given

iv.   Depression—see Chapter VI, *Psychiatric/Psychological Symptoms and Diagnoses*

v.   Despair/loss of meaning—see *Spiritual Aspects of Care* in this chapter

vi.   Fear and worry

   (a)   Possible etiologies—fear of or perceived abandonment, feeling a burden, uncontrolled pain and symptoms, inadequate resources (personal, healthcare, community, financial), dependency, fear of dying and death, and future ability of survivors to manage

vii. Guilt—feelings of remorse for an actual or perceived wrongdoing and/or an actual or perceived something that should have been done. Both patients and caregivers can experience guilt.[18] Guilt can be an emotional reaction to a loss[19]

   (a)   Possible etiologies—unresolved issues, feelings of failure, troubled relationships, existential/spiritual turmoil, dependence on others

   (b)   Interventions

      (i)   Forgiveness—feelings of guilt are often accompanied by the desire for repentance by asking for forgiveness, which is deeper than forgetting, diminishing the harm, or condoning the behavior; patients and caregivers may need assistance and even prompting in talking to someone to say "I'm sorry;" steps that may assist the person include acknowledging that harm was done, to feel worthy of being forgiven, forgive oneself, and to fully embrace the experience of the other who was involved.[20,21] Benefits of granting forgiveness include decreased symptoms of depression, resolving of angry feelings, and improved quality of life. Assist those being asked for forgiveness to understand the importance of granting forgiveness[21]

      (ii)   Active listening—listen for the person's individual feelings of guilt; support the person's dignity by being sensitive to his/her feelings; avoid asking directly about feelings of guilt as this may be seen as intrusive. Instead, help the person to understand that guilt is a common reaction (e.g., "Some people often have feelings of guilt after the one they have been caring for dies . . . it may help to talk about these feelings if you are feeling this way.")[18,22]

      (iii) Sometimes feeling of guilt requires professional counseling[23]

      viii. Sleep disturbance—see Chapter VI, *Psychiatric/Psychological Symptoms and Diagnoses*

      ix. Suicidal/homicidal ideation/wish for hastened death

        (a) Suicide—see Chapter VI, *Psychiatric/Psychological Symptoms and Diagnoses*

        (b) Homicidal ideation—thoughts of killing another person; take all comments seriously, clarify emotion expressed, take measures to ensure safety

        (c) Wish for hastened death—includes a patient's passive wish for death (no active plans), requesting assistance with hastening death, to a developed plan to commit suicide[24]

        (d) Possible etiologies—may be transient or persistent; depression, psychiatric illness, despair, uncontrolled symptoms, need for control, hopelessness, perceived loss of dignity, sense of self as "burden," delirium, misuse or abuse of medications

B. Interventions—the shared responsibility of the IDT and the individualized responsibility of the team clinician whose expertise and relationship establish their role as the primary provider of psychosocial care

   1. Are individualized and based on an ongoing assessment of the unique and potentially different needs of the patient, family, and caregiver

   2. Provided in collaboration and consultation with IDT who have a shared knowledge base as well as individual areas of expertise

   3. Include medical management and education as well as advocacy, psychosocial, spiritual, complementary techniques, and expressive therapies, which may be provided by nurse, social worker, physician, or chaplain

   4. Balance respect for patient, family, and caregiver pace and adaptation with the team's need to provide information, educate, and foster shared decision-making

   5. Are developmentally- and culturally-sensitive

   6. Reinforce aspects of experience that remain stable at the same time that patient, family, and caregiver cope with change caused by illness progression and changing goals of care

   7. Presuppose that psychological and spiritual suffering cannot be totally alleviated

   8. May be delivered in person, via phone, email, or other ways given patient and family needs and geographical distances

   9. Include counseling and referral to interdisciplinary colleagues as appropriate and within keeping with the preferences of the patient and family (e.g., social worker, chaplain, music, art, massage therapist), and involve modalities such as individual, supportive group, or family counseling

IV. Spiritual Aspects of Care

A. Follow guidelines for spiritual care as written in Domain 5: Spiritual, Religious, and Existential Aspects of Care from the *Clinical Practice Guidelines for Quality Palliative Care*[4]

1. Guideline 5.1—The interdisciplinary team assesses and addresses spiritual, religious, and existential dimensions of care

2. Guideline 5.2—A spiritual assessment process, including a spiritual screening, history questions, and a full spiritual assessment as indicated is performed. This assessment identifies religious or spiritual/existential background, preferences, and related beliefs, rituals, and practices of the patient and family; as well as symptoms, such as spiritual distress and/or pain, guilt, resentment, despair, and hopelessness

3. Guideline 5.3—The palliative care service facilitates religious, spiritual, and cultural rituals or practices as desired by patient and family, especially at and after the time of death

B. Spiritual interdisciplinary team members ideally include an officially credentialed clergy

1. Team members do not impose their personal beliefs, preferences, or rituals on the patient and/or family

2. Team members approach spiritual aspects of care with dignity and respect for the beliefs of the patient and family

C. Spiritual Assessment—the beginning of spiritual care

1. Definition of spirituality—"the aspect of humanity that refers to the way individuals seek and express meaning and purpose and the way they experience their connectedness of the moment to self, to others, to nature, and/or to the significant or sacred"[25]

2. Spirituality can be described as

   a) The search for ultimate meaning and purpose of life, which may involve connection to a higher power

   b) The capacity to persevere with hope in the face of challenges in quality of life

   c) A way to describe the organizing center in a person's life

3. Definitions of words related to spirituality

   a) Religion—organized, codified, and often institutionalized beliefs and practices that express one's spirituality. Can be described as the formal expression of one's spirituality[26]

   b) Religiosity—the quality of being religious, piety, devoutness[27]

   c) Faith—the acceptance, without objective proof, of something (e.g., God)[26]

4. Spiritual distress

   a) Common concerns, which can cause spiritual distress

      i. Alienation from the religious or spiritual community

      ii. Lack of access to religious or spiritual rituals or contact with faith of choice

      iii. Existential distress, despair, anxiety related to the struggle to find meaning in the experience of illness, suffering, death, and dying

      iv. Need to reconcile with God, others, and self

      v. Spiritual beliefs opposed by family, peers, and/or healthcare professionals vi.　Loss of hope or meaning

        (a)　Possible causes—grief, disability, emotional overload, fear of death, depression, uncontrolled symptoms

      vii.　Unresolved spiritual issues

        (a)　Possible causes—guilt, regret, lack of meaning, loss of sense of self, problematic relationships, fear of unknown, wish or need for forgiveness

5.　Use a two-tiered approach to spiritual assessment[26]

  a)　Brief assessment

    i.　Sample questions

      (a)　What is giving you the strength to cope with your illness now?

      (b)　What spiritual beliefs and practices are important to you as you cope with your illness?

      (c)　Do you have someone to talk to about religious matters?

      (d)　Is faith/religion/spirituality important to you in this illness?

      (e)　Has faith been important to you at other times in your life?

  b)　Utilize screening tools when possible[14,26]

    i.　FICA[28] most widely used

      (a)　**F**aith, belief, meaning

      (b)　**I**mportance and influence

      (c)　**C**ommunity

      (d)　**A**ddress in care

    ii.　Maugens' SPIRIT[26,29]

      (a)　**S**piritual belief system (religious affiliation)

      (b)　**P**ersonal spirituality (beliefs and practices)

      (c)　**I**ntegration with a spiritual community

      (d)　**R**itualized practice and restrictions

      (e)　**I**mplications for medical care

      (f)　**T**erminal events planning (advance directives, clergy)

    iii.　Anandarajah and Hight's HOPE[26,30]

      (a)　**H** = sources of hope, meaning, strength, peace, love, and connection

      (b)　**O** = organized religion

      (c)　**P** = personal spiritual and religious practices

      (d)　**E** = effects on medical care and end-of-life issues

    6. Explore spiritual and existential, meaning of life, values, and beliefs

       a) Use life review, dignity therapy, and other spiritual exploration questions

    7. Incorporate patient's spiritual leader/guide into process if requested

D. Interventions

1. Explore and acknowledge feelings of spiritual suffering

2. Listen, pray, caring presence, touch

3. Encourage verbalization and elicit patient, family, and caregiver values, relationships, fears, hopes, and unfinished business

4. Enhance sense of meaning and value to include respect for the full life experience of the individual and family

5. Work with chaplains, spiritual counselors, and team members to determine most appropriate way to assist with issues of forgiveness, hopelessness, mending fractured relationships, withholding of nutrition and/or hydration when appropriate, etc.

6. Evaluate for depression—consider antidepressants and multidimensional interventions such as counseling, cognitive behavioral interventions if prognosis and goals of care permit

7. Explore priorities and achievable goals to broaden the scope of hope and hope-related activities beyond cure of illness as the only acceptable and meaningful outcome

8. Encourage life review/reminiscence

    a) Look through photo albums

    b) Reflect on memories of life events

    c) There are several interview guides available publically

9. Explore the value of rituals

    a) Facilitate practice of rituals

    b) Work with the patient and family, chaplains, spiritual counselors to provide requested prayers, readings, hymns, pastoral visits

10. Remember physical symptoms are sometimes difficult to relieve if spiritual distress is present and spiritual distress is exacerbated by unrelieved physical symptoms

11. Spiritual competency for professionals can be enhanced by education

V. Cultural Aspects of Care

A. Assessment—requires consideration of the reality that cultural beliefs, values, and practices infuse professional caregiver experience as well as the experience of the patient, family, and caregiver. Professionals have the responsibility to

1. Develop a knowledge base about the major cultures served in the programs in which they work while understanding this is not a finite knowledge base that can be mastered

2. Develop general understanding of historical and current healthcare disparities related to race, culture, class, gender, and sexual orientation

3. Understand concept of cultural humility as a professional—ongoing practice of self-awareness and self-critique that addresses power imbalance inherent in medical system[31]

    a) Understanding power imbalance considers patient experience through the lens of race, class, ethnicity, gender, sexuality, nation, language, (dis)ability, education level, etc.

4. Seek avenues for ongoing learning and awareness-building as an individual professional and for the team

5. Adapt and accommodate assessment and interventions to respect cultural and spiritual variation

6. Utilize patient-centered interviewing and communication strategies, honoring the patient and family's agenda and communication style

7. Understand that it is the clinician and team's responsibility to work through challenges and misunderstandings that can evolve when the culture of the healthcare professional differs from the culture of the family[32]

8. Avoid using family as translators as families translate through the filter of their own emotional and cognitive reactions, and clinicians cannot know what is being said or understood

9. Avoid stereotyping—do not assume all people from a certain country, region, or nationality hold the same beliefs

10. Explore how assimilation, acculturation, and generational differences influence family member's customs, language, beliefs, and attitudes. Persons who have been in the United States for several generations may no longer follow the same customs as those who have recently immigrated and customs do not remain static

11. Know the areas of healthcare that can be impacted by cultural and/or religious beliefs and values including

    a) Time orientation—emphasis on past versus present or future

    b) Decision-making style—self-determination/autonomy versus family, community decision-making

    c) Family roles in communication/decision-making—patriarchy/matriarchy, role of children

    d) Ideas about causation of illness

    e) Preferences and comfort with concept of advance care planning

    f) Appropriateness of clothing, food preferences, traditional remedies

    g) Issues related to privacy, gender, eye contact, personal space

    h) Communication styles and preferences—truth telling, direct, nonverbal, respect for silence

    i) Taboos, rituals, and healing practices

    j) Treatment decisions such as nutrition/hydration, discontinuing treatments, organ donation

    k) Customs and belief systems related to death, transitions, afterlife, etc.

    l) Expectations and perceptions of healthcare relationships (e.g., egalitarian, hierarchical, informal, paternalistic)

    m) Practices and behaviors related to illness, pain, treatments, suffering, and end of life

VI. Patient and Family Education

A. The knowledge or skill obtained or developed by a learning process; an instructive or enlightening experience[33]

1. Assess patient and caregiver strengths and limitations as well as emotional (e.g., depression, anxiety), cognitive (e.g., fears, worries), cultural, and physical (e.g., fatigue, insomnia, other symptoms) factors to determine appropriateness, ability, and readiness to integrate and carry out specific tasks

2. Teach primary caregivers specific techniques for patient care—medication administration, dressing changes, position changes, safety, etc.

3. Language and cultural variations may require adaptation of teaching tools and approaches

4. Identify and consider individualizing factors that impact ability, style, or environment of learning

    a) Personal factors—patient or caregiver illiteracy and/or innumeracy, learning disabilities, impairments of vision or hearing, preferred learning style

    b) Environmental challenges—noise, frequent interruptions, lack of privacy, general chaos

    c) Family dynamics and/or cultural factors, which impact appropriateness of asking family members to provide care (e.g., in some cultures, it is not *proper* for a daughter to provide personal care for her father)

    d) Language differences and communication challenges (i.e., inability to speak, read and/or write English; no available bilingual professionals, no teaching materials in preferred language, sensory deficits)

5. Seven steps to effective teaching that can be applied to patient and family[34]

    a) State the purpose/goal/objective of the learning experience

    b) Determine the needs of the learner, to match content and presentation to learner's needs

        i.   Assess language and cultural differences, readiness, and motivation of learner

        ii. Assess literacy, numeracy level, if appropriate

        iii. Assess visual and hearing needs

    c) Devise a plan or a method of presenting the material to the learner; include members of the IDT in the planning and as instructors

    d) Provide time for the learner to clarify content

        i.   Discuss using their own words

        ii. Questions

        iii. Observe

        iv. Demonstrate

        v.   Example

        vi. Supplement with appropriate written and visual materials

      vii.   Utilize technological advances in educational methodology—Internet sites, blogs, YouTube, social media, online learning. See Chapter II, *Interdisciplinary Collaborative Practice in the Hospice and Palliative Settings*, for suggestions on how to determine if an Internet site if reputable

    e)   Schedule time for the learner to practice the newly acquired knowledge or skills

      i.   Joint visits

      ii.   Patient/caregiver practice

      iii.   Observation

    f)   Schedule time for the learner's new skills to be evaluated. Involve other IDT members if doing so enhances the comfort of the learner

      i.   Review

      ii.   Observation/return demonstration—if an in-person visit is not feasible, consider telehealth and/or Internet-based means of observations (e.g., Skype, FaceTime)

      iii.   Verbal recall

    g)   Assess health literacy and adapt principles of teaching to provide the skills needed[35]

      i.   Up to 50% of all prescription and over-the-counter medications are administered incorrectly

      ii.   Refer to AHRQ Health Literacy Toolkit (www.ahrq.gov/qual/literacy/index.html), especially the "brown bag" medication review technique

      iii.   Utilize health literacy assessment tools such as Newest Vital Sign (NVS),[36] Rapid Estimate of Adult Literacy in Medicine-Short Form (REALM-SF)[37]

      iv.   Present no more than 3 to 5 key points with each patient visit

      v.   Utilize "teach back" methods to assure comprehension

      vi.   Use visual aids when available

6.   Assess primary caregiver's ability to provide care

    a)   Verbalization of understanding of instructions and willingness to provide care

    b)   Return demonstration of technique(s) taught

    c)   Observe, support, and positively reinforce actual care during patient contact (i.e., visits to home, palliative care unit, acute care setting)

    d)   Conduct ongoing proactive assessment of caregiver physical and emotional status as over time caregiver's fatigue, mood, and physical abilities change (a reality that may go unrecognized or unarticulated by the caregiver)

    e)   Assess volunteers and/or professional care providers for compassion fatigue and address as indicated

7.   Instruct patient, family, and caregiver on

    a)   End stage disease processes (see Chapter III, *Patterns of Disease Progression*)

    b)   Pain and symptom management (see Chapter IV, *Pain Management*, and Chapter V, *Symptom Management*)

c)   Signs and symptoms as death nears (see Chapter X, *Care of the Patient and Family in the Final Days*)

d)   Seven dimensions of nearing death[38]

    i.   Redefining—shifting from what used to be to what is now

    ii.   Burdening—when patients see themselves as purposeless, dependent, and immobile

    iii.   Struggling with paradox—of living while dying

    iv.   Contending with change—relationships, roles, and in socialization and work patterns

    v.   Searching for meaning—patients turn inward and reflective; especially spiritually

    vi.   Living day by day—especially if the individual is able to find meaning in this experience, trying to live each day to the fullest

    vii.   Preparing for death—leaving legacies for loved ones

VII. Advocacy

A.   Definition—promoting "patient and family values, wishes, and preference of care, legal and ethical decision-making, and improves access to care and community resources by influencing or formulating health and social policy"[39, p. 23]

B.   Assess needs for changes in levels of palliative/hospice care and/or IDT services

1.   Assess patient, family, and caregiver needs at each contact

2.   Encourage family and caregiver to report changes in patient status as well as changes in their own physical and emotional state when they occur

3.   Encourage all team members who have patient/family contact to assess needs and report changes in patient condition, and in the physical and emotional state of the caregiver and family

4.   Facilitate effective communication between patient, family, and care providers; sit down, minimize personal distractions, take a couple of deep breaths to focus self

5.   Observe expressions, body language, etc. Pay attention when they do not reflect what is being said

6.   Communicate in terms the listener understands—verbal and nonverbal

7.   Be sure you understand what the speaker intended to communicate (e.g., solicit feedback), be an active listener

C.   Encourage and support patient and family as the unit of care in sharing their individual decision-making style regarding illness-related decisions and treatment options (i.e., empower patient and family; inquire about cultural dimensions)

D. In collaboration, members of the IDT, including the patient's own provider and with consideration of individual and cultural differences, inform patient/family of treatment options available to them

1. Assist the patient/family in clarifying their goals versus focusing on specific treatments and/or interventions

2. Discuss with patient/family each option with consideration of both physical and psychological benefits and burdens for patient, caregiver, and family members

3. Answer questions truthfully and as completely as possible

    a) Utilize available resources as needed

    b) Seek input from primary physician and other IDT members

    c) Assure full disclosure

    d) Clarify misunderstandings, as a treatment may not change the progression of the disease, but could add to burden

    e) Offer "what if?" questions to ensure all perspectives are considered

    f) Assure truth telling is the philosophy of all[11,12]

4. Support the patient/family in the decision-making process

    a) Acknowledge their right and ability to make the decision

    b) Reassess decisions as medical and/or psychosocial situation changes

    c) Be nonjudgmental, maintaining an awareness of nonverbal messages and tone of voice

    d) Ensure that needs of children, adolescents, and extended family are met all along the continuum of illness, and that expert clinical help is provided to assist family members of all generations. Utilize IDT members specifically educated in this area (see Chapter VIII, *Palliative Care Across Care Settings*)

    e) Advocate for patient/family wishes and preferences

E. Make referrals for IDT consults for interventions to augment the expertise of the members of the core IDT

1. Therapy services—physical therapy, speech therapy, occupational therapy

2. Counseling services—spiritual, dietary, bereavement

3. Psychology/psychiatry counseling, crises intervention, group intervention, resources

4. Complementary and alternative modalities—massage therapy, aromatherapy, pet therapy, music, and other expressive therapies

F. Participate in the shared process of advance care planning (e.g., advance directives, preferences about life-sustaining treatment, do not resuscitate [DNR] status)

1. Inform patient of the teams' desire to understand and respect their preferences (right of self-determination), recognizing that cultural and individual beliefs may be based in a different value system

a)   Identify the decision-maker and/or healthcare agent selected by the patient if the patient is no longer decisional

b)   In some cases, the decision-maker designated by legal statute may not be the decision-maker designated by family or culture

c)   Be familiar with your state's advance directives laws, rules, and regulations and forms

2.   Assess decision-making preferences of patient and family

a)   Information and education may be helpful for some and not for others

b)   In some family settings the presence and participation of elders, clergy, healers, etc. are essential, and decision-making is a family or larger group process

3.   Provide information and education to assist the patient/family in the decision-making process; individualize according to cultural and family belief systems that may be incongruous with advance care planning concepts

4.   Ask "what if?" questions to assure patient/family are able to anticipate future issues

5.   Assure patient/family of continued care in the most appropriate setting as long as they meet admission criteria and desire care by the agency

6.   Engage in opportunities to advocate for palliative care in public policy on the local, state, and federal levels, following the Hospice and Palliative Nurses Association (HPNA) Public Policy Guiding Principles[40]

VIII. The Environment of Care

A.   **Assessment—implicit in an assessment of the environment of care is the acknowledgment and respect for the clinician responsibility that accompanies any invitation to enter the home or living space of a patient**

1.   Assess patient/family/caregiver ability to respond to emergencies, including fire, power failure, weather, and other natural disasters

2.   Assess family/caregiver physical and psychological/cognitive ability to provide assistance with patient's activities of daily living

3.   Recognize that one's home has psychological significance and changes or additions such as medical equipment have the potential to change a home into a medical setting

a)   Evaluate need for durable medical equipment and assistive devices

4.   Perform a systematic safety assessment with an emphasis on prevention of falls, infection control, fire prevention, proper storage of medications, use and storage of oxygen, firearm safety

a)   Assess adequacy of electricity, heat, indoor plumbing, smoke alarms

5.   Recognize need to modify or supplement plan of care to accommodate psychological/socioeconomic factors and resource needs

a)   Based on assessment, collaborate with the interdisciplinary team and refer to social worker or other community resources, if appropriate

6.　Education and assessment

   a)　Inform patient/family/caregiver how and when to access hospice/palliative care services 24 hours a day, 7 days a week, 365 days a year, by providing appropriate contact phone numbers

   b)　Instruct patient/family/caregiver on the procedure to obtain medications, equipment, and supplies from agency or healthcare provider

   c)　Educate about current and potential symptoms creating a proactive care plan with the goal of avoiding crises and unnecessary distress for patient, family, caregiver, and staff

   d)　Monitor disposal of supplies/equipment (e.g., needles, syringes, dressings, or other medical waste)

      i.　Instruct patient, family, and caregiver on proper use, storage, and disposal of supplies/equipment

   e)　Refer to the agency's policies/procedures related to delivery and/or pick up of biohazardous medical waste, disposal of discontinued medications, etc.

      i.　Monitor controlled substances[41,42]

      ii.　Assure patient adherence in use as prescribed

      iii.　Consider use of contracts with patients with history of addiction or medication diversion

      iv.　Explore risk factors for diversion with family and caregivers

      v.　Explore unrelieved pain to assure adherence

         (a)　Ask patient and/or caregiver to complete journal of medications administered for 1 week

         (b)　Count tablets/capsules/other dosage forms with each visit to validate journal

         (c)　Explore miscounts further

            (i)　See Chapter IV, *Pain Management*, for further information

         (d)　Diversion

            (i)　Definition—selling or trading prescription pain medication by patients, family, healthcare workers, and anyone who comes in contact with or transports controlled substances for illicit purposes[42,43]

            (ii)　Explore further if

               a.　No constipation, especially when laxatives are not being taken

               b.　Pain management record or journal does not match medications remaining

               c.　Pain continues to be unrelieved

               d.　Drug shortages are unexplained

vi.   Soiled dressings should be discarded using a double bagging technique

vii.   Sharps disposal in appropriate container labeled per local municipality protocol

f)   Enhance patient/family/caregiver comfort in handling medication

g)   Medication administration

   i.   Instruct patient, family, and caregiver on the agency's policies and procedures related to medications (e.g., over the counter, prescriptions, controlled substances)

   ii.   Provide patient, family, and caregiver instruction regarding appropriate medication use (i.e., medication name, dosage, schedule, indications, and side effect profile) and document in the patient medical record. Provide in writing whenever possible

   iii.   Suggest the use of assistive devices (e.g., pill boxes, counting and/or measuring devices) to ensure patient is following medication orders correctly

   iv.   Evaluate instances of problematic over or under use of medication which may be due to

      (a)   Misunderstanding of directions

      (b)   Patients' self-medicating in an effort to manage undertreated symptoms

      (c)   Medications being withheld due to fears of side effects, worry about addiction, or hastening death

      (d)   Financial concerns impacting medication availability

      (e)   Substance abuse

         (i)   Do a risk assessment that includes history, home environment, IDT observations, patterns of medication management, and comprehensive symptom assessment

         (ii)   Distinguish from pseudoaddiction (relief-seeking that mimics drug-seeking behavior but emanates from unrelieved symptoms)

         (iii)   Ongoing observation, consultation, and assessment with IDT and patient, family, and caregiver to work toward the goal of altering the care plan to safely and effectively treat symptoms and addictive disease if diagnosed

         (iv)   Consult with an addiction specialist, if appropriate

         (v)   Follow the agency/institutional protocol if substance abuse/diversion is suspected

h)   Handling of medications at time of death in the home setting

   i.   Inform family/caregiver of legal requirement regarding disposition of controlled substances and inform supervisor if family and caregiver refuse disposal as per policy

   ii.   Destroy drugs in the presence of a witness

   iii.   Document outcomes as per agency policy

i) Assess for neglect and abuse (of patient, family, and caregiver) in collaboration with members of the IDT. The presence of any of these indicators does not necessarily mean the individual is abused (e.g., caregiver physically unable to care for the patient); it should alert the nurse to the need for ongoing assessment and discussion with the other members of the IDT. However, if evidence of abuse exists, immediate action by the IDT is expected

   i. Potential physical indicators include

      (a) Unexplained or neglected injuries and/or those incompatible with history

      (b) Evidence of inadequate care (e.g., poor hygiene, disheveled/inappropriate clothing)

      (c) Evidence of inadequate or inappropriate administration of medication

      (d) Dehydration and/or malnourishment without illness-related cause

      (e) Lack of bandages on injuries, stitches when indicated, or evidence of unset bones

      (f) Cuts, lacerations, puncture wounds, burns, scald lines

      (g) Bruises, welts, discoloration (e.g., bilateral on upper arms, morphologically similar to an object, clustered in one general area, evidence of physical restraints)

   ii. Potential behavioral indicators in patient, family, or caregiver include

      (a) Fear, withdrawal, flinching, helplessness, hesitation to talk openly, implausible stories, ambivalence/contradictory statements not due to mental dysfunction, resignation, non-responsiveness

      (b) Aggressive behavior toward patient or aggressive behavior toward caregiver that may emanate from anger, frustration at being sick, feeling dependent or trapped, or a reflection of prior abuse history

      (c) Patient/family/caregiver disclosure of abuse or observation of physical or emotional abuse or neglect

   iii. Potential behavioral indicators on part of family/caregiver

      (a) Patient/client not given the opportunity to speak for self or to be alone with team members

      (b) Family declines visits from members of the IDT

      (c) Absence of necessary, available assistance, attitudes of indifference or anger toward patient

      (d) Family and caregiver blames patient for their illness or incapacitation

   iv. Interventions

      (a) Confer with members of the IDT especially the social worker. Signs of neglect and abuse have multilevel etiologies such as

         (i) Caregiver fatigue and depression

         (ii) Patient anger, rage, helplessness, or prior history of abuse in family

(iii) Patient's inability or unwillingness to cooperate with family/caregivers

(iv) Inadequate symptom management (e.g., pain, delirium)

(v) Increased stress—financial, physical, emotional

(vi) Psychiatric illness, alcoholism, drug abuse, cognitive impairment in patient or family

(b) Report according to applicable state law

(i) If possible, inform patient/caregiver that a report is being made

IX. Grief and Loss

A. Theory and Concepts

1. Definitions

   a) Grief is a normal reaction to loss, and an essential part of dealing with loss, especially loss in death[44,45]

   b) Mourning is the cultural ritual and social response to grief

   c) Anticipatory grief precedes the death and results from the expectation of death[46]

   d) Disenfranchised grief refers to a bereavement experience that is not socially endorsed or supported (e.g., death of a homosexual partner, death of an ex-spouse)[47]

   e) Complicated grief is a state of chronic, ineffective bereavement characterized by persistent yearning, recurrent intrusive thoughts of the person who died, preoccupation with sorrow including ruminative thoughts, excessive bitterness, alienation from previous social relationships, difficulty accepting the death, and perceived purposelessness of life[48]

      i. To meet diagnostic criteria for complicated grief, the death must have occurred over 6 months ago

      ii. Symptoms must be present for 1 month and cause significant functional impairment

   f) Grief support is provided by friends, family, health and mental health professionals, and spiritual care professionals to facilitate a normal grief process

   g) Grief therapy includes specialized techniques to address complicated grief, or grief in the setting of depression, anxiety, or difficult life circumstances (e.g., multiple losses)[49]

B. Grief Processs

1. Early (acute) grief is characterized by disbelief, intense sadness, loneliness, longing to be with the deceased (perhaps even fleeting desire to die to be with the deceased)

2. Sorrow may be broken by periods of positive memories and emotions

3. Crying, irritability, and poor concentration are common

4. Somatic distress includes appetite changes, sleep disturbance, fatigue, restlessness

5.   Normal grief evolves as the finality of the loss and the adjustments to life without the deceased are gradually made

   a)   Grief becomes integrated into the present and future life

   b)   Interest and engagement in life resume

   c)   Thoughts and memories of the deceased continue but do not dominate

6.   Grief is highly individualized. Each person responds to grief differently according to the

   a)   Nature of the loss *to the person*

   b)   Grieving person's personality

   c)   Norms within the grieving person's culture and family

   d)   Other stressors in the grieving person's life

   e)   Grieving person's history of coping with other losses

7.   Children and adolescents grieve differently than adults and grief support should be age-appropriate (see Table 7-1)

C.   Grief in the Dying Patient

1.   Dying patients experience grief as they anticipate the dying process and personal mortality[52,53]

2.   Patients who are psychologically aware of their terminal status and consider themselves "at peace" have less distress[54]

3.   Active listening and honest communication facilitate healthy grief in dying patients

4.   Encouraging a life review/reminiscence process where the patient reflects on the life lived and its meaning is often helpful

5.   Dignity in care (dignity therapy)[55]

Table 7-1. Children's Understanding of Death[50,51]

Age	Think	Common Behaviors in Reaction to Grief	Things that May be Helpful
Before 3	A wish can cause death and undo it Recognize death by 3	Crying Separation anxiety Attachment to primary caregiver	Want physical contact that is close and constant
3 to 6 years	Think that someone can be both dead and alive Death can be temporary and reversible Death, separation, and sleep are thought to be the same Do not think that they will die Know death is irreversible	Fear of sleep Potential for misplaced guilt	Physical contact Reassurance Gentle cuing to understand
6 to 12 years	By 7 years most have an understanding that death is irreversible and universal Earlier in phase, grasp on external causes of death, not internal Very interested in the specifics of death—burial, what happens to the body after burial, coffins By 12 can think of own death, but will think that it is connected with older age	Concerns regarding separation and being isolated Do not want to lose body integrity or control	Body treated with careful respect Correct information—dolls, drawings may be helpful
12 years and older	Think about consequences and results of death Effect of death on world around them Future orientation allows them to think about own death in the future, but not as something that could happen now May think of death as "heroic" or "tragic"	Acting out or risk-taking Do not want to deal with a problem directly If individual knows that they are dying, may not follow medical instructions, keep to themselves, express anger, and want to get married now as they will not be alive to marry later	Support from family and peers Privacy but not desertion Document their life and story Help to recognize maladaptive behaviors Help with understanding that love and sorrow are part of being an adult and a child

D.   Grief Support for the Patient's Family and Caregivers

1.   Provide death vigil support[56]

2.   Encourage acceptance of individual differences in family members' grief behaviors and emotions

3.   Provide information on agency care of the patient upon death and funeral practices

4.   Visit at time of death to facilitate notification, pronouncement, and transportation

5.   Demonstrate sensitivity to cultural and/or religious bereavement practices

6. Facilitate transition into bereavement care

7. Participate in closure activities

   a) Condolence call made by appropriate member(s) of IDT

   b) Sign sympathy card for family/caregivers

   c) Attend funeral/memorial service, if appropriate

8. Participate in personal or IDT process to assist in integration of loss[57]

9. Provide emotional support for family/caregivers as a natural extension of the clinical relationship

   a) Help family/caregivers explore the significance of the loss

   b) Help family/caregivers express feelings, lingering questions, and reminiscences

   c) Assist in practical aspects of life without the deceased

   d) Interpret and affirm normal grief

10. Assess family for risk of complicated grief and refer for appropriate bereavement care[58]

X. Intimacy Relationship Issues

A. **Relationship issues can be new and a direct result from living with a serious illness or being in a relationship with a person with a serious illness. Relationship issues may not be new, but are further complicated by the illness. For some, the diagnosis of a serious illness may be the impetus to repair the relationship**

B. **Intimacy is a universal need of all people to be in close personal relationships with others that can include but is not limited to sexuality. Intimacy, a source of communication and emotional connections and support, is closely linked to how people cope with difficult situations. Relationships that lack intimacy or have never had intimacy are at risk for breaking down[59,60]**

C. **All humans are sexual beings and express their sexuality in their own individual way, not just by sexual intercourse. Sexuality includes self-acceptance, respect, gender identification, and feelings of belonging to and involvement in one's culture as well as sexual desire and functioning. Difficulties with sexual health can impact quality of life[59,60]**

D. **Challenges to Sexual Health**

   1. Physical changes related to the illness and its care can impact how a patient views themselves or their partner (e.g., scars, mastectomies, weight loss, ascites) and their ability for sexual functioning (e.g., prostate surgery, fatigue, pain, incontinence)[59,60]

   2. Psychosocial issues can include dealing with body image changes, realization that you cannot have children or more children, concern with how your partner feels

   3. Hospitalization and changes in living arrangements (e.g., an adult child moving into the home to assist with caregiving, transfer to a long-term care facility) also impact the patient and/or their partner's sexual expression (e.g., lack of privacy and alone time, shared rooms, staff interruptions, single hospital beds)[59]

4. Assessing for problems related to sexual issues can begin with asking "Do you have any concerns about your sexual health?"[59]

E. **Interventions to support the patient and their relationship partner are based on the nature of the issue and can range from simply providing more privacy to consulting with other disciplines/experts as needed[59,60]**

CITED REFERENCES

1. Coyle N. Introduction to palliative care. In: Ferrell BR, Colye N, eds. *Oxford Textbook of Palliative Nursing*. 3rd ed. New York, NY: Oxford University Press; 2010:3-11.

2. Perrin KO. Communicating with seriously ill and dying patients, their families, and their health care practitioners. In: Matzo M, Sherman D, eds. *Palliative Care Nursing: Quality Care to the End of Life*. 4th ed. New York, NY: Springer Publishing Company; 2015:169-188.

3. Levine C. *Always on Call: When Illness Turns Families into Caregivers*. New York, NY: United Hosptial Fund; 2004.

4. National Consensus Project for Quality Palliative Care. *Clinical Practice Guidelines for Quality Palliative Care*. National Consenus Project, 2013. www.nationalconsensusproject.org/NCP_Clinical_Practice_Guidelines_3rd_Edition.pdf. Accessed October 13, 2014.

5. Hospice and Palliative Nurses Association (HPNA). *The Nurse's Role in Advance Care Planning*. [Position Statement]. 2013. hpna.advancingexpertcare.org/education/position-statements/. Accessed October 20, 2014.

6. Derby S, O'Mahony, Tickoo R. Elderly patients. In: Ferrell BR, Coyle N, eds. *Oxford Textbook of Palliative Nursing*. 3rd ed. New York, NY: Oxford University Press; 2010:713-743.

7. Brandt DS, Shinkunas LA, Gehlbach TG, Kaldjian LC. Understanding goals of care statements and preferences among patients and their surrogates in the medical ICU. *J Hosp Palliat Nurs*. 2012;14(2): 126-132.

8. Physicians Orders for Life-Sustaining Treatment Paradigm (POLST). *POLST and Advance Directives*. 2012. www.polst.org/advance-care-planning/polst-and-advance-directives/. Accessed September 8, 2014.

9. Quill TE, Bower KA, Holloway RG, et al. *Primer of Palliative Care*. 6th ed. Chicago, IL: American Acadamy of Hospice and Palliative Medicine; 2014.

10. Curtis JR. Caring for patients with critical illness and their families: the value of the integrated team. *Resp Care*. 2008;53(4):480-487.

11. Finn JJ. *A Palliative Ethic of Care*. Sunbury, MA: Jones & Bartlett; 2006.

12. Fallowfield LJ, Jenkins VA, Beveridge HA. Truth may hurt but deceit hurts more: communication in palliative care. *Palliat Med*. 2002;16(4):297-303.

13. Waldrop DP, Meeker MA. Communication and advanced care planning in palliative and end-of-life care. *Nurs Outlook*. 2012;60(6):365-369. doi: 10.1016/j.outlook.2012.08.012.

14. Schaffer MA, Norlander LK. *Being Present: A Nurse's Resource for End-of-Life Communication*. Indianapolis, IN: Nursing Knowledge International; 2009.

15. National Palliative Care Research Center (NPCRC). *About Palliative Care*. 2013. www.npcrc.org/content/15/About-Palliative-Care.aspx. Accessed October 10, 2014.

16. LanguageLine Solutions®. *Over-the-Phone Interpreting*. 2015. www.languageline.com/solutions/interpretation/telephone-interpretation/. Accessed January 6, 2015.

17. National Palliative Care Research Center (NPCRC). *Caregiver Assessment*. 2013. www.npcrc.org/resources/resources_show.htm?doc_id=376172.

18. Harstäde CW, Andershed B, Roxberg Åsa, Brunt D. Feelings of guilt—experiences of next of kin in end-of-life care. *J Hosp Palliat Nurs*. 2013;15(1):33-40.

19. D'Antonio J. Caregiver grief and anticipated mourning. *J Hosp Palliat Nurs.* 2014;16(2):99-104.

20. Ferrell B. Forgiveness in palliative nursing. *J Hosp Palliat Nurs.* 2012;14(8):501.

21. Exline JJ, Prince-Paul M, Root BL, Peereboom KS, Worthington Jr. EL. Forgiveness, depressive symptoms, and communication at the end of life: a study with family members of hospice patients. *J Palliat Med.* 2012;15(10):1113-1119.

22. Melhado LW, Byers JF. Patients' and surrogates' decision-making characteristics: withdrawing, withholding, and continuing life-sustaining treatments. *J Hosp Palliat Nurs.* 2011;13(1):16-28.

23. Byock I. *The Four Things that Matter Most.* New York, NY: Free Press; 2004.

24. Olden M, Pessin H, Lichtenthal WG, Breitbart W. Suicide and desire for hasten death in the terminally ill. In: Chochinov HM, Breibart W. *Handbook of Psychiatry in Palliative Medicine.* 2nd ed. New York, NY: Oxford University Press; 2009:101-112.

25. Puchalski C, Ferrell B, Virani R, et al. Improving the quality of spiritual care as a dimension of palliative care: the report of the Consensus Conference. *J Palliat Med.* 2009;12(10):885-904.

26. Taylor EJ. Spritual assessment. In: Ferrell BR, Coyle N, eds. *Oxford Textbook of Palliative Nursing.* 3rd ed. New York, NY: Oxford University Press; 2010:647-661.

27. The Free Dictionary. Religiosity (definition of). *The Free Dictionary.* 2014. www.thefreedictionary. com/religiosity. Accessed October 10, 2014.

28. Puchalski C, Romer AL. Taking a spiritual history allows clinicians to understand patients more fully. *J Palliat Med.* 2000;3(1):129-138.

29. Maugens TA. The SPIRITual history. *Arch Fam Med.* 1996;5:11-16.

30. Anandarajah G, Hight E. Spirituality and medical practice: using HOPE questions as a practice tool for spiritual assessment. *Am Fam Physician.* 2001;63(1):81-89.

31. Tervalon M, Murray-Garcia J. Cultural humility versus cultural competence: a critical distinction in defining physician training outcomes in multicultural education. *J Health Care Poor Underserved.* 1998;9(2):117-125.

32. Stark D. Teamwork in palliative care: an integrative approach. In: Altilio T, Otis-Green S, eds. *Oxford Textbook of Palliative Social Work.* New York, NY: Oxford University Press; 2011:415-424.

33. Houghton Mifflin Company. Education. *The American Heritage® Dictionary of the English Language.* 4th ed. Chicago, IL: Houghton Mifflin Company; 2009.

34. Leonard DJ. Workplace education: adult education in a hospital staff development department. *J Nurs Staff Development.* 1993;9:68-73.

35. Roett MA. Help your patient "get" what you just said: a health literacy guide. *J Fam Pract.* 2012;61(4):190-196.

36. Pfizer. *The Newest Vital Sign: A Health Literacy Assessment Tool.* 2011. www.pfizer.com/files/health/ nvs_flipbook_english_final.pdf. Accessed September 8, 2014.

37. Agency for Healthcare Research and Quality (AHRQ). *Health Literacy Measurement Tools: Fact Sheet.* 2009. www.ahrq.gov/professionals/quality-patient-safety/quality-resources/tools/literacy/. Accessed September 8, 2014.

38. Davies B. Supporting families in palliative care. In: Ferrell BR, Coyle N, eds. *Oxford Textbook of Palliative Nursing.* 3rd ed. New York, NY: Oxford University Press; 2010:614-618.

39. Dahlin CM, Sutermaster DJ, eds; Hospice and Palliative Nurses Association, American Nurses Association. *Palliative Nursing: Scope and Standards of Practice—An Essential Resource for Palliative and Hospice Nurses.* Silver Spring, MD: nursesbooks.org; 2014.

40. Hospice and Palliative Nurses Assocation (HPNA). *HPNA Public Policy Guiding Principles.* 2014. hpna.advancingexpertcare.org/advocacy/guiding-principles/. October 20, 2014.

41. Walsh AF, Broglio K. Pain management in advanced illness and comorbid substance use disorder. *J Hosp Palliat Nurs.* 2010;12(1):8-14.

42. Starr TD, Rogak LJ, Casper DJ, Kirsh KL, Passik SD. Palliative care for patients with substance abuse and patients with personality disorders. In: Chochinov HM, Breibart W, eds. *Handbook of Psychiatry in Palliative Medicine.* 2nd ed. New York, NY: Oxford University Press; 2009:122-138.

43. Drug Enforcement Administration (DEA). *Disposal of Controlled Substances.* 2014. www.federalregister.gov/articles/2014/09/09/2014-20926/disposal-of-controlled-substances. Accessed September 9, 2014.

44. Wright PM, Hogan NS. Grief theories and models: applications to hospice nursing practice. *J Hosp Palliat Nurs.* 2008;10(6):350-356.

45. Hallenbeck J. Grief and bereavement. 2nd ed. *Fast Facts and Concepts.* 2009; 32. www.eperc.mcw.edu/EPERC/FastFactsIndex/ff_032.htm. Access October 10, 2014.

46. Kehl KA. Recognition and support of anticipatory mourning. *J Hosp Palliat Nurs.* 2005;7(4):206-211.

47. Doka KJ. Disenfranchised grief in historical and cultural perspective. In: Stroebe MS, Hansson RO, Schut MH, Stroebe W, eds. *Handbook of Bereavement Research and Practice: Advances in Theory and Intervention.* Washington, DC: American Psychological Association; 2008:223-240.

48. Claxton R, Reynolds CF. Complicated grief. 2nd ed. *Fast Facts and Concepts.* 2012; 254. www.eperc.mcw.edu/EPERC/FastFactsIndex/ff_254.htm. Accessed October 10, 2014.

49. Craig L. Prolonged grief disorder. *Oncol Nurs Forum.* 2010;37(4):401-406.

50. Faulkner KW. Children's understanding of death. In: Armstrong-Daily A, Zarbock S, eds. *Hospice Care for Children.* 3rd ed. New York, NY: Oxford University Press; 2009:9-23.

51. Chrastek J, Eull D. *Just in Time Guide: A Primer for Pediatric Palliative Care at Home.* Pittsburgh, PA: Hospice and Palliative Nurses Association; 2010.

52. Block SD. Perspectives on care at the close of life. Psychological considerations, growth, and transcendence at the end of life: the art of the possible. *JAMA.* 2001;285(22):2898-2905.

53. Knight SJ, Emanuel L. Processes of adjustment to end-of-life losses: a reintegration model. *J Palliat Med.* 2007;10(5):1190-1198.

54. Ray A, Block SD, Friedlander RJ, Zhang B, Maciejewski PK, Prigerson HG. Peaceful awareness in patients with advanced cancer. *J Palliat Med.* 2006;9(6):1359-1368.

55. Chochinov HM. *Dignity in Care: Approach.* 2010. www.dignityincare.ca/en/approach.html. Accessed October 10, 2014.

56. Waldrop DP. Caregiving and support: caregiving systems at the end of life: how informal caregivers and formal providers collaborate. *Fam Soc (J Contemp Soc Serv).* 2006;87(3):427-437.

57. Lobb EA, Oldham L, Vojkovic S, et al. Frontline grief: the workplace support needs of community palliative care nurses after the death of a patient. *J Hosp Palliat Nurs.* 2010;14(4):225-233.

58. Milberg A, Olsson EC, Jakobsson M, Olsson M, Friedrichsen M. Family members' perceived needs for bereavement follow-up. *J Pain Symptom Manage.* 2008;35(1):58-69.

59. Matzo M. Sexual health and intimacy. In: Matzo M, Sherman DW, eds. *Palliative Care Nursing: Quality Care to the End of Life*. 4th ed. New York, NY: Springer Publishing Company; 2015:129-146.

60. Matzo M, Pope LE, Whalen J. An integrative review of sexual health issues in advanced incurable disease. *J Palliat Med*. 2013;16(6):686-691.

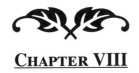

CHAPTER VIII

PALLIATIVE CARE ACROSS CARE SETTINGS

Sherra Stewart-Rego, RN, BSN, MPH, CHPN®
Dena Jean Sutermaster, RN, MSN, CHPN®

I. **Communication—Essential Skills for Teams in the Provision of Quality Hospice and Palliative Care Across Care Settings**

   A. **Effective communication with healthcare providers across the healthcare continuum is key to the delivery of quality hospice and palliative care[1]**

      1. Effective communication is a fundamental nursing intervention and essential for patient advocacy

      2. Communication is 80% nonverbal (e.g., eye contact, body language, presence, intonation, gestures)

      3. Attentive listening and silence are important communication skills

         a) Do not interrupt

         b) Do not anticipate what will be said

         c) Do not change the subject

         d) If unsure what to say, say nothing

   B. **Effective communication facilitates teamwork within and across multiple care settings[1]**

      1. Demonstrates respect among team members, acknowledging the unique knowledge, skills, and insights each individual contributes to the care of the patient

      2. Leads to consensus regarding goals and objectives of care

      3. Delineates responsibility with shared accountability

      4. Respects the patient and family

   C. **Thorough communication has been shown to lead to improved outcomes for patients and families when care is closely coordinated[2]**

      1. Patient and family goals are clearly identified

      2. Patient and family preferences are supported

3. Patient and family values are respected

4. Clinical information is correctly and completely communicated

D. Conflicts Are Inevitable[1]

1. Conflicts can be productive, affording opportunities for understanding different perspectives, facilitating discussion, growth

2. Conflicts can arise from

    a) Complex ethical issues and differing opinions about what is best for patients and their families

    b) Blurring of professional roles

    c) Power struggles between ranks

    d) Differing/conflicting regulatory compliance requirements among healthcare providers

3. Conflict resolution is necessary to maintain healthy, positive teams, professional relationships, and to **promote positive patient outcomes**

4. Strategies for managing conflicts[1]

    a) Examine your emotions—is it personal?

    b) Identify the problem

    c) Find common points that can be agreed upon

    d) Agree that the conflict exists and talk about it

    e) Seek advice from other colleagues

    f) Advocate for the patient's goals and preferences

E. Developing effective communication skills, whether with colleagues or patients and families, requires skill-based learning and practice[3]

1. Self-assessment of communication strengths and weaknesses

2. Regular assessment of interdisciplinary team communication processes

3. Utilize role play exercises to practice skills

4. Ask a colleague to critique an interaction

II. Collaboration Across Care Settings

A. Palliative, which includes hospice, and end-of-life care is provided in a variety of settings in order to meet the needs of persons with serious or life-threatening illness and their families

1. Because nearly 60% of persons receiving hospice care die in places other than private residences, the ability to collaborate with other healthcare providers is key in providing quality hospice and palliative care. The following statistics represent places of death of hospice patients[4]

    a) Patient's place of residence (66.6%)

        i. Private residence (41.7%)

      ii.   Long-term nursing facility (17.9%)

      iii.   Residential facility (7.0%)

   b)   Hospice inpatient facility (26.4%)

   c)   Acute care hospital (7.0%)

B. Persons receiving palliative care may transition back and forth between care settings and levels of care during the course of their illnesses

1. *Home to hospital or inpatient hospice* for acute symptoms unable to be managed in the home

2. *Hospital to nursing facility* for short-term rehabilitation prior to returning to the home setting

3. Hospital/skilled nursing facility (SNF) to home after acute/subacute stays

4. Home or hospital to an assisted living or skilled nursing facility if patient can no longer safely remain at home

C. Transition between healthcare settings requires collaboration among healthcare providers, patients, and families[5]

1. Complete transfer of patient information across settings can help avoid inefficiencies that lead to inappropriate and expensive interventions at end of life

2. Proper communication at discharge can improve patient/family understanding and compliance regarding medication management, medical follow-up instructions, safety, and other important care issues

3. Provider accountability in collaboration across healthcare settings can improve patients' and families' knowledge and ability to navigate the healthcare system

4. Adequate collaboration can reduce incidence of unnecessary and costly re-hospitalizations

D. Collaboration Between Levels of Care Should Include

1. Collaboration with the patient and family in developing the plan of care, taking into account patient goals and preferences

2. Nurse-to-nurse hand-off communication—includes direct communication with emergency department and intensive care unit (ICU) staff regarding goals of care for patients transferred with acute conditions

3. Collaboration with physicians and other providers (i.e., advanced practice registered nurses, physician assistants), specialty clinic staff (e.g., oncology, hemodialysis, disease management case managers)

4. Collaboration with staff of skilled nursing, assisted living, group home facilities, home care agencies, area agencies on aging, and other providers within the extended health services community

5. Collaboration with members of the hospice/palliative interdisciplinary team

E.   **Documenting collaboration is essential to demonstrate interdisciplinary involvement—one of the hallmarks of palliative care**

F.   **Nurses are in a unique position to improve palliative care across care settings by ensuring communication of patient/family needs and goals of care between interdisciplinary team members across the continuum**

III. Hospice

A.   **Hospice care is a covered benefit under Medicare, commercial insurance, Veterans' benefits, and, in most states, Medicaid. The Medicaid Hospice Benefit closely models the Medicare Hospice Benefit in terms of eligibility, coverage, and regulatory compliance. Benefits and coverage vary among commercial and other non-Medicare insurers[6]**

B.   **Medicare Hospice Benefit: Eligibility and Benefit Election/Certification[6]**

1.   To be eligible for hospice services under Medicare an individual must

a)   Have Medicare Part A Hospital Insurance, and

b)   Be certified as terminally ill by a physician. Terminal illness, as defined in Chapter 9 of the Medicare Benefit Policy Manual, means an individual has a life expectancy of 6 months or less, if the illness follows its usual course.

2.   An individual who meets Medicare Hospice Benefit criteria accesses their benefit by signing an election form. This signifies that the individual understands the benefit, that the care provided is comfort-focused and not curative or primarily life prolonging, and that certain other Medicare coverage related to the terminal illness is waived

3.   Medicare Hospice Benefit Certification/Recertification/Face-to-Face (F2F)

a)   When an individual elects the hospice benefit, a hospice must obtain verbal or written certification of terminal illness from an individual's attending physician *and* the hospice physician. The initial certification must be obtained no later than 2 days after the start of the certification period, although it may be obtained up to 15 days prior to the election of the hospice benefit. For each subsequent certification period, only the hospice physician is required to recertify the individual as terminally ill, and this recertification must be obtained up to 15 days before, but no later than 2 days after, the start of the new certification period. The first and second certification periods are for 90-day periods. Every subsequent certification period is 60 days. There is no limit on the number of times an individual may be recertified as long as they continue to meet eligibility criteria

b)   Beginning with the third certification period, a hospice physician or nurse practitioner must document a F2F encounter with an individual in order to recertify terminal illness. The F2F can occur at any time in the 30-day period preceding the start of the new certification period. Failure to conduct a F2F encounter will render an individual ineligible for the hospice benefit

C.   **Medicare Hospice Benefit: Covered Services[6]**

1.   Services of members of the interdisciplinary team (IDT). The IDT process provides the foundation for hospice and palliative care

      a) Nurse

      b) Physician

      c) Social worker

      d) Certified nursing assistant/hospice aide/homemaker

      e) Physical, occupational, speech therapy

      f) Counseling

            i. Dietary

            ii. Pastoral

            iii. Bereavement

2. Medical supplies/durable medical equipment

3. Medications for conditions related to the primary hospice diagnosis and related conditions. Effective July 2014, medications in four categories—analgesics, antiemetics, laxatives, and antianxiety drugs that are NOT related to the hospice primary diagnosis or related conditions, and therefore not paid for by the hospice provider—will require prior authorization by the patients Medicare Part D drug plan in order to be covered by Medicare[7]

D. Medicare Hospice Benefit—Levels of Care[8]

1. Routine home care—most hospice care is provided in an individual's home, whether that is a private residence, nursing home, assisted living facility, or other residence. Care at this level includes the services of the interdisciplinary team: nurse, physician, social worker, therapist(s), chaplain, certified nursing assistant/hospice aide, and volunteer(s). Nursing support is available 24 hours a day, 7 days a week

2. Continuous care—up to 24 hours of predominantly nursing care daily that is provided at home, assisted living, or nursing facility during a period of crisis. This level of care is intended to be short-term for situations requiring management of acute pain or other symptoms. When a caregiver who has been providing a skilled level of care for an individual becomes unable or unwilling to continue providing that care that may precipitate a crisis; however, continuous care would not be appropriate in situations where there are no acute pain management or other skilled needs

3. General inpatient care—this level of care is provided in a hospital, skilled nursing facility, or hospice inpatient facility and is intended for the short-term management of pain or other symptoms that cannot reasonably be provided in the home setting. Requires the availability of a registered nurse 24 hours a day. The interdisciplinary team continues to be accountable for the professional management of the patient's care in accordance with the hospice plan of care. A daily visit from one of the team members is recommended. Once symptoms are managed, an individual must return to a lower level of care[9]

4. Respite care—inpatient care that is available to provide a needed rest for a caregiver who has become exhausted and/or unable to care for an individual at home. This level of care is provided in an inpatient setting for up to 5 calendar days. While an individual may have more than 1 respite stay during a certification period, these episodes cannot be back-to-back. Multiple episodes of respite care during a certification period may signal a need for alternate care arrangements for the hospice patient

5. **Important**—transitioning between levels of care often involves transitions between care environments. In these instances, **the hospice maintains professional management responsibility for the care of the hospice patient**

E. **Medicare Hospice Benefit—Conditions of Participation—Overview[8]**

1. Conditions of participation (CoPs) are uniform standards healthcare providers must adhere to in order to participate in Medicare/Medicaid and receive federal funding. They are developed by the Centers for Medicare & Medicaid Services (CMS) for ensuring quality, safe care for beneficiaries

2. The Medicare Hospice Benefit CoPs were first written in 1983 when legislation creating the Medicare Hospice Benefit was enacted, and were updated in 2008

F. **Medicare Hospice Benefit Conditions of Participation—Hospice care in a hospital, skilled nursing facility (SNF)/nursing facility (NF), or intermediate care facility for individuals with intellectual disabilities (ICF/IID). Medicaid and several states refer to these facilities as ICF/MR (intermediate care facilities for individuals with mental retardation) and refer to the same facility[8]**

1. CoPs for short-term inpatient care—general inpatient care and respite care

    a) General inpatient care (GIP)—GIP-level care can be provided in Medicare certified hospitals, hospice facilities, or skilled nursing facilities and is intended for symptom management and pain control that cannot be achieved in other settings. The criteria for this level of hospice care are described in Section III.D.3. of this chapter

    b) Respite care—can be provided in Medicare certified hospitals, hospices, or skilled nursing facilities. This type of care is intended to be no longer than 5 consecutive days at any given time and is provided to relieve a primary caregiver who is temporarily unable to meet a patient's needs. Respite stays of 5 days or less *may* be provided more than once each certification period, however, repeated requests for caregiver respite may indicate a patient requires relocation to another environment of care

2. CoPs for hospice care in SNF/NF or ICF/IID facilities

    a) In 2008, the CoPs were revised to focus on the quality of hospice care programs and outcomes of that care. A large focus area of the revision, found in §418.112, seeks to clarify the contracted "relationship between nursing facilities and hospices"[10]

    b) Section §418.112, published in Title 42 of the Code of Federal Regulations,[11] sets forth 3 standards for the delivery of hospice care in skilled nursing and other nursing facilities (SNF/NF), and intermediate care facilities for individuals with intellectual disabilities (ICF/IID)

        i.   Patients receiving hospice care in SNF/NF and ICF/IID settings must meet the same eligibility criteria as recipients in other settings

        ii. The hospice must assume "responsibility for professional management" of the hospice services provided in these care settings

        iii. The hospice and the SNF/NF or ICF/IID must have signed, written agreements specifying, in accordance with the standard, how hospice services will be provided

3. *Why this is important*—when hospices contract with nursing facilities to provide hospice care, there is often confusion about which the patient/resident "belongs to." The answer is, both

   a) Each party has different responsibilities with regard to the care of the patient, as spelled out in the written agreement between the parties

   b) *Professional management* means that it is the *hospice's* responsibility to oversee and ensure that the hospice plan of care is adhered to, that the hospice is notified of changes in the resident's condition, and that the hospice interdisciplinary team makes decisions about changes in the resident's hospice plan of care, including levels of care, for the patient

   c) Although this provision speaks to SNF/NF or ICF/IID facilities, professional management applies to all settings in which hospice patients receive care

4. Important provisions under §418.112[10] *Conditions of Participation: Hospices that provide hospice care to residents of a SNF/NF or ICF/IID*, include

   a) Hospices and SNF/NF or ICF/IID staff have a specified manner in which to communicate and document communication to ensure that residents' needs are met 24 hours/day

   b) The SNF/NF or ICF/IID staff immediately notifies the hospice of any significant change in condition of the patient, if the patient requires transfer to another facility, or if the patient dies

   c) The hospice is responsible for decisions regarding the appropriate course of the hospice care, including transfers between levels of care

   d) The SNF/NF or ICF/IID is responsible to furnish room, board, and other services a primary care person would normally provide if the patient resided at home

   e) The hospice is responsible for services related to the terminal illness as specified in the plan of care

   f) Hospice "must report all alleged violations involving mistreatment, neglect, or verbal, mental, sexual, and physical abuse including injuries of unknown source, and misappropriation of patient property by anyone unrelated to the hospice" within 24 hours

   g) The hospice is responsible to ensure that SNF/NF or ICF/IID staff receives orientation and training regarding hospice philosophy, pain and symptom management, principles of death and dying, patient rights, and documentation requirements. The training and name of person providing the training must be documented

   h) When GIP for the management of acute symptom management is provided in a SNF/NF or ICF/IID, the hospice must ensure 24-hour nursing services that meet the patient's needs are furnished in accordance with each patient's plan of care, and that a patient receives direct care from a registered nurse (RN) on every shift

IV. Palliative Care in the Hospital Setting

   A. History of Hospitals as Place of Death

      1. In the first half of the 20th century, most Americans died at home. It was not until mid-century that technological advances in medicine resulted in a shift to hospitals as the site of death for the majority of U.S. decedents. That trend continued, peaking between 1980 and 1992 with approximately 74% of persons in the United States dying in hospitals and other institutional settings. Since the mid-1990s the pendulum has begun to slowly reverse as the hospice movement in the United States has gained momentum[12]

      2. In 2010, 715 000 or approximately 29% of all deaths occurred in hospitals.[13,14] Of hospice patient deaths, in 2013, 7.0% died in hospitals, down from 7.4% in 2011 and 11.4% in 2010[4,15]

   B. Inherent Problems with End-of-Life Care in Hospitals

      1. Acute care focuses on prolonging life

         a) Medicalized/specialist perspective on goals of care

         b) Inadequate communication/consideration of patient/family wishes

      2. Sense of failure among acute care staff when death is near or when a patient dies

      3. Difficult to promote a peaceful dying experience

         a) Patients may endure unnecessary suffering

         b) Lack of patient choice over where and how to die

         c) Lack of support for families

   C. End-of-Life Care in the Emergency Department (ED)

      1. Presentation to the ED often presumes patient and family are making an "active solicitation for help"[16]

      2. Uncertainty of prognosis, especially in end stage chronic illness, is often confusing to patients, families, and ED staff in the face of an acute exacerbation of symptoms

      3. The culture of the ED is not conducive to end-of-life discussions. Often ED staff has little patient information and lacks time to develop relationships to elicit goals of care and informed decision-making[16]

   D. Dying in the Intensive Care Unit (ICU)

      1. Approximately 20% of Americans die in ICUs[17,18]

      2. ICUs offer life-prolonging and disease stabilization therapies

      3. Environment of care can be chaotic and loud with suboptimal privacy, limited visiting hours for family, and a focus on technology

      4. ICU staff and patients/families may have different opinions about the efficacy or futility of treatments[18]

      5. Family communication of medical condition is often suboptimal and confusing

      6. Patients often unable to advocate for themselves; medical decision-making can fall to poorly prepared surrogates

E.   Palliative Care Services in Hospitals

1.   Like hospice care, palliative care can be provided in a variety of settings, but most palliative care teams are hospital-based. Palliative care is appropriate from the time of diagnosis of a serious or life-threatening illness and throughout its course. Palliative care team members

   a)   Communicate with specialists and other healthcare providers to provide continuity of care while patients undergo concurrent disease-directed treatment

   b)   Provide expert symptom management to optimize comfort

   c)   Offer guidance with healthcare decision-making

   d)   Provide emotional and spiritual support

   e)   Advocate for patient/family preferences

2.   According to the 2011 *Report Card of the Center to Advance Palliative Care*, the prevalence of palliative care services in United States hospitals continues to evidence annual growth[19]

   a)   There are currently over 1600 palliative care programs in hospitals throughout the country

   b)   Only 54% of public hospitals and less than 40% of sole community hospitals have palliative care services in place. This impacts the delivery of palliative care to low income and rural Americans[19]

   c)   Reimbursement

      i.   Palliative care physicians and advanced practice clinicians can bill for palliative care consultations and follow-up visits

      ii.   In some settings, licensed clinical social workers can bill directly for their services

      iii.   Other costs incurred by hospitals for palliative care programs are not reimbursed by Medicare, Medicaid, or other insurers. Currently, there is no reimbursement for other interdisciplinary team members such as chaplains

3.   Research has demonstrated the efficacy of palliative care teams in improving outcomes for persons with serious and advanced illness[18,20,21]

   a)   Earlier clarification of patient/family preferences

   b)   Earlier implementation of palliative plan of care

   c)   Improved pain and symptom ratings

   d)   Improved levels of patient/family satisfaction

   e)   Decreased levels of anxiety and depression in the bereavement period

   f)   Decreased lengths of stay in ICUs

   g)   Cost avoidance/decreased costs

   h)   Increased likelihood to be transferred home with hospice services

   i)   Improved bereavement patterns in caregivers have been seen with earlier access to hospice

F.   Hospice General Inpatient Care in Hospitals

   1.   Based on the 2007 hospice discharge data, 27% of patients enrolled in hospice utilized general inpatient services, either in hospitals or hospice inpatient/residential facilities (HIRFs).[22] In 2011, that number had dropped to 23% of hospice enrollees[23]

   2.   Medicare Hospice Benefit CoPs have clarified eligibility criteria[22] for short-term GIP-level of care. The National Hospice and Palliative Care Organization (NHPCO) GIP Tip Sheet[9] states to be considered appropriate for GIP-level care a patient must have

      a)   Pain or symptom crisis not managed by treatment changes in the current setting or that require frequent medication adjustment and monitoring

      b)   Intractable nausea and vomiting

      c)   Advanced open wounds requiring changes in treatment and close monitoring

      d)   Unmanageable respiratory distress

      e)   Delirium with behavior issues

      f)   Sudden decline necessitating intensive nursing intervention

      g)   Imminent death ONLY if skilled nursing needs are present

   3.   The hospice interdisciplinary team, in collaboration with hospital staff and the patient and family, develop the hospice inpatient plan of care

   4.   GIP hospice care is intended to be short-term. The hospice plan of care must include discharge planning to other settings

   5.   Thorough documentation of the necessity for GIP-level care is important at all phases of care

G.   Education and Advocacy

   1.   The difficulty of prognostication in chronic disease contributes to late referrals to palliative care. Physicians and healthcare providers require education and tools to assist in the identification of patients in need of palliative care

   2.   Reluctance of healthcare providers to illicit goals of care and to communicate truthfully about their status and prognosis with their patients often results in increased ED visits and hospital admissions near the end of life. Communication strategies for a successful goals of care discussion should be a component of healthcare provider education

   3.   Early involvement of palliative care teams has been shown to improve pain and symptom control, increase patient and family satisfaction, improve the likelihood of hospice referrals upon discharge, and decrease ICU lengths of stay and hospital costs.[2,20] Advocacy for the establishment of palliative care services in low-income and rural area hospitals is important to improve end-of-life care for vulnerable populations

V.   Community Palliative Care

A.   Outpatient palliative care can be given in an ambulatory care setting, patient's home, nursing facility, assisted living facility, and via telephone support.[24] Though new, community palliative care is gaining momentum

   1.   May be a consultative model and/or be the first point of contact[24]

B.   Delivered by an interdisciplinary team of healthcare professionals (e.g., advance practice clinicians, nurses, physicians, social workers), patient and family who are at the center, and community caregivers[24]

C.   Benefits can include increased caregiver and patient satisfaction, decreased hospitalizations, improved quality of life, optimal symptom management, improved continuity of care, earlier advance care planning discussions, smooth transitions between healthcare settings, and decreased healthcare costs[24]

D.   Challenges include finding resources (e.g., staff, location for offices and/or clinic); lack of knowledge of palliative care by potential referrers, patients, and family; different preferences for management of patients by primary team and palliative team

VI.   Long-Term Care Services

A.   This section focuses on the common elements of providing care on a long-term basis to individuals with serious or life-threatening illness, which is palliative care. The elements of care that are unique to each setting are in their own section, noting that most palliative long-term care (LTC) research has focused on nursing homes and nursing home residents[25]

1.   Definition—"health and supportive services provided to people unable to practice self-care . . . [and] includes personal care, social services, room and board, transportation, and medical and rehabilitative care."[25, p. 1180] LTC services can assist individuals to maintain or improve an optimal level of functioning and quality of life[26]

2.   Though the terms *long-term care* and *nursing home* are often used interchangeably, LTC actually includes care provided in personal residences, community support services (e.g., adult day care service centers, transportation services, home care agencies), and facility-based programs (e.g., nursing homes/facilities, assisted living facilities, board and care communities, continuing care retirement communities)[25,27]

3.   *Resident* is the term used for a person who lives in a nursing home or assisted living facility

4.   Though a patient can receive hospice care for years, it is not usually considered long-term care as it is generally short-term care.[27] Residents in long-term care facilities can elect to have hospice care when they are eligible. Many LTC providers also provide hospice either through their own facility or by contracting with hospices[26]

5.   In 2012, there were over 8 million participants/day receiving LTC services. See Chart 8-1 for the distribution by type of LTC services

6.   LTC agencies and facilities are subject to state and/or federal regulation and oversight[28]

Chart 8-1. Distribution of Long-Term Care Participants by Type of Care Provided[26]

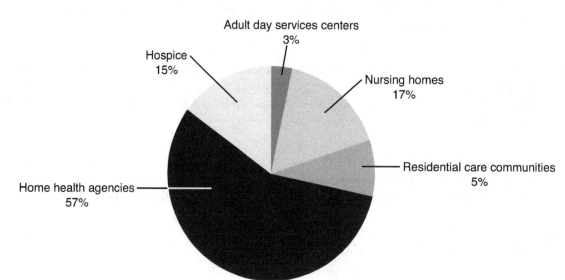

B.   Payment for Long-Term Care Services[27]

1.   Medicare—pays for skilled care and rehabilitative care in a nursing home for a maximum of 100 days or skilled home health/in-home services following a hospital stay of 3 days. See Table 8-1 for average costs of LTC

   a)   Skilled care—"nursing care such as help with medications and caring for wounds, and therapies such as occupational, speech, respiratory, and physical therapy. Skilled care usually requires the services of a licensed professional such as a nurse, doctor, or therapist"[27]

   b)   Examples of reasons for skilled nursing care in a nursing home—recovering from surgery (e.g., joint replacement), or acute medical conditions (e.g., major infection, heart failure)[28]

   c)   Generally the goal is for the resident to return to where he/she had lived before hospitalization

   d)   Medicare does not pay for non-skilled assistance with activities of daily living (ADLs)/custodial care, though Medicare Part B may pay for certain LTC services (e.g., enteral nutrition)[28]

2.   Medicaid—pays for largest amount of non-skilled LTC services, though residents must meet the state's eligibility requirements—need assistance in 2 or more activities of daily living (ADLs) and financial (i.e., income and assets level below a certain level)[28]

   a)   If initially not eligible, a resident "pays/spends down" his/her own assets to meet Medicaid financial eligibility criteria[27]

3.   Programs for All-Inclusive Care of the Elderly (PACE®)[29]

   a)   Interdisciplinary coordinated care for individuals 55 years of age or older who qualify (i.e., certified to need nursing home care as per their state, able to live safely in their community, live in a PACE® service area)

---

b) The program's goal is to assist individuals to maintain their independence in their homes for as long as possible

c) Services include medical and supportive services (e.g., physician and nursing services, laboratory and x-ray testing), adult day care, meals, home healthcare, personal care, prescription drugs, social services, medical specialists (e.g., audiology, dentistry, optometry, podiatry, speech therapy), respite care, transportation, caregiver support, and hospital and nursing home care when necessary

d) Paid for by Medicare, Medicaid, private pay, or a combination, depending on financial situation

e) PACE® can provide end-of-life care. If a participant specifically wants to elect the hospice benefit from a certified hospice organization, the participant must voluntarily disenroll from the PACE® program

4. Private health insurance—varies by plan, though usually similar to Medicare

5. Older Americans Act—can provide funds for home and community-based services to assist low- and moderate-income individuals who are at high risk for nursing home placement[30]

6. U.S. Department of Veterans Affairs (VA)—see section on Veterans

7. LTC insurance—reimburses policyholders a daily amount based on the plan the individual selected and paid into. Many plans have limits on how long or how much will be paid

8. Private pay—resident's own assets (e.g., savings, investments, reverse mortgages, life insurance options, annuities)

9. Other possible sources of paying for LTC—disability insurance (may replace some of lost wages, but does not pay for LTC services), automobile insurance, court settlement (see Table 8-1)

Table 8-1. Average Costs of Long-Term Care in the United States[27]

Setting	Cost	Average Annual Costs
Home	Homemaker services—$19/hour	$32 032–$56 056
	Home health aide—$21/hour	$34 320–$57 200
	Adult day healthcare center—$67/day	Up to $33 639
Assisted living facility	One-bedroom unit—$3293/month	Up to $72 000
Nursing home	Semi-private room—$205/day or $6235/month	$47 538–$270 845
	Private room—$229/day or $6965/month	$55 360–$255 891

C. **Advance Directives**

1. Ideally all adults would complete an advance directive and routinely review and update it as needed

2. Decision-making is more difficult for families and healthcare providers when individuals receiving LTC services have not expressed their wishes for the type and amount of medical care they would want (e.g., resuscitation, artificial nutrition and hydration, hospitalization). Patients with neurocognitive disorders (e.g., dementia, delirium) can participate in advance directive discussions, however someone else will need to be the ultimate decision-maker

3.   Most nursing home residents and their families prefer less aggressive medical care[25]

4.   In addition to advance directives, many states now provide a signed medical order called a Physician/Provider/Medical Order for Life-Sustaining Treatment (POLST/MOLST) form. This form documents what type of medical care patients and/or their surrogate medical decision-maker prefer

5.   For more on advance directives, see Chapter IX, *Advance Care Planning and Goals of Care*

D.   Prevention of Unnecessary Transfers to the Hospital

1.   In 2011, one-quarter of Medicare nursing home residents were admitted to the hospital at least once. Hospitalization or rehospitalization is necessary when residents require acute care services, though some hospitalization could be avoided.[28] Reasons for hospital admission include

    a)   Clinical—septicemia (13.4%), pneumonia (7%), congestive heart failure (5.8%), urinary tract infections (5.3%), and aspiration pneumonia (i.e., food, vomitus; 4%) were the 5 most common reasons for hospitalization[28]

    b)   Nonclinical—availability and training of nursing home staff, resident and family member preferences, physician availability and preference[28]

2.   Risks for hospitalization or rehospitalization—recent hospitalization, congestive heart failure, hypercarbia in residents with chronic obstructive pulmonary disease (COPD), poor renal function, clinical instability, and depression[31]

3.   Lower rates of hospital readmission—geriatric assessment and nurse practitioner involvement[31]

4.   Negative impact of hospital transfers—disruption to care plans, disorientation, stress and iatrogenic illness (e.g., adverse events), financial costs (e.g., lack of Medicare reimbursement for hospital readmissions within 30 days of discharge, physician services, co-pays)[28]

5.   Transfers are complicated when vital information about the resident is not communicated to the emergency and admitting medical providers in the hospital[28]

E.   Family Transitions from Primary Caregiver to Family Member of Resident

1.   The decision to admit a loved one to a LTC facility is difficult

    a)   For family members—feelings of guilt or abandonment due to inability to care for a loved one, not wanting to give up caregiving activities

    b)   For the resident—loss of independence, loss of home, living in a strange place, new routines, having a roommate(s)

2.   Support for families of LTC residents include the need for information, symptom management of loved ones, and emotional support[32]

F.   Reason for Need of Long-Term Care Services

1.   Needing assistance with ADLs is the most common reason for beginning LTC services

2.   Cognitive impairment from Alzheimer's disease and other types of dementia are a major impetus for persons needing LTC services

Table 8-2. Use of Long-Term Care by Persons with Cognitive Impairment[33]

Setting	Approximate percentage of individuals who have cognitive impairment, Alzheimer's disease, or another form of dementia
Home care	37%
Adult day care services	≥ 50%
Assisted living	42%
Nursing home	64%

    a)   A large number of individuals who use LTC services have cognitive impairment.[33] See Table 8-2

G. Nursing Assistants

    1.   Nursing assistants provide the majority of hands-on care in LTC agencies, especially assisted living and nursing homes[34]

        a)   Certified nursing assistants (CNAs) working in a facility that receives Medicare or Medicaid payment must attend a Centers for Medicare & Medicaid Services (CMS) certified educational program and participate in yearly continuing education

            i.   This is different from being certified by the Hospice and Palliative Credentialing Center (HPCC) as a Certified Hospice and Palliative Nursing Assistant (CHPNA®). Certification focuses specifically on the individual and is an indication of current competence in a specialized area of practice. It is highly valued and provides formal recognition of basic hospice and palliative nursing assistant knowledge. Nursing assistants who have 500 hours in the most recent 12 months or 1000 hours of practice in the most recent 24 months in hospice and palliative nursing assistant practice under the supervision of a registered nurse[35]

        b)   Work under the supervision of a nurse as per state regulations

        c)   Care is mostly limited to providing assistance with ADLs

            i.   Nursing assistants can also provide some nonpharmacological methods of pain and symptom management[36]

                (a)   Consistency in caregivers

                (b)   Maintain resident dignity (e.g., providing choices)

                (c)   Treat each resident as an individual

                (d)   Relaxation and distraction (e.g., music, life-reviews, meaningful activities)

            ii.   Some states permit specialized types of care with additional education in certain circumstances (e.g., administering oral medication in assisted living, wound care)

        d)   As nursing assistants spend more time with the resident than any other healthcare provider in LTC, they provide valuable information and insights into resident's palliative care needs. Thus, they should be considered valuable members of the interdisciplinary team and included in team meetings[36,37]

e) Barriers to nursing assistants being full members of the team[37]

   i. Often little to no formal education

   ii. Limited access to continuing education

   iii. Unable to attend team meetings or care conferences given work schedules

   iv. A pattern of high work burden, job dissatisfaction, and decreased job commitment and morale leading to staff turnover, all of which can result in poor quality of care

     (a) Nursing assistant turnover is associated with residents' weight loss[38]

   v. Inability to obtain certification from Hospice and Palliative Certification Center (e.g., lack of financial resources to pay for study materials and testing fee, limited study time, limited experience with formalized testing, language barrier)

VII. Long-Term Care in the Community

A. Home Care Services

1. Short-term—provided by a home health agency following an acute health incident, that may or may not have required hospitalization, to patients who cannot easily leave their home. Home care includes in-home care by nurses, nursing assistants, therapies (e.g., physical, occupational), etc. with a rehabilitation goal of bringing the individual as close as possible to their pre-incident function. Once goals have been met, the patient is discharged. Home care is usually paid for by Medicare, Medicaid, or private insurance.

2. Long-term—provided by unpaid caregiver (e.g., family, friend) and/or privately paid caregivers (e.g., nurse, home health or home care aide, therapists) with the goal of keeping the person in their home as long as safely possible.[27] With proper education, unpaid and paid caregivers can provide some form of palliative care. See Table 8-3 for assessment of an individual's ability to remain living in his/her own home

Table 8-3. Assessment of an Individual's Ability to Remain Living in His/Her Own Home[27]

	Below are questions to ask—when answering questions, consider present and future needs. Note: For any negative answers • Can family/friends help? • Can person or someone else afford to pay for help/services/improvements?
ADLs/Instrumental activities of daily living (IADLs)	• Is the person capable of doing all or some of his/her own personal care? • Are home delivered meals available? • Does the person have opportunity for socialization and exercise? • Are assistive devises needed (e.g., grabbers/reachers, elevated toilet seats, utensils with padded grip, hearing aids)? • Is person capable of doing housework and yard chores?
Condition of home	• Is the bathroom and shower/bathtub accessible? • Are doorways wide enough for wheelchair and other equipment? • Are modifications needed to prevent falls and to make the living area more accessible (e.g., entry ramps, grip bars in shower, medical alert system, hand rails, adequate lighting, first floor bathroom)? • If the person is renting, will the property owner permit modifications to be made? • If the person owns a home that is subject to tenant agreements, are the modifications permitted?
LTC services/ Community resources	• Are adult day care centers nearby? • Are medical facilities nearby? • Is there convenient and affordable public transportation? If so, is the person capable of using public transportation? If so, can the person afford public transportation? • Is there someone to drive person on errands and appointments?
Financial issues	• Can the person afford to continue to live in his/her home (e.g., rent/ mortgage, groceries, upkeep, extra help)? • Does the person qualify for financial help (e.g., local Area Agency on Aging, Title III of Older American Act)?

ADLs—bathing, dressing, transferring to/from bed and/or chair, eating, caring for incontinence

IADLs—light housework, preparing and cleaning up after meals, taking medication, shopping for groceries and clothes, using the telephone, managing money, taking care of pets, using communication devices, getting around in the community, responding to emergencies (e.g., fire, fire alarms)

B.   Adult Day Care Services

1.   Services provided during the day at a community-based center. Programs address the individual needs of functionally- or cognitively-impaired adults. These structured, comprehensive programs provide social and support services in a protective setting during any part of a day, but not 24-hour care. Many adult day service programs include health-related services.[27] Palliative care can be provided in this setting

   a)   There are over 4800 adult day programs in the United States[26]

   b)   Participation can be full (80%) or partial day, 5 days a week (46%) or less, some programs offer services during weekends and evenings[39]

c) Three types of adult day care centers[39]

    i. Social—provides meals, recreation, and some health-related services

    ii. Medical/health—provides social activities along with intensive health and therapeutic services

    iii. Specialized—provides services to specific populations (e.g., dementia, developmental disabilities)

        (a) Dementia services—cognitive stimulations (90%), memory training programs

4. Although there is variation, most centers offer[39]

a) Social interaction and planned activities based on the individual's ability to participate

b) Home to center and back home again transportation

c) Meals and snacks, with attention to dietary needs

d) Assistance with ADLs

e) Exercise and mental interaction—80% offer physical activity programs for cardiovascular disease and diabetes

f) Interdisciplinary professional services (e.g., nursing [80%]; social work [50%]; case management [60%]; physical, occupational, and speech therapy [50%])

g) Caregiver support programs—educational programs (70%), caregiver support groups (58%), individual counseling (40%)

5. Benefits of adult day care services include potential to delay nursing home placement, enhanced quality of life for caregivers (e.g., lower exposure to stressors, reduction of burden on family caregivers), respite care, and enable caregivers to continue working[39,40]

C. **Supportive Services—Indirectly related to palliative care as transportation and meal services may allow an individual to remain as independent as possible**

1. Transportation

a) Once an individual is no longer able to be independent in their own transportation (e.g., cannot drive, ride, or have access to bus routes) or families/friends are not able to take the person in their vehicle (e.g., nonambulatory individuals requiring wheelchairs), alternative transportation is needed

b) Careful discussion and assessment are needed to determine if the individual is able to utilize alternative transportation alone

c) Alternative transportation varies in hours of service, availability of an escort to assist with navigating from the vehicle to the destination, availability of wheelchair transportation

d) Types of alternative transportation

    i. Door-to-door—reservation is made in advance to take the individual from their home to where and when he/she wants to go (e.g., shopping, appointments, entertainments, religious services), usually requires a fee[41]

        (a) Taxies—can be very costly if used on a regular basis and may not be available in all locations (e.g., rural areas), location determines if advance reservations are needed, hours of service

    ii.   Fixed route—scheduled transportation along a set route, usually requires a fee[41]

    iii.   Ridesharing programs—scheduled transportation to a specific place (e.g., appointments, nutrition sites, senior centers)[41]

2.   Meal services

    a)   For some individuals capable of living at home, assistance with meals may be needed if family/friends are not able meet all of the person's nutritional needs

    b)   Types of meal services

        i.   Well-balanced nutritious meals delivered to the individual's home by community-based services such as Meals on Wheels, usually inexpensive; subsidies are often available based on income[42]

        ii.   Meals provided as one of the services offered by a home health agency, cost depends on the level of care needed[42]

        iii.   Group meals provided at local care facilities (e.g., adult day care, senior centers); includes added advantage of socialization, cost varies based on other services provided; if transportation is not included, arrangements will need to be made at the person's expense[42]

        iv.   Hiring someone independently or through a home care service to cook meals in the person's home. Individual can assist with meal planning and preparation as able, providing both socialization and participation. Arrangements for purchasing groceries are needed and can be costly

VIII. Long-Term Care in Facilities

A. Group Homes and Institutional Settings (also called Board and Care Homes)

1.   Residential private homes designed to provide housing, meals, housekeeping, personal care services, and support to frail or disabled residents. At least 1 caregiver is onsite at all times. In many states, group homes are licensed or certified and must meet criteria for facility safety, types of services provided, and the number and type of residents they can care for. Group homes are often owned and managed by an individual or family involved in their everyday operation[27]

2.   Individuals with intellectual and developmental disabilities (IID) afflict nearly 5 million people in the United States[43]

    a)   Intellectual disability is defined as a disability characterized by significant impairment in intellectual functioning (IQ scores at or below 70), and in adaptive behaviors, and which has an onset before age 18[44]

    b)   Developmental disability is defined as severe or chronic disability that results from mental or physical impairment that begins before adulthood and that includes intellectual disability and conditions such as cerebral palsy, epilepsy, and autism.[45] Persons with developmental disability may or may not have subaverage IQ scores

3.   In the past 30 years, average life expectancy for persons with IID has approached that of the non-IID population[46]

    a)   Parental caregivers are no longer outliving their children with IIDs and this trend is expected to continue

    b)   The number of individuals with intellectual and developmental disabilities receiving long-term care services is nearly 600 000 and that number is expected to increase to over 700 000 by 2020

    c)   Currently over 340 000 IID persons reside in group homes or other institutional settings

4.   People with IID are as likely as the general population to suffer from serious or life-threatening illnesses such as heart disease, diabetes, and cancer

    a)   Persons with IID may be at increased risk for certain health problems that result from the underlying cause of their disability. For example, persons with cerebral palsy may have increased risk for swallowing disorders and aspiration pneumonias

    b)   Persons with Down syndrome have been noted to have earlier onset Alzheimer's disease more than the general population[47]

5.   Barriers to the provision of hospice and palliative care to persons with IID[48–50]

    a)   Late diagnosis of adverse health conditions as a result of

        i.   Decreased cognitive capacity; inability to understand health status

        ii.   Impaired communication ability; inability to verbalize complaints of pain and other symptoms

        iii.   Lack of recognition of symptoms by caregivers as a result of cognitive and communication limitations

    b)   Knowledge deficits exist among healthcare providers that lead to decreased access to end-of-life care for IID individuals

        i.   Lack of familiarity of IID caregivers in community and institutional settings, as well as at home, regarding hospice and palliative care

        ii.   Hospice and palliative care providers are often not well versed in the unique needs of the IID population. This may result in decreased outreach and quality of care

    c)   Ethical issues of autonomy, competence, and surrogate healthcare decision-making can create legal barriers affecting

        i.   Decisions to treat

        ii.   Decisions to withhold treatment

        iii.   Advance directives and do not resuscitate (DNR) status

6.   Strategies for providing quality hospice and palliative care for persons with IID

    a)   Develop trusting collaborative relationships with healthcare providers/caregivers in group home/institutional settings

    b)   Communication techniques that promote involvement of IID patients in the plan of care as much as possible[51]

        i.   Consult with caregivers about what comforts/frightens the individual

        ii.   Show interest in objects important to patient (e.g., dolls, toys)

        iii.   Allow extra time for explanation

iv.   Speak directly to patient (direct eye contact may not be recommended for autistic patients)

v.   Speak to adults as adults

vi.   Use of short, clear sentences

vii.   Use of pictures and diagrams

viii.   Use therapeutic touch if person is comfortable with being touched

ix.   Ask patient to repeat what they have heard

c)   Provide education regarding signs and symptoms that may indicate a palliative care evaluation is necessary

i.   New diagnosis of serious or life-threatening illness

ii.   Changes in level of functioning

iii.   Changes in behavior

iv.   Decreased activity

v.   Decreased appetite

vi.   Increased sleeping

vii.   Indicators of pain or other symptoms

d)   Collaborate with all members of the hospice IDT to develop a plan of care that addresses all domains of care for the IID patient

i.   Assess, manage, treat, and evaluate pain and other symptoms[52,53]

(a)   Allow time for comprehensive assessment

(b)   Utilize self-report when possible

(c)   Utilize validated scales such as the Non-Communicating Child Pain Checklist (NCCPC), or the Non-Communicating Adult Pain Checklist (NCAPC)

(d)   Utilize caregiver feedback

(e)   Recognize that achieving comfort may require a trial and error approach

ii.   Physical therapy/occupational therapy (PT/OT) can promote optimal functioning, assess for customized equipment needs

iii.   Speech therapists, in consultation with the nutritionist, can make recommendations for dietary consistency modifications, nutritional and adaptive equipment needs[47]

iv.   Social workers provide psychosocial support to patients, caregivers, family members, surrogate decision-makers, and other residents[54]

v.   Arts and music therapy can decrease depression, facilitate grieving, and improve quality of life for IID individuals[55]

vi.   Spiritual care needs of persons with IID are similar to the general population[55]

vii.   Support the bereavement needs of healthcare providers, family members, and, importantly, residents in the group home/institutional setting[55]

7. Goals for improvement in the delivery of palliative care for persons with IID in all settings are based on shared expertise of healthcare providers[48-50]

   a) Collaborative relationships between group home/institutional healthcare providers/caregivers and the palliative care interdisciplinary team are essential for quality end-of-life care

   b) Reciprocal education for healthcare providers

   c) Implementation of measures of success for the care of persons with IID

   d) Involvement of ethics committees to address complex issues facing healthcare providers and surrogate decision-makers

   e) Increased advocacy at the state and federal level to ensure persons with IID have access to palliative care

   f) Development of research initiatives to increase the body of knowledge of hospice and palliative care for persons with intellectual and developmental disabilities

B. Assisted Living

1. "Residential living arrangement that provides individualized personal care, assistance with activities of daily living, help with medications, and services such as laundry and housekeeping. Facilities may also provide health and medical care, but care is not as intensive as care offered in a nursing home. Types and sizes of facilities vary, ranging from small homes to large apartment-style complexes. Levels of care and services also vary. Assisted living facilities allow people to remain relatively independent"[27]

2. Facility and population characteristics

   a) Does not have skilled 24-hour nursing care onsite

   b) Respite care cannot be provided in an assisted living facility, because Medicare requires 24-hour nursing care availability at respite sites unless the individual or family pays privately

   c) Residents report an emphasis on healthy "aging in place" and curative therapies[56]

   d) Residents can often coordinate necessary specialized care from outside teams that travel to the site. This outpatient care can provide continuity when patients move between ambulatory facilities and facilities with around-the-clock skilled nursing care

   e) In some cases, an integrated care team and multiple levels of care (e.g., nursing home, memory care) are available as a part of the care services associated with that facility. Other assisted living facilities will transfer patients who need more intensive nursing care to other facilities as necessary

   f) Like nursing homes, assisted living facilities vary in size, staffing, relationships with local hospitals and outpatient providers, etc. Optimal palliative care delivery varies and is best created with input from assisted living and hospice teams

3. Patient, family, and provider perspectives on end-of-life care in assisted living[56]

   a) Patients in assisted living facilities report

      i. Minimal discussion about end-of-life choices with caregivers or adult children

      ii. A desire for information and discussion about legal and financial decisions

b) A similar desire to learn about medical interventions at the end of life

c) Family members report

    i. A desire for high-quality care that supports the comfort of the patient

    ii. Aging and symptoms of chronic disease can interfere with discussions about end of life

    iii. They would benefit from more information about the patient's options and medical situation

d) Assisted living staff report

    i. A need to begin educational outreach early

    ii. Financial or property concerns were raised more frequently than end-of-life or quality-of-life concerns

    iii. They did not always feel prepared to support discussions of end-of-life concerns with patients

C. Nursing Homes

1. There are 15 700 nursing homes in the United States, with less than 1% not participating in Medicare and Medicaid programs.[26,57]

2. Population and facility characteristics

a) A nursing home resident is most likely to be a white, widowed female between 75 and 84 years of age.[58] See Table 8-4 for demographics of nursing home residents

b) Most nursing home residents are admitted following an acute care hospital stay or from their private residence and had been living with family members or alone[58] (see Table 8-4)

c) Some nursing homes primarily focus on skilled care and rehabilitation of patients with a care goal of returning the individuals to their home, some primarily focus on LTC of residents who will not live independently again, and most offer a combination of services (> 90%)[27,28]

d) Optimal palliative care systems will vary and are best created with input from both nursing home and available consultants including palliative care and hospice teams[59]

Table 8-4. Snapshot of U.S. Nursing Home Residents*[57,58]

Characteristic			
U.S. nursing home residents	• > 1.4 million	• 0.5% of U.S. population	
Gender	• Female: 67.2%	• Male: 32.8%	
Age	• 0–30 years old: 0.5% • 31–64 years old: 14.4%	• 65–74 years old: 14.6% • 75–84 years old: 27.5%	• 85–95 years old: 35.3% • 95+ years old: 7.6%
Race/Ethnicity	• White, non-Hispanic: 78.9% • Black, non-Hispanic: 13.8%	• Hispanic or Latino: 4.9% • Asian: 1.7% • American Indian/ Alaska Native: 0.4%	• More than 1 race: 0.3% • Native Hawaiian/Pacific Islander: 0.1%
Needing assistance with ADLs	• 0–3 ADLs: 40.3%	• 4 ADLs: 36.8%	• 5 ADLs: 23%
Cognitive impairment	• None–mild: 35.2%	• Moderate: 26.2%	• Severe: 38.6%
Reporting of pain in previous 5 days	• None: 63.4%	• Mild/infrequent: 21.3%	• Moderate or severe: 15.3%
Clinical measures	• Incontinent: 37.2% • Antipsychotic use: 25.5%	• Feeding tube: 5.9% • Pressure ulcers: 5.9%	• Unintended weight loss: 5.9% • Any restraint use: 2.2%
Falls since admission or most recent MDS assessment	• No falls: 83.1%	• 1+ fall without injury: 11.5%	• 1+ fall with injury: 5.4%
Place of residence before admission to nursing home	• Acute care hospital: 36% • Private/semiprivate residence: 29%	• Other nursing home: 11% • Hospital-based skilled nursing facility: 9%	• Assisted living, board and care, or group home: 8% • Other institution: 4% • Unknown: 3%

Key: ADLs = activities of daily living; MDS = Minimum Data Set
*Data represents the U.S. nursing home population on December 31, 2011.

3. Need for palliative care in nursing homes

   a) Common medical diagnoses and conditions of nursing home residents include serious or life-threatening illness that would benefit from palliative care (e.g., diseases of the circulatory system, mental diagnoses, diseases of the nervous system and sense organs,[58] delirium, cancer[38])

   b) Pain is reported by 36.6% to 45% of nursing home residents[57,60]

      i. Nursing home residents have a high rate of untreated pain and may not report pain, believing it to be an expected part of aging[60]

      ii. Medication for nonpain symptoms of chronic life-limiting illness is underprovided[61]

      iii. Palliative care working groups and palliative care educational interventions may reduce the frequency of reports of pain[60]

iv. Barriers to effective pain and symptom management in nursing homes[25,36]

(a) Regulatory guidelines

(b) Staff's lack of knowledge and education

(c) Unclear goals of care

(d) Access to pain management therapies

(e) Limited policies and procedures to guide palliative care

(f) Staffing ratios (e.g., nurse-to-patient; CNA-to-patient)

c) Nursing home residents are at an increased risk for suffering[36]

i. Pain

ii. Often experience loss more than others with serious or life-threatening illness (e.g., independence)

iii. Diminishing quality of life related to dependence on others

iv. Unfamiliar routines

v. Inadequate symptom management with curative/restorative care goals

d) Variation of quality end-of-life care in nursing homes[62]

e) Many deaths occur in nursing homes, with 40% of the elderly projected to die in nursing homes in 2020[63]

4. Models of palliative care in nursing homes[25,64]

a) External palliative care consultation service—on request by an attending physician, a palliative care provider can consult on resident care. Educational support, end-of-life discussions, and other clinical care can also be provided through contract to the nursing home

b) Hospice partnerships—nursing homes can partner with palliative/hospice providers to provide specialist care on request

c) Facility-based teams and hospice units—in-house palliative care services can be provided by the nursing home

5. Barriers to palliative care in nursing homes

a) Nursing homes have high staff turnover and are usually understaffed[65]

b) Regulations can impede palliative care by considering normal signs of decline, such as loss of appetite with accompanying weight loss, as markers of poor or inadequate care, even though these symptoms are normal and expected in many chronic conditions[65]

c) Medicare reimbursement requirements and payment incentives can make it easier to pay for care that is not palliative, even if that care is not consistent with goals of care[65]

d) Nursing home staff do not generally have specialist education in palliative care[65]

e) A facility focus on rehabilitative care can make it more difficult to initiate discussions of palliative care or end-of-life care goals[56]

    f)   Barriers to hospice in nursing homes[63]

        i.   Conflicts between hospice and nursing home staff can arise over philosophy of care, so that clinical goals are in opposition to each other and priorities do not match

        ii.   The hospice plan of care may not be implemented as planned, including errors or time delays in medication ordering and delivery

        iii.   Regulatory conflict between nursing home and hospice providers can interfere with appropriate care

        iv.   Nursing home staff may view their end-of-life care as appropriate and hospice support as unnecessary

6.   Hospice care in the nursing home

    a)   Hospice care is for terminally-ill residents approaching end of life[66]

    b)   Nursing home residents have a longer average stay in hospice than enrollees in other settings, perhaps because they are more likely to have conditions with variable prognoses like dementia[61,67,68]

    c)   Nursing home residents have a significant need for symptom management and family support at the end of life[63]

    d)   Quality of care improves with hospice for those dying in nursing homes[68,69]

        i.   Fewer hospitalizations—patients prefer to die at home, and the facility is their home

        ii.   Symptom and pain management is improved

        iii.   Families report higher satisfaction with care at end of life

        iv.   Lower number of residents with feeding tubes

    e)   Hospice is not utilized for the majority of residents who die in nursing homes[68]

7.   Best practices for hospice in nursing homes

    a)   The best outcomes are achieved when teams from both providers collaborate with the patient to determine how to best meet patient goals of care[59]

    b)   Successful collaborations often feature[59]

        i.   A shared understanding between nursing home and hospice and a common goal established at the administrative level

        ii.   Consistent relationships between nursing homes and hospice facilities

        iii.   Establishment of a formal liaison

        iv.   Consistent use of strategies and tools for communication

        v.   Formal and informal educational outreach by hospice

        vi.   Nursing home staff who identify potential hospice needs

        vii.   Hospice staff with 24/7 availability

    c)   The nursing home must designate a clinical member of the interdisciplinary care team to coordinate with the hospice providers and the patient and family

8. Initial and periodic resident assessments in nursing homes using the Minimum Data Set (MDS) are required by CMS[70]

a) The MDS is "a core set of screening, clinical, and functional status elements, including common definitions and coding categories, which form the foundation of a comprehensive assessment for all residents of nursing homes certified to participate in Medicare or Medicaid. The items in the MDS standardize communication about resident problems and conditions within nursing homes, between nursing homes, and between nursing homes and outside agencies."[71, p. 6] See Table 8-6 at the end of the chapter for the 18 assessment sections

b) MDS assessments are completed electronically at specified times (e.g., admission, quarterly, annual, significant change, discharge, etc.) for a specific time period, which varies per section for all nursing home residents regardless of payer

   i. Combinations of MDS elements create triggers, which prompt staff to further assess residents who may be at risk for developing specific functional problems

c) MDS data is linked to reimbursement from Medicare and Medicaid as well as monitoring the quality of care given to nursing home residents

   i. The public has access to information (e.g., characteristics, staffing, quality care measures) about each certified nursing home at www.medicare.gov/nursinghome compare/search.html

d) A registered nurse must conduct or coordinate the assessment. Most nursing homes use registered nurse assessment coordinators (RNACs) in this position

   i. Nursing homes have flexibility to determine who else participates in the process

   ii. Ideally all staff should be consulted to ensure an accurate assessment of each resident

D.   Continuing Care Retirement Communities

1. Multiple levels of care on one campus including independent (retirement) living homes/ apartments, assisted living facilities, skilled nursing and rehabilitation units, and nursing home care

2. Hospice and palliative care can be provided at any level of living spaces

3. Benefits that can be offered

a) Flexibility in care, for example

   i. Residents in independent living apartments can arrange for in-home nursing assistant care

   ii. Independent living apartments can be kept available for a resident who needs to spend time in skilled and/or rehabilitation unit, if they are expected to recover to be able to live independently again

b) Offer community environment and many activities for each level of care

c) Medical and dental care often onsite

d) Ease of transition from level of care to the next

4. Burdens

    a) Can be very costly to the residents/family

    b) Long-term commitment may be needed

IX. Vulnerable Populations—Offenders

A. Facility and Population Characteristics

1. Prisons are required to provide appropriate medical care to offenders who are incarcerated at the facility

2. Care is generally provided onsite, though depending on the care required, moving inmates to an offsite correctional medical facility or hospital may be necessary

3. Inmates are more likely to have preexisting illnesses (including mental illness) and/or a history of or current chemical dependency than the populations served in nursing homes or assisted living facilities

4. Aging of inmates

    a) Incarcerated male and female older adults "age" faster than non-incarcerated adults due to a number of factors (see Table 8-5)[72,73]

        i. Increased vision and hearing impairments (as compared to non-incarcerated adults) could be the cause of rule violations

    b) The number of older incarcerated adults is growing at fast rate[72]

    c) Older incarcerated adults require more healthcare services than their younger counterparts[72]

    d) Cognitive impairment presents unique challenges in prison populations

        i. Limited ability to follow prison rules

        ii. Higher risk of psychological and economic victimization[72,74]

        iii. Offenders with dementia may no longer be able to comprehend the reason for their punishment[72,75]

Table 8-5. Contributing Factors to Faster Aging of Incarcerated Adults[72,76,77]

Functional	Health-Related	Higher Rates of Medical Conditions	Psychosocial
• Limited access to healthcare prior to incarceration • Functional impairments occurring earlier • Poor health practices throughout life • Lack of functional assistance (e.g., grab bars, level handles)	• Early onset of multiple chronic medical conditions, averaging ≥ 3 • Undiagnosed and/or untreated mental illness • Vision and hearing impairment • Incontinence • High rate of falls • Cognitive impairment • Substance abuse • Posttraumatic stress disorder • Previous traumatic brain injuries • End stage liver disease	• Hypertension • Diabetes mellitus • Pulmonary disease	• Unmet psychosocial needs • Feelings of being abandoned by God • Depression • Guilt • Worry • Psychological stress

5. Grief and mourning in the prison setting is complicated by a number of factors, which can lead to unresolved grief

   a) Dying offenders fear dying alone and being remembered only for the offenses they committed[73]

   b) Offenders, especially women, who have been incarcerated with the same people over a period of time develop bonds, which creates a community experience of loss when one of the inmates dies[73]

   c) Transfer to infirmary/prison hospital or hospice, isolates dying offenders from the support of their long-term fellow inmates as special permission is needed to visit[73]

   d) Variation exists in how offenders are notified of the deaths of family and friends.[73] Offenders are not usually permitted to attend mourning rituals (e.g., visitation at the funeral home, funeral and burial services)

   e) Notification of deaths from natural causes within the prison is often via informal channels[73]

   f) Public grieving of inmates may be curtailed to avoid appearing vulnerable[73]

6. Release of offenders to the community

   a) 600 000 to 700 000 offenders are released each year[72]

   b) Former offenders, especially older ones, transitioning to community living have a high rate of use of emergency departments and hospitalizations

      i. As medical benefits (e.g., Medicare, Medicaid) make take several months to be applied for or reinstated,[72] hospice care can be delayed

      ii.   Generally released offenders are only given a several weeks' supply of medications[72]

      iii.   Goals of prison discharge planning include reducing acute medical events, declining status requiring hospitalization, and costs as well as provide social service referrals and resources[78]

   c)   Compassionate release—early release of eligible, seriously ill offenders allowing them to die outside of prison[75]

      i.   Eligibility guidelines vary, requirements include that the offender must have a terminal or severely debilitating medical condition (or their functional status is such the justification for incarceration is undermined) from which they are expected to die from soon and that cannot be appropriately cared for within the prison, and does not pose a threat to society[75]

      ii.   The process starts with a written appeal then four levels of review resulting in an approximately 7% dying of offenders being awarded a compassionate release[75]

      iii.   Compassionate release is complicated by offenders who do not have a place to live due to estrangement from family and/or friends and were homeless prior to incarceration[73]

      iv.   Any offender who could potentially be awarded a compassionate release should be receiving palliative care[75]

      v.   Compassionate release offers significant savings costs to the prison system, though once out of prison healthcare will most likely be paid for by Medicare/Medicaid[75]

B. Palliative Care for Offenders

1.   Palliative care is the standard of care for terminally ill offenders and includes pain management[73]

2.   "Families of choice," included in decision-making and care, may include fellow inmates[79]

3.   Barriers

   a)   Decreased trust of the prison healthcare system by offenders (e.g., experiences of indifference to healthcare needs, providers lack of compassion and humanity),[73] and decreased staff support from security, may pose obstacles to appropriate care by the interdisciplinary team[79]

   b)   The high prevalence of chronic illness and the "aging" of offenders

   c)   Provider access to and support of patients can be restricted by or conflict with the rules followed by prisons to secure and manage offenders[80]

   d)   Prison staff have little prior experience or education supporting palliative care and palliative care providers have little prior experience with facilities for incarceration[80]

      i.   Staff may see an offender's politeness as trying to manipulate[73]

   e)   Drugs used for pain relief can also have illicit uses; the need for prisons to control access to drugs can inhibit their availability to patients and can delay implementation of changes in prescriptions.[80] Staff may question an offender's reports of pain, thinking that the offender is drug-seeking[73]

    f)   Prison environments are more punitive or rehabilitative than therapeutic[80]

    g)   Custodians of offenders may view suffering as appropriate care for offenders[80]

    h)   Friends and family are generally restricted in their ability to visit patients[81]

    i)   Offenders may not wish to share information that would support palliative care with providers if those providers are also prison authorities[81]

    j)   Volunteers may experience obstacles related to security and prison rules (e.g., offenders are not allowed to touch each other)[81,82]

4.   Hospice care in prisons

    a)   Though not subject to Medicare regulations, hospices in prisons follow similar guidelines as able

    b)   Care is provided in a section of the prison hospital by prison healthcare staff

    c)   Programs vary widely in how the program is organized

    d)   Offender hospice volunteer caregiver programs

        i.   All volunteers receive continuing education in hospice and palliative care appropriate to their responsibilities[79]

        ii.   In correctional facilities, volunteer offenders support the hospice program by providing needed care, expecting that other inmates will care for them when they need end-of-life care[79]

        iii.   Some prisons allow offenders to be hospice volunteers caring for fellow inmates on hospice. This volunteer work is above and beyond their assigned job and is not reflected in their record

        iv.   Offender volunteer aides provide physical care and support as do paid community nursing assistants (e.g., bathing, incontinence care, postmortem care). Additionally, offender caregivers protect the belongings of the patient and protect the patient from predatory abuse[74]

        v.   Offender volunteer caregivers improved the quality of care to dying offenders[74]

        vi.   Offender volunteer caregivers reported finding their own humanity and found value in being able to atone for their past offenses[74]

X. Vulnerable Populations—Veterans

A.   For the purposes of this section, a Veteran is anyone who has served in the military regardless of eligibility for Department of Veteran Affairs (VA) benefits

B.   Unique Veteran Issues

1.   One-fourth of all U.S. citizens who die each year are Veterans[83,84]

2.   Most Veterans do not receive VA benefits

3.   Posttraumatic stress disorder (PTSD)—though PTSD is not unique to Veterans, Veterans report PTSD 2.4 to 4.3 times more than the general population.[85] See Chapter VI, *Psychiatric/Psychological Symptoms and Diagnoses*, for more information about PTSD

4. End of life

    a) Sources of agitation and restlessness

        i. PTSD may present when terminal diagnosis is given or when actively dying as these may trigger memories and emotions of military experiences (e.g., combat, trauma)[84]

        ii. Life review is important for closure, though it may lead to anxiety, guilt, anger, and sadness in Veterans. Allow time for the Veteran to tell his/her story and for the family to listen[83]

        iii. Avoidance behaviors are common in Veterans[83] and may result in the Veteran coping by ignoring problems, which may appear as nonadherence. Isolation may result from avoidance behaviors as Veterans push away caregivers, family, and friends[83]

    b) Veterans are often comforted by being around other Veterans with a shared history of military service[86]

5. Pain management—as stoicism is valued in the military culture, it is important to build trust with Veterans so that they will report pain and know that their reports will be believed[83]

6. Female Veterans—there are 2 271 222 female Veterans; 10.3% of all U.S. Veterans.[87] The role of women in the military has greatly changed over time. Women are now in combat zones and exposed to the same physical and psychological traumas of war[83]

7. Homeless Veterans

    a) On a single night in 2012, there were 62 619 homeless Veterans accounting for 13% of all homeless adults, this is a decrease from 17.2% in 2009. Slightly more homeless Veterans were in shelters than unsheltered. Almost half of homeless Veterans were located in major cities[88]

    b) Of homeless Veterans living in shelters, the majority (88%) are 31 to 61 years of age, with 6% being 62 years of age and older[89]

    c) VA offers services to assist homeless Veterans, at-risk Veterans (e.g., very low-income, recently released from incarceration), and their families to recover from homelessness and live as self-sufficiently and independently as possible[90]

    d) Assistance includes community supportive services, vocational assistance job development and placement, transitional housing, permanent housing with continued support[90]

8. Incarcerated Veterans—benefits may be affected, outreach and case management is available for Veterans after release from prison[90]

C. VA Benefits

1. Through the VA, Veterans may be eligible for healthcare benefits at more than 1500 sites. Basic eligibility for VA benefits includes serving in the active military, naval, or air service and released under conditions other than a dishonorable discharge[90]

a) Potentially eligible service men and women include those who served in the U.S. Air Force, Army, Marines, Navy; World War II (WWII)-era Filipino Veterans (e.g., Old Philippine Scouts, Commonwealth Army Veterans); WWII-era Merchant Marine seamen; World War I (WWI) or WWII allied Veterans; World War Service groups (e.g., Woman Air Force Service Pilots [WASPs], Women's Army Auxiliary Corp [WAAC]); a complete listing can be found at www.va.gov/opa/publications/benefits_book/benefits_chap10.asp

2. The presence of service-related injuries and income level determine what VA benefits a Veteran is eligible to receive. All Veterans are encouraged to enroll in the VA healthcare system to determine if they are eligible for benefits. Though it is outside of the scope of this chapter to review all of the complex VA benefits, below is an overview of VA benefits that a Veteran may be eligible for that specifically pertain to the care of Veterans with serious or life-threatening illnesses[90]

    a) Preventative, acute, and chronic care at VA hospitals and community clinics[90]

    b) Disability compensation—monetary benefits paid to Veterans who are disabled by an injury or illness that was incurred or aggravated during active military service[90]

        i. Disability compensation for presumptive conditions—certain chronic diseases (e.g., multiple sclerosis, diabetes mellitus, arthritis) may be considered service-connected. Amyotrophic lateral sclerosis (ALS) is a presumptive condition if the Veteran served a minimum of 90 consecutive days. See Table 8-7 at the end of the chapter for information specific to former prisoners of war, Vietnam Veterans exposed to Agent Orange, Veterans exposed to ionizing radiation, and Gulf War Veterans[90]

    c) Prescription and nonprescription medication via VA pharmacy; private and Medicare supplemental health insurances may be billed; co-pay may apply[90]

    d) Reimbursement of healthcare travel costs[90]

    e) Mental healthcare treatment and residential rehabilitation (e.g., domiciliaries)—prior enrollment is not needed for mental health emergencies (e.g., suicidal, homicidal, symptoms of PTSD)[90]

    f) Nursing home care at VA owned and operated community living centers (CLCs), State Veterans Homes that are owned and operated by the states but receive VA funding if meet VA standards, and community nursing homes through a contract with the VA[90]

    g) Caregiver programs and services (e.g., income- and community-based care, respite care, caregiver education and training programs, family support services, travel)[90]

    h) Hospice care—all *enrolled* Veterans are eligible for hospice if they meet the clinical need for the service. Hospice care may be provided by the VA or an organization with a VA contract[91]

    i) Hospice volunteers with a service history provide Veteran-to-Veteran support through the Last Watch/No Veteran Dies Alone project[92]

    j) Burial in a VA national cemetery for Veterans, spouses, and dependents (e.g., gravesite, grave-liner, opening and closing of the grave, headstone or marker, perpetual care as part of a national shrine, burial flag, military funeral honors, financial assistance with funeral and burial [if not at a national cemetery])[90]

D. Communicating with Veterans

1. Most importantly just be present and listen

2. To determine if he/she served, simply ask "Did you serve in the military?"—some may not consider themselves Veterans (e.g., those who did not see combat, dishonorably discharged, etc.)

    a) If the answer is yes, it is appropriate to thank them for their service

    b) Sometimes the answer may be "No, but I wanted to, but . . ."—listen to these stories as well

3. Let the Veteran guide the conversation—if the Veteran wants to talk, he/she will

    a) Do not ask

        i. Questions about killing—even when necessary, many Veterans will always have difficulty with knowing they have killed someone

        ii. About being a hero—most Veterans, even those who received medals, do not consider themselves to be a hero

        iii. If their time in the military was like a movie or as bad as it looked in the movie—most movies are far from the reality and everyone's experience was unique

4. All Veterans have been impacted by the time they served in the military

E. Veteran End-of-Life Issues[93]

1. Culture influences how Veterans and others respond to each other and their environment. Military service is an acquired culture that continues to affect the Veteran throughout his/her life.[94] The military connection can have both a positive and a negative influence on Veterans with a serious or life-threatening disease and at end of life. For caregivers to provide holistic care to Veterans, understanding the cultural context is important. Some aspects will be a source of strength while others may be a source of distress

    a) Military service creates a

        i. Key impact in the lives of many Americans as they evolve from youth to adulthood. The experience may be something that is difficult for family and caregivers to accurately understand

        ii. Military values include loyalty, duty, selfless service, honor, integrity, and personal courage

        iii. One of the important aspects of military life is the development of stoicism. Stoicism is the ability to diminish the outward show of emotion, appearing indifferent to pain, grief, joy, and pleasure. Veterans have been known to have inconceivable stoicism in the event of illness.[94] Stoicism may also extend to suffering during a serious or life-threatening illness or at end of life and may lead to the underreporting of pain or symptoms

    b) Combat influences impact how a Veteran perceives illness and end of life

        i. Veterans are less likely to request life-prolonging medical treatment

        ii. Veterans often prefer for others to assist in completing advance directives

          iii.   Veterans prefer frank conversations with physicians and caregivers

          iv.   Pet therapy can provide a source of comfort for those having experienced combat

    c)   Different fears

          i.   Many have a fear of being alone when they die. Many Veterans have neither family nor close friends near to be with them at end of life. Approximately 65% of dying Veterans are not married and have poor support systems. Many of the Veterans develop psychological distress at end of life because of these circumstances.[94] The Veteran has learned of the strength of many and the power and wisdom of the group[94]

          ii.   Caution should be taken to not generalize Veterans recognizing that individual preferences supersede group norms[94]

F.   Veterans Health Administration[82]

1.   The VA provides palliative care to individuals who meet the service requirements established by the U.S. military, including home, domiciliary, respite, and nursing home care

2.   Every VA Medical Center is supported in palliative care provision by interdisciplinary consultant teams, national office program staff, and regional leaders

3.   An extensive electronic medical recordkeeping system supports continuity of care across the VA system

4.   Veterans may have health conditions related to service, including those stemming from exposure to nuclear, chemical, and biological agents, and those stemming from trauma

5.   Veterans have a higher rate of mental health conditions, such as PTSD, than the average palliative/hospice patient[95]

XI. Vulnerable Populations—Urban Poor

A.   Definition

1.   An income below the poverty threshold or level, which varies by size of family and is updated yearly[96]

2.   Examples of 2013 poverty thresholds[97]

    a)   Individual $\geq$ 65 years of age living alone—$11 173/year

    b)   A family of three people—$18 552/year

    c)   A family of six people—$31 932/year

B.   U.S. Population Below the Poverty Level

1.   48.5 million or 15.9%[96]

2.   Large metropolitan areas—37.7% of the population are below the poverty line[96]

C. **Effects of Poverty on Serious or Life-Threatening Illness**

1. Decreased health literacy[98,99]

2. Increased morbidity and mortality due to unhealthy lifestyle factors (e.g., poor nutrition, smoking, obesity), and poor socioeconomic status[100]

3. Increased hospitalizations. Use of the ED in lieu of a primary healthcare provider[101]

4. Increased suffering due to marginalization/social isolation[100]

D. **Barriers to Hospice and Palliative Care for the Poor[98–104]**

1. Lack of health insurance leading to

   a) Decreased access to care, notably preventive care

   b) Poor continuity of care

   c) Lack of coordination of care

   d) Inability to afford medication and other treatments

2. Mistrust of the healthcare system

3. Cultural and religious beliefs, which may inform the meaning of suffering

4. Language barriers

5. Transportation availability/affordability

6. Behavioral issues (e.g., no-show for appointments, substance abuse, opioid and other prescription abuse, psychiatric illness)

7. Lack of a primary healthcare provider to make referral

8. Lack of a formal caregiver and social support system

9. Substandard housing conditions; unreliable phone service and other utilities; unsafe neighborhoods

E. **Strategies for providing quality hospice and palliative care to the inner city poor[99,102–105]**

1. Increasing health literacy regarding hospice and palliative care. A 2008 study[98] showed no difference in racial/ethnic acceptance of hospice and palliative care services when compared with whites after a video education intervention. This may indicate that barriers to palliative care thought to arise from issues of trust, culture, and religion may be overcome by educational initiatives

2. Establishing trusting relationships based on

   a) Respect for persons

   b) Consistency in approach

   c) Providing material assistance (e.g., supplies, equipment, food)

   d) Having realistic expectations about what can be accomplished

3. Promoting racial and ethnic diversity in the palliative care workforce through training programs and hiring practices

4. Improved communication and collaboration with other healthcare providers to improve continuity of care across the continuum

5. Familiarity with community resources that are preexisting in neighborhoods

6. Remove stigma of providing care in crime-prone neighborhoods by utilizing escorts to ensure safety of healthcare workers

7. Use of inpatient palliative care consultation services to increase education and dispel myths about palliative care

8. Advocacy for better housing, insurance coverage, and community-based primary care services to improve quality of life for persons in inner city neighborhoods

XII. Vulnerable Populations—Homeless

A. Definition of Homelessness

1. Homelessness is being without a permanent home

2. Subcategories of homelessness[88]

   a) Chronically homelessness—continuously homeless for > 1 year or ≥ 4 episodes of homelessness in the last 3 years and has a disability

   b) Sheltered homeless—staying in emergency shelters, transitional housing programs, or safe havens

   c) Unsheltered—living in places not meant for human habitation (e.g., the streets, campgrounds, abandoned buildings, vehicles, parks)

3. Homelessness is often the result of a downward spiraling series of events—for example: poor health/health crisis of one of the members of the family → loss of job and/or ability to work accompanied by loss of healthcare insurance → loss of housing → limited personal support → homelessness[106]

B. On a single night in 2012, there were 633 782 homeless people in the United States[88]

1. 16% were chronically homeless

2. 62% were homeless as individuals (e.g., single adults, unaccompanied youths); 38% were homeless as persons in families (i.e., at least 1 adult and 1 child)

3. 62% were sheltered and the other 38% were unsheltered

C. Characteristics of Homeless Persons

1. As people come to be homeless from a variety of circumstances, their life before they were homeless (or if they have been homeless their entire lives) must be taken into account when planning care

2. With an average life expectancy of 41 years, homeless persons are 3 to 4 times more likely to die before those with adequate housing[106]

   a) Fair or poor health was reported by 46% of homeless people and can include co-occurring physical, psychiatric, substance use, and social problems[106–108]

b)   38% of homeless persons report having multiple chronic conditions (e.g., > 2 of the following: asthma, cancer, chronic bronchitis, diabetes, emphysema, heart problems, human immunodeficiency virus [HIV]/acquired immune deficiency syndrome [AIDS], hypertension, liver conditions, stroke, weak/failing kidneys)[106]

c)   Whether preexisting and/or related being homeless, severe mental illness (25%), including depression, and alcohol dependence (11%) are common[106]

d)   Homeless people are exposed to infectious diseases (e.g., tuberculosis, HIV, influenza, common cold), violence, extreme weather conditions[106]

e)   Major and minor injuries resulting from accidents or violence, can be difficult to heal due to lack of the ability to keep clean, bandage supplies, adequate rest, and good nutrition. These wounds can quickly become infected[106]

f)   Lack of healthcare leads to visits to emergency departments and hospitalizations, which do not improve overall health when the patient goes back to being homeless. Stable housing can improve health more than healthcare[106]

3.   Obtaining additional support is difficult. Social services income support is usually only available to those with dependent children living in very low-income households. Usually only small children, pregnant women, and those with a proven permanent disability can apply for Medicaid, which takes an average of 22 months to obtain, if found to be eligible[106]

4.   Twenty-one percent of homeless people have reported not having enough food. Of those who rely on soup kitchens and shelters, meals are often high in salt, sugar, and starch that lack balanced nutritional content. Lack of dental care leads to poor nutrition as well[106]

D.   Challenges of Providing Palliative Care to the Homeless

1.   Just as most people prefer to die at home, so do the homeless who consider their home to be where they are and feel comfortable (e.g., shelter, streets, substandard housing) and with the people they consider to be family[107,109]

a)   Hospitals and inpatient hospices may not be able to accommodate the homeless person's wish to continue smoking and other addictions and have their friends nearby[107]

2.   Flexibility is needed when planning palliative care for homeless persons, especially those with current drug and/or alcohol use, mental illness, and behavior issues[109]

3.   Pain relief interventions are hindered in many ways

a)   Substance abuse is very common.[106,107] See Chapter IV, *Pain Management*, for further information regarding treating pain in a person with a history of current or active substance abuse

b)   Protection of medications from being stolen requires a method of safe storage that the individual can access safely when needed[109]

4.   Homeless persons often fear and mistrust the healthcare system and many have never dealt with mainstream healthcare[107]

5. Mental illness can hinder discussion about the homeless person's care and advance directives[107]

6. Healthcare power of attorney and surrogate medical decision-makers may be difficult to designate/locate

7. Palliative care can be provided at homeless shelters[24,108]

XIII. Vulnerable Populations—Rural Dwellers

A. Definitions of Rural

1. U.S. Census Bureau—areas of less than 50 000 people or clusters of less than 2500 people[110] and less than 1000 people per square mile.[111] According to the 2010 U.S. Census, there are over 59.4 million rural dwellers in the United States making up 19.3% of the population[110]

2. U.S. Office of Management and Budget (OMB)—a city with less than 50 000 or more inhabitants or an urbanized area with less than 50 000 inhabitants and a total metropolitan statistical area (MSA) population of less than 100 000 (75 000 in New England). This definition includes the county of the central city and any surrounding counties that have economic and social ties with the central county[111]

3. Economic Research Service (ERS)/U.S. Department of Agriculture (USDA)—use codes to indicate degree of urbanization. Nonmetro codes are 4 (i.e., urban population of 20 000 or more, adjacent to a metro area) to 9 (i.e., completely rural or urban population of fewer than 2500, not adjacent to a metro area)

B. Characteristics of Rural Dwellers Related to Health and End of Life

1. Though each rural community is different, there are some characteristics of people who live in rural areas that pertain to palliative care.[112] Long and Weinert's seminal work on rural nursing theory described key concepts of understanding rural health needs and rural nursing practice—health is viewed as the ability to work; despite needing to travel long distances for healthcare (e.g., average 50 miles for routine healthcare), rural dwellers to not consider themselves isolated; self-reliance and reliance on healthcare providers; lack of anonymity; rural dwellers prefer to receive care from insiders/old-timers rather than outsiders/newcomers.[113] Lee and McDonagh found both support and nonsupport for these initial key concepts[114]

2. People

    a) Unlike the previous vulnerable populations, rural dwellers including both the patient and some if not all of their healthcare providers

    b) Due to small populations, rural healthcare practitioners are likely to know or be related to the dying person they are providing care,[112] which can complicate boundaries between personal and professional relationships[115]

    c) Family care providers in rural settings are more likely to have relocated in order to provide care than family in urban settings[116]

d) Rural elderly tend to be older, poorer, and have fewer physicians and dentists available for care[117]

    i. Rural dwellers, especially elders, wish to be connected to their community, want to have the freedom to control their level of independence, and feel isolated from much needed resources.[118] These 3 concepts can be conflicting when the rural dweller has a serious or life-threatening illness. For example, if a rural dweller lives in a community where the resources to treat her cancer are not available, she must go to an urban medical center thus losing her connection with her community and is no longer in control of her level of independence

3. Use of healthcare

a) Those who live in rural and remote areas have less access to palliative care, want to remain in their communities, and do not want to receive end-of-life care in urban centers.[119] This may explain why rural dwellers tend to delay seeking healthcare until very ill,[118,120] resulting in less frequent use of hospice and, when used, elect hospice care later in the disease course[115]

b) Few rural communities have formal palliative care programs despite having disproportionately higher elderly and chronically ill populations.[121] Only 20% of hospitals with 50 or fewer beds have palliative care programs[121]

c) As many are self-employed, they are less likely to have employer-provided healthcare, prescription, and drug coverage and Medicaid.[117] It is too soon to know if the Affordable Care Act will increase the numbers of rural dwellers who have health insurance

C. **Challenges to Rural Palliative Care**[112,115,116,122]

1. Many of the challenges of providing palliative care in rural areas are related to distance and remoteness[122]

2. Patient to healthcare services[122]

a) Depending on the remoteness and size of the town, there may or may not be healthcare services close by. If there are healthcare services close by, they may be limited. Travel to a metropolitan medical center, possibly in another state, may be needed for services such as major surgery, chemotherapy, and radiation therapy

b) Those who do need to travel for healthcare, usually need to travel with a support person

c) Financial hardships are incurred due to the cost of travel (e.g., gasoline, lodging, meals) when away from home. For patients with farms and ranches, being away may require hiring additional help to take over the work (e.g., feeding livestock, milking cows, watering crops) that the patient and/or their travel companion would have done

d) Due to distances to travel for healthcare, rural dwellers may not be able to make it home to die and are more likely to die in a hospital[118]

3. Home care/hospice nurse and other healthcare professionals to patient[122]

a) The distance between clients can be substantial, adding commuting time, impeding information sharing, and complicating scheduling of the care team members[116]

    i. Especially difficult for the hospice nurse to make a crisis or death visit as the hospice and nurse may be located in another town[122]

b)   Limited access to medications and supplies (e.g., incontinence briefs, dressing materials), durable medical equipment, and therapies

c)   Assessing for potential needs and preplanning, as much as possible, are imperative[122]

d)   With the need to cover a wide geographical area, nurses may experience emotional and physical isolation making team development activities (e.g., debriefing, memorial services) very important, even if by phone or video conferencing[24,122]

e)   Professional caregivers not from the community may be seen as "outsiders"

f)   Continuing education

　　i.   Educational resources and opportunities are difficult to access and infrequently scheduled, necessitating the need create opportunities for continuing education and use of online learning[112]

　　ii.   Few opportunities for networking with fellow providers to share knowledge; feelings of isolation due to geographical distances

　　iii.   Informal and even formal meetings between members of the care team are less frequent, because scheduling meetings when providers are serving a geographically dispersed caseload is a low priority[112]

g)   There is a general lack of access to specialized palliative care services. Some areas may have only a small number of physicians and nurses, who by necessity must be generalists. Some very small towns, may have only one nurse and one physician/advance practice clinician[118,121,123]

　　i.   As palliative care is a small percentage of his/her practice, staying current in palliative care as well as other areas is challenging[118]

　　ii.   With practice coverage challenges, opportunities for education (e.g., attend conferences, network with colleagues) and self-care (e.g., vacations) may be few[118,123]

　　iii.   To provide appropriate care, palliative care providers may often work alone and/or perform multiple roles, undertaking cross-training[115,121]

h)   Because they are members of a smaller community, rural palliative care providers are more likely to have social ties or nonprofessional relationships to their patients and the families, which can both strengthen and complicate therapeutic relationships[112,115]

i)   Telehospice, or the use of a telephone to connect with patients, and other ways to provide care remotely, such as web-based monitoring devices, can help support patients in rural areas when in-person providers are scarce or difficult to access[124]

4.   Both healthcare professionals and patients

a)   Barriers to adequate pain management in rural settings are similar to those in urban settings (e.g., lack of knowledge of pain management, fear of addiction)[125]

b)   Winter weather can amplify challenges of distance and remoteness[122]

c)   Members of rural communities report having a greater sense of connectedness (e.g., well-developed social networks, teams with strong interpersonal relationships), which can result in the entire community assisting with problem solving leading to better coordination of palliative care[122]

d)   Confidentiality is challenging as autonomy and privacy can be limited when caring for and being cared by people who live and work in a close knit community[122]

e)   Technology can assist in overcoming the challenge of distance—communicating via phone or video conference when an in-home visit is not imperative or necessary[122] as well as providing web-based education[123]

Table 8-6. Minimum Data Set 3.0 Assessment Areas[71]

Sections		Assessment
A	Identification information	Obtain key information to uniquely identify each resident, nursing home, and reasons for assessment
B	Hearing, speech, and vision	Document the resident's ability to hear, understand, and communicate with others and whether the resident experiences visual, hearing, or speech limitations and/or difficulties
C	Cognitive patterns	Determine the resident's attention, orientation, and ability to register and recall information
D	Mood	Identify signs and symptoms of mood distress
E	Behavior	Identify behavioral symptoms that may cause distress or are potentially harmful to the resident, or may be distressing or disruptive to facility residents, staff members, or the environment
F	Preferences for customary routine and activities	Obtain information regarding the resident's preferences for his/her daily routine and activities
G	Functional status	Assess the need for assistance with activities of daily living (ADLs), altered gait and balance, and decreased range of motion
H	Bladder and bowel	Gather information on the use of bowel and bladder appliances, the use of and response to urinary toileting programs, urinary and bowel continence, bowel training programs, and bowel patterns
I	Active disease diagnosis	Code diseases that have a relationship to the resident's current functional, cognitive, mood or behavior status, medical treatments, nursing monitoring, or risk of death
J	Health conditions	Document health conditions that impact the resident's functional status and quality of life
K	Swallowing and nutritional status	Assess conditions that could affect the resident's ability to maintain adequate nutrition and hydration
L	Oral/dental status	Record any oral or dental problems present
M	Skin conditions	Document the risk, presence, appearance, and change of pressure ulcers as well as other skin ulcers, wounds, or lesions. Also include treatment categories related to skin injury or avoiding injury
N	Medications	Record the number of days that any type of injection, insulin, and/or select medications were received by the resident
O	Special treatments and procedures	Identify any special treatments, procedures, and programs that the resident received during the specified time periods
P	Restraints	Record the frequency that the resident was restrained by any of the listed devices at any time during the day or night
Q	Participation in assessment and goal setting	Record the participation of the resident, family, and/or significant others in the assessment, and to understand the resident's overall goals
R	Care area assessment (CAA) summary	Document triggered care areas, whether or not a care plan has been developed for each triggered area, and the location of care area assessment documentation

Table 8-7. "Presumptive" Disability Benefits for Certain Groups of Veterans[126]

What is "Presumptive" Service Connection?

VA presumes that specific disabilities diagnosed in certain Veterans were caused by their military service. VA does this because of the unique circumstances of their military service. If one of these conditions is diagnosed in a Veteran in one of these groups, VA presumes that the circumstances of his/her service caused the condition, and disability compensation can be awarded. Go to www.VA.gov for more information.

What Conditions are "Presumed" to Be Caused by Military Service?

Veterans in the groups identified below—Entitlement to disability compensation may be presumed under the circumstances described and for the conditions listed.

Veterans within 1 year of release from active duty—Veterans diagnosed with chronic diseases (e.g., arthritis, diabetes, hypertension) are encouraged to apply for disability compensation.

Veterans with continuous service of 90 days or more—Veterans diagnosed with amyotrophic lateral sclerosis (ALS; Lou Gehrig disease) at any time after discharge or release from qualifying active service is sufficient to establish service connection for the disease, if the Veteran had active, continuous service of 90 days or more.

Former Prisoners of War

(1) Imprisoned for any length of time, ***and*** disability at least 10% disabling

- Psychosis
- Any of the anxiety states
- Dysthymic disorder
- Organic residuals of frostbite
- Posttraumatic osteoarthritis
- Heart disease or hypertensive vascular disease and their complications
- Stroke and its residuals

(2) Imprisoned for at least 30 days, ***and*** disability at least 10% disabling

- Avitaminosis
- Beriberi
- Chronic dysentery
- Helminthiasis
- Malnutrition (including optic atrophy)
- Pellagra
- Any other nutritional deficiency
- Irritable bowel syndrome
- Peptic ulcer disease
- Peripheral neuropathy
- Cirrhosis of the liver

Vietnam Veterans (Exposed to Agent Orange)

Served in the Republic of Vietnam between 1/9/62 and 5/7/75

- Acute and subacute peripheral neuropathy*
- AL amyloidosis
- Chloracne or other acneform disease similar to chloracne*
- Type 2 diabetes
- Ischemic heart disease
- Parkinson's disease
- Porphyria cutanea tarda*
- Cancers (i.e., multiple myeloma, chronic lymphocytic leukemia, B-cell leukemias, Hodgkin's disease, non-Hodgkin's lymphoma, prostate cancer, respiratory cancers [lung, bronchus, larynx, trachea], soft-tissue sarcoma [other than osteosarcoma, chondrosarcoma, Kaposi's sarcoma or mesothelioma])

*Must become manifest to a degree of 10% or more within a year after the last date on which the Veteran was exposed to an herbicide agent during active military, naval, or air service

Atomic Veterans (Exposed to Ionizing Radiation)

Participated in atmospheric nuclear testing; occupied or was a prisoner of war in Hiroshima or Nagasaki; service before 2/1/92 at a diffusion plant in Paducah, KY, Portsmouth, OH, or Oak Ridge, TN; or service before 1/1/74 at Amchitka Island, AK

- All forms of leukemia (except for chronic lymphocytic leukemia)
- Cancer of the thyroid, breast, pharynx, esophagus, stomach, small intestine, pancreas, bile ducts, gall bladder, salivary gland, urinary tract (kidneys, renal pelves, ureters, urinary bladder and urethra), brain, bone, lung, colon, ovary
- Bronchiolo-alveolar carcinoma
- Multiple myeloma
- Lymphomas (other than Hodgkin's disease)
- Primary liver cancer (except if cirrhosis or hepatitis B is indicated)

Gulf War Veterans (Undiagnosed Illness)

Served in the Southwest Asia Theater of Operations during the Gulf War with condition at least 10% disabling by 12/31/11. Included are medically unexplained chronic multisymptom illnesses defined by a cluster of signs or symptoms that have existed for 6 months or more, such as

- Chronic fatigue syndrome
- Fibromyalgia
- Irritable bowel syndrome
- Any diagnosed or undiagnosed illness that the Secretary of Veterans Affairs determines warrants a presumption of service connection

Signs or symptoms of an undiagnosed illness include fatigue, skin symptoms, headaches, muscle pain, joint pain, neurologic symptoms, respiratory symptoms, sleep disturbance, gastrointestinal symptoms, cardiovascular symptoms, weight loss, menstrual disorders

CITED REFERENCES

1. Dahlin C. Communication in palliative care: an essential competency for nurses. In: Ferrell BR, Coyne N, eds. *Oxford Textbook of Palliative Nursing*. 3rd ed. New York, NY: Oxford University Press; 2010:107-133.

2. National Quality Forum. *A National Framework and Preferred Practices for Palliative and Hospice Care Quality: A Consensus Report*. Washington, DC: National Quality Forum; 2006. www. qualityforum.org/Publications/2006/12/A_National_Framework_and_Preferred_Practices_for_ Palliative_and_Hospice_Care_Quality.aspx. Accessed October 14, 2014.

3. Malloy P, Virani R, Kelly K, Munevar C. Beyond bad news: communication skills of nurses in palliative care. *J Hosp Palliat Nurs*. 2010;12(3):166-174.

4. National Hospice and Palliative Care Organization (NHPCO). *NHPCO's Facts and Figures: Hospice Care in America*. 2014. www.nhpco.org/sites/default/files/public/Statistics_Research/2014_Facts_ Figures.pdf. Accessed December 16, 2014.

5. Golden R, Shier G. What does "care transitions" really mean? *J Am Soc Aging*. 2013;36(4):6-12.

6. Centers for Medicare & Medicaid Services (CMS). *Medicare Benefit Policy Manual Chapter 9— Coverage of Hospice Services Under Hospital Insurance*. 2012. www.cms.gov/Regulations-and- Guidance/Guidance/Manuals/Downloads/bp102c09.pdf. Accessed May 2, 2014.

7. Centers for Medicare & Medicaid Services (CMS). *Part D Payment for Drugs for Beneficiaries Enrolled in Medicare Hospice*. 2014. www.cms.gov/Medicare/Medicare-Fee-for-Service-Payment/ Hospice/Downloads/2014-PartD-Hospice-Guidance-Revised-Memo.pdf. Accessed October 14, 2014.

8. Centers for Medicare & Medicaid Services (CMS). Medicare and Medicaid Programs: Hospice Conditions of Participation. *Fed Regist*. 2008;73(109):32088-32220.

9. National Hospice and Palliative Care Organization (NHPCO). *Managing General Inpatient Care for Symptom Management*. 3rd ed. 2012. www.nhpco.org/sites/default/files/public/regulatory/GIP_Tip_ GIP_Sheet.pdf. Accessed August 5, 2014.

10. Centers for Medicare & Medicaid Services (CMS). 42 CFR Part 418. Medicare and Medicaid Programs: Hospice Conditions of Participation. *Fed Regist*. 2008;73(109):32088-32220.

11. Centers for Medicare & Medicaid Services (CMS). *Title 42 Public Health-Part 418 Hospice Care*. 2014. www.ecfr.gov/cgi-bin/text-idx?c=ecfr&rgn=div5&view=text&node=42:3.0.1.1.5&idno=42. Accessed October 14, 2014.

12. Wilke DJ. *Epidemiology of Death and Dying in the United States*. 2003. www.tneel.uic.edu/tneel-ss/ demo/impact/frame1.asp. Accessed September 12, 2013.

13. Hall MJ, Levant S, DeFrances CJ. *Trends in Inpatient Hospital Deaths: National Hospital Discharge Survey, 2000–2010. NCHS Data Brief, No. 118*. Hyattsville, MD: National Center for Health Statistics; 2013.

14. Murphy SL, Xu J, Kochanek KD. Deaths: final data for 2010. *Natl Vital Stat Rep*. 2013;61(4):1-17.

15. National Hospice and Palliative Care Association (NHPCO). *NHPCO Facts and Figures: Hospice Care in America*. 2012. www.nhpco.org/sites/default/files/public/Statistics_Research/2012_Facts_ Figures.pdf. Accessed April 28, 2014.

16. Chan G. End-of-life models and emergency department care. *Acad Emerg Med*. 2004;11(1):79-86.

17. Papadimos TJ, Maldonado Y, Tripathi RS, Kothari DS, Rosenberg AL. An overview of end-of-life issues in the intensive care unit. *Int J Crit Illn Inj Sci.* 2011;1(2):138-146. doi: 10.4103/2229-5151.84801.

18. Cox S, Handy JM, Blay A. Palliative care in the ICU. *The Intensive Care Society.* 2012;13(4):320-326.

19. Center to Advance Palliative Care (CAPC). *A State-by-State Report Card on Access to Palliative Care in Our Nation's Hospitals.* 2011. www.capc.org/reportcard/findings. Accessed October 14, 2014.

20. Walker KA, Mayo RL, Camire LM, Kearney CD. Effectiveness of integration of palliative medicine specialist services into the intensive care unit of a community teaching hospital. *J Palliat Med.* 2013;16(10):1237-1241.

21. Nelson JE, Bassett R, Boss R, et al. Models for structuring a clinical initiative to enhance palliative care in the intensive care unit: a report from the IPAL-ICU project (improving palliative care in the ICU). *Crit Care Med.* 2010;38(9):1765-1772.

22. Chung K, Burke SC. Characteristics of hospice patients utilizing hospice inpatient/residential facilities. *Am J Hosp Palliat Care.* 2013;30(7):640-647.

23. Office of Inspector General (OIG). *Medicare Hospice: Use of General Inpatient Care, OEI-02-10-00490.* 2013. oig.hhs.gov/oei/reports/oei-02-10-00490.pdf. Accessed October 14, 2014.

24. Gibson S, Bordofsky M, Hirsch J, Kearney M, Solis M, Wong C. Community palliative care: one community's experience providing outpatient palliative care. *J Hosp Palliat Nurs.* 2012;14(7):491-499.

25. Ersek M, Carpenter JG. Geriatric palliative care in long-term care settings with a focus on nursing homes. *J Palliat Med.* 2013;16(10):1180-1187.

26. Harris-Kojetin L, Sengupta M, Park-Lee E, Valverde R. *Long-Term Services in the United States: 2013: Overview.* Hyattsville, MD: National Center for Health Statistics; 2013. www.cdc.gov/nchs/data/nsltcp/long_term_care_services_2013.pdf. Accessed April 22, 2014.

27. U.S. Department of Health and Human Services (DHHS). *Find Your Path Forward.* 2014. longtermcare.gov/. Accessed April 9, 2014.

28. Department of Health and Human Services, Office of Inspector General (OIG). *Medicare Nursing Home Resident Hospitalization Rates Merit Additional Monitoring.* 2013. oig.hhs.gov/oei/reports/oei-06-11-00040.pdf. Accessed April 24, 2014.

29. Centers for Medicare & Medicaid Services (CMS). *Pub. 100-11 Programs of All-Inclusive Care for the Elderly (PACE®) Manual.* 2011. www.cms.gov/Medicare/Health-Plans/pace/downloads/R1SO.pdf. Accessed April 9, 2014.

30. Administration on Aging (AoA). *Older Americans Act and Aging Network: Frequently Asked Questions (FAQ).* 2013. www.aoa.gov/AoARoot/AoA_Programs/OAA/resources/Faqs.aspx. Accessed March 26, 2014.

31. Berkowitz RE, Jones RN, Rieder R, et al. Improving disposition outcomes for patients in a geriatric skilled nursing facility. *J Am Geriatr Soc.* 2011;59(6):1130-1136.

32. Gibson M, Gorman E. Contextualizing end-of-life care for ageing Veterans: family members' thoughts. *Int J Palliat Nurs.* 2010;16(7):339-343.

33. Alzheimer's Association. *2014 Alzheimer's Disease Facts and Figures.* Chicago, IL: Alzheimer's Association; 2014. www.alz.org/downloads/Facts_Figures_2014.pdf. Accessed May 9, 2014.

34. Head BA, Washington KT, Myers J. Job satisfaction, intent to stay, and recommended job improvements: the palliative nursing assistant speaks. *J Palliat Med.* 2013;16(11):1356-1361.

35. National Board for Certification of Hospice and Palliative Nurses (HPCC). *NA Overview*. 2014. hpcc.advancingexpertcare.org/competence/na-chpna/. Accessed October 20, 2014.

36. Carpenter JG, Berry PH. Refractory cancer pain in a nursing home resident. *J Hosp Palliat Nurs*. 2012;14(8):516-521.

37. Wholihan D, Anderson R. Empowering nursing assistants to improve end-of-life care. *J Hosp Palliat Nurs*. 2013;15(1):24-32.

38. Duncan JG, Bott MJ, Thompson SA, Gajewski BJ. Symptom occurrence and associated clinical factors in nursing home residents with cancer. *Res Nurs Health*. 2009;32:453-464.

39. National Adult Day Services Association (NADSA). *About Adult Day Services*. 2014. nadsa.org/learn-more/about-adult-day-services/. Accessed April 22, 2014.

40. Zarit SH, Kim K, Femia EE, Almeida DM, Savla J, Molenaar PC. Effects of adult day care on daily stress of caregivers: a within-person approach. *J Gerontol B Psychol Sci Soc Sci*. 2011;66(5):538-546. doi: 10.1093/geronb/gbr030. Epub June 3 2011.

41. FamilyCare American, Inc. *National Caregivers Library: Transportation and the Elderly*. 2013. www.caregiverslibrary.org/caregivers-resources/grp-transportation/transportation-and-the-elderly-article.aspx. Accessed April 23, 2014.

42. FamilyCare American, Inc. *National Caregivers Library: Meal Services*. 2013. www.caregiverslibrary.org/caregivers-resources/grp-home-care/hsgrp-nutrition/meal-services-article.aspx. Accessed April 23, 2014.

43. University of Colorado. *The State of the States in Developmental Disability*. 2013. www.stateofthestates.org/documents/UnitedStates.pdf. Accessed April 27, 2014.

44. American Association on Intellectual and Developmental Disabilities (AAIDD). *Definition of Intellectual Disability*. 2013. aaidd.org/intellectual-disability/definition#.U16E3ZpOXq4. Accessed April 27, 2014.

45. State of California Department of Developmental Services (DDS). *Information about Developmental Disabilities*. 2014. www.dds.ca.gov/general/info_about_dd.cfm. Accessed April 28, 2014.

46. Braddock D. Summary of national trends: the state of the states in developmental disabilities. *Public Hearing Populations in Need of LTSS and Service Delivery Issues*. 2013. ltccommission.lmp01.lucidus.net/wp-content/uploads/2013/12/July-17-Official-Testimony.pdf. Accessed December 11, 2014.

47. Rosenzweig L. Serving the aging developmentally disabled population. *Topics in Clinical Nutrition*. 2008;23(2):98-102.

48. Hahn JE, Cadogan MP. Development and evaluation of a staff training program on palliative care for persons with intellectual and developmental disabilities. *J Policy Pract Intellect Disabil*. 2011;8(1):42-52.

49. Stein GL. Providing palliative care to people with intellectual disabilities: services, staff knowledge and challenges. *J Palliat Med*. 2008;11(9):1241-1248.

50. Cross H, Cameron MA, March S, Tuffrey-Wijne I. Practical approaches toward improving end-of-life care for people with intellectual disabilities: effectiveness and sustainability. *J Palliat Med*. 2012;15(3):322-326.

51. Chew KL, Iacono T, Tracy J. Overcoming communication barriers: working with patients with intellectual disabilities. *Aust Fam Physician*. 2009;38(1-2):10-14.

52. Breau L, Burkitt C. Assessing pain in children with intellectual disabilities. *Pain Res Manag*. 2009;14(2):116-120.

53. Lotan M, Moe-Nilssen R, Ljunggren AE, Strand LI. Measurement properties of the non-communicating adult pain checklist (NCAPC): a pain scale for adults with intellectual and developmental disabilities, scored in a clinical setting. *Res Dev Disabil.* 2010;31(2):367-375.

54. Tuffrey-Wijne I, Hogg J, Curfs L. End-of-life and palliative care for people with intellectual disabilities who have cancer or other life-limiting illness: a review of the literature and available resources. *J Appl Res Intellect Disabil.* 2007;20:331-344.

55. Ailey SH, O'Rourke M, Breakwell S, Murphy A. Supporting a community of individuals with intellectual and developmental disabilities in grieving. *J Hosp Palliat Nurs.* 2008;10(5):285-292.

56. Schaffer MA, Keenan K, Zwirchitz F, Tierschel L. End-of-life discussion in assisted living facilities. *J Hosp Palliat Nurs.* 2012;14(1):13-24.

57. Centers for Medicare & Medicaid Services (CMS). *Nursing Home Data Compendium: 2012 Edition.* 2012. www.cms.gov/Medicare/Provider-Enrollment-and-Certification/CertificationandComplianc/Downloads/nursinghomedatacompendium_508.pdf. Accessed March 26, 2014.

58. Jones AL, Dwyer LL, Bercovitz AR, Strahan GW; National Center for Health Statistics. The National Nursing Home Survey: 2004 overview. *Vital Health Stat.* 2009;13(167):1-164.

59. Miller SC. A model for successful nursing home-hospice partnerships. *J Palliat Med.* 2010;13(5):525-533.

60. Long CO, Morgan BM, Alonzo TR, Mitchell KM, Bonnell DK, Beardsley ME. Improving pain management in long-term care: the campaign against pain. *J Hosp Palliat Nurs.* 2010;12(3):148-155.

61. Rodriguez KL, Hanlon JT, Perera SS, Jaffe EJ, Sevick MA. A cross-sectional analysis of the prevalence of undertreatment of nonpain symptoms and factors associated with undertreatment in older nursing home hospice/palliative care patients. *Am J Geriatr Pharmacother.* 2010;8(3):225-232.

62. Thompson SA, Bott M, Gajewski B, Tilden VP. Quality of care and quality of dying in nursing homes: two measurement models. *J Palliat Med.* 2012;15(6):690-695.

63. Martz K, Gerding A. Perceptions of coordination of care between hospice and skilled nursing facility care providers. *J Hosp Palliat Nurs.* 2011;13(4):210-221.

64. Center to Advance Palliative Care (CAPC). *Improving Palliative Care in Nursing Homes.* 2008. www.capc.org/capc-resources/capc_publications/nursing_home_report.pdf. October 14, 2014.

65. Meier DE, Lim B, Carlson MD. Raising the standard: palliative care in nursing homes. *Health Aff.* 2010;29(1):136-140. doi: 10.1377/hlthaff.2009.0912.

66. Weckmann MT, Freund K, Bay C, Broderick A. Medical manuscripts impact of hospice enrollment on cost and length of stay of a terminal admission. *Am J Hosp Palliat Care.* 2013;30(6):576-578.

67. Huskamp HA, Stevenson DG, Grabowski DC, Brennan E, Keating NL. Long and short hospice stays among nursing home residents at the end of life. *J Palliat Med.* 2010;13(8):957-963.

68. Unroe KT, Sachs GA, Hickman SE, Stump TE, Tu W, Callahan CM. Hospice use among nursing home patients. *J Am Med Dir Assoc.* 2013;14(4):254-259.

69. Mukamel DB, Caprio T, Ahn R, et al. End-of-life quality-of-care measures for nursing homes: place of death and hospice. *J Palliat Med.* 2012;15(4):438-446.

70. Carpenter JG. Physical aspects of care. In: Stafford C, ed. *Core Curriculum for the Long-Term Care Nurse.* Pittsburgh, PA: Hospice and Palliative Nurses Association; 2012:11-58.

71. Centers for Medicare & Medicaid Services (CMS). *Long-Term Care Facility Resident Assessment Instrument User's Manual. Version 3.0.* Washington, DC: CMS; 2013.

72. Williams BA, Goodwin JS, Bailargeon J, Ahalt C, Walter LC. Addressing the aging crisis in U.S. criminal justice health care. *J Am Geriatr Soc.* 2012;60(6):1150-1156.

73. Loeb SJ, Penrod J, Hollenbeak CS, Smith CA. End-of-life care and barriers for female inmates. *J Obstet Gynecol Neonatal Nurs.* 2011;40(4):477-485.

74. Loeb SJ, Hollenbeak CS, Penrod J, Smith CA, Kitt-Lewis E, Crouse SB. Care and companionship in an isolating environment: inmates attending to dying peers. *J Forensic Nurs.* 2013;9(1):1-15.

75. Williams BA, Sudore RL, Greifinger R, Morrison RS. Balancing punishment and compassion for seriously ill prisoners. *Ann Intern Med.* 2011;155(2):122-126.

76. Williams BA, Stern MF, Mellow J, Safer M, Greifinger RB. Aging in correctional custody: setting a policy agenda for older prisoner health care. *Am J Public Health.* 2010;102(8):1475-1481.

77. Phillips LL, Allen RS, Harris GM, Presnell AH, DeCoster J, Cavanaugh R. Aging prisoners' treatment selection: does prospect theory enhance understanding of end-of-life medical decisions? *Gerontologist.* 2011;51(5):663-674.

78. May JP, Hamid N. Enhancing continuity of care through medical discharge planning in a large urban jail system. *Correctional Health Today.* 2009;1(1):43-48.

79. Stone K, Papadopoulos I, Kelly D. Establishing hospice care for prison populations: an integrative review assessing the UK and USA perspective. *Palliat Med.* 2012;26(8):969-978. doi: 10.1177/0269216311424219. Epub October 12, 2011.

80. Turner M, Payne S, Barbarachild Z. Care or custody? An evaluation of palliative care in prisons in North West England. *Palliat Med.* 2011;25(4):370-377.

81. Wood FJ. The challenge of providing palliative care to terminally ill prison inmates in the UK. *Int J Palliat Nurs.* 2007;13(3):131-135.

82. Shreve S. Hospice and palliative care by the VA, beyond the VA. *Am Soc Aging.* 2010;34(2):49-56.

83. Erickson-Hurt C. Care of Veterans. In: Dahlin CM, Lynch MT, eds. *Core Curriculum for the Advanced Practice Hospice and Palliative Registered Nurse.* 2nd ed. Pittsburgh, PA: Hospice and Palliative Nurses Association; 2013:545-566.

84. Running A, Shumaker N, Clark J, Dunaway L, Tolle LW. Veteran preferences for end-of-life care. *Int J of Older People Nurs.* 2009;4:41-47. doi 10.1111/j.1748-3743.200888.00134.x.

85. Gradus JL. *Epidemiology of PTSD.* Washington DC: National Center for PTSD; 2014. www.ptsd.va.gov/professional/PTSD-overview/epidemiological-facts-ptsd.asp. Accessed May 5, 2014.

86. Gibson M, Gorman E. Contextualizing end-of-life care for ageing Veterans: family members' thoughts. *Int J Palliat Nurs.* 2010;16(7):339-343.

87. Department of Veterans Affairs. *Fact Sheet: Woman Veterans Population.* Washington DC: Office of Public Affairs Media Relations; 2013.

88. U.S. Department of Housing and Urban Development, Office of Community Planning and Development (ONECPD). *The 2012 Point-in-Time Estimates of Homelessness: Volume I.* 2012. www.onecpd.info/resources/documents/2012AHAR_PITestimates.pdf. Accessed May 6, 2014.

89. National Center for Veterans Analysis and Statistics. *Profile of Sheltered Homeless Veterans for Fiscal Years 2009 and 2010.* 2012. www.va.gov/vetdata/docs/SpecialReports/Homeless_Veterans_2009-2010.pdf. Accessed May 6, 2014.

90. U.S. Department of Veterans Affairs. *Federal Benefits for Veterans, Dependents, and Survivors.* Washington, DC: Department of Veterans Affairs; 2013. www.va.gov/opa/publications/benefits_book.asp. Accessed May 5, 2014.

91. U.S. Department of Veterans Affairs. *Geriatrics and Extended Care: Hospice and Palliative Care.* 2014. www.va.gov/GERIATRICS/Guide/LongTermCare/Hospice_and_Palliative_Care.asp#. Accessed May 6, 2014.

92. Gerber PS. Last watch: developing an inpatient palliative volunteer program for U.S. Veterans in hospice. *Omega.* 2013;67(1-2):87-95.

93. Deja K, Samuels C, Schauer CJ. Special needs of the Veteran. In: Stafford C, ed. *Core Curriculum for the Long-Term Care Nurse.* Pittsburgh, PA: Hospice and Palliative Nurses Association; 2012:158-170.

94. Emanuel LL, Hauser JM, Bailey FA. *EPEC for Veterans: Education in Palliative and End-of-Life Care for Veterans.* Chicago, IL and Washington, DC: U.S. Department of Veterans Affairs; 2010.

95. Casarett D, Pickard A, Bailey A, et al. A nationwide VA palliative care quality measure: the family assessment of treatment at the end of life. *J Palliat Med.* 2008;11(1):68-75.

96. Bishaw A. *American Community Survey Briefs: Poverty: 2010 and 2011.* Washington DC: U.S. Census Bureau; 2012:1-8.

97. U.S. Department of Commerce. *Preliminary Estimate of Weighted Average Poverty Thresholds for 2013.* Washington, DC: Bureau of the Census; 2014. www.census.gov/hhes/www/poverty/data/threshld/index.html. Accessed May 12, 2014.

98. Volandes A, Paasche-Orlow M, Gillick M, et al. Health literacy not race predicts end-of-life care preferences. *J Palliat Med.* 2008;11(5):754-762.

99. O'Mahony S, McHenry J, Snow D, Cassin C, Schumacher D, Selwyn PA. A review of barriers to utilization of the Medicare Hospice Benefits in urban populations and strategies for enhanced access. *J Urban Health.* 2008;85(2):281-290.

100. Francoeur RB Payne R, Raveis VH, Shim H. Palliative care in the inner city: patient religious affiliation, underinsurance, and symptom attitude. *Cancer Supplement.* 2007;109(2):425-434.

101. Hughes A. Poor, homeless, and underserved populations. In: Ferrell BR, Coyle N. *Oxford Textbook of Palliative Nursing.* 3rd ed. New York, NY: Oxford University Press; 2010:745-755.

102. Born W, Grenier KA, Sylvia E, Butler J, Ahluwalia JS. Knowledge, attitudes, and beliefs about end-of-life care among inner city African Americans and Latino/Hispanic Americans. *J Palliat Med.* 2004;7(2):247-256.

103. Enguidanos S, Vesper E, Goldstein R. Ethnic difference in hospice enrollment following inpatient palliative care consultation. *J Hosp Med.* 2013;8(10):598-600. doi: 10.1002/jhm.2078. Epub September 10, 2013.

104. Gibson R. Palliative care for the poor and disenfranchised: a view from the Robert Wood Johnson Foundation. *J R Soc Med.* 2001;94(9):486-489.

105. Dy SM, Reder EA, McHale JM, Clayton RR, Silva C. Caring for patients in an inner-city home hospice: challenges and rewards. *Home Health Care Management & Practice.* 2003;15(4):291-299.

106. National Health Care for the Homeless Council (NHCHC). *Homelessness & Health: What's the Connection?* 2011. www.nhchc.org/wp-content/uploads/2011/09/Hln_health_factsheet_Jan10.pdf. Accessed May 8, 2014.

107. Collier R. Bringing palliative care to the homeless. *Canadian Med Assoc J.* 2011;183(6):E317-E3128. doi: 10.1503/cmaj.109-3756.

108. Podymow T, Turnbull J, Coyle D. Shelter-based palliative care for the homeless terminally ill. *Palliat Med.* 2006;20(2):81-86.

109. MacWilliam J, Bramwell M, Brown S, O'Connor M. Reaching out to Ray: delivering palliative care services to a homeless person in Melbourne, Australia. *Int J Palliat Nurs.* 2014;20(2):83-88.

110. United States Census Bureau. *2010 Census Urban and Rural Classification and Urban Area Criteria.* 2013. www.census.gov/geo/reference/ua/urban-rural-2010.html. Accessed March 25, 2014.

111. Reynnells L, John PL, Rural Information Center. *What is Rural?* 2013. www.nal.usda.gov/ric/ricpubs/what_is_rural.shtml. Accessed April 24, 2014.

112. Arnaert A, Seller R, Wainwright M. Homecare nurses' attitudes toward palliative care in a rural community in Western Quebec. *J Hosp Palliat Nurs.* 2009;11(4):202-208.

113. Long KA, Weinert C. From rural nursing: developing the theory base. *Sch Inq Nurs Pract.* 1989;3:113-127.

114. Lee HJ, McDonagh MK. Updating the rural nursing theory base. In: Winters CA, ed. *Rural Nursing: Concepts, Theory, and Practice.* 4th ed. New York, NY: Springer Publishing Co., LLC; 2013:16-34.

115. Robinson CA, Pesut B, Bottorff JL, Mowry A, Broughton S, Fyles G. Rural palliative care: a comprehensive overview. *J Palliat Med.* 2009;12(3):253-258.

116. Brazil K, Kaasalainen S, Williams A, Rodriguez C. Comparing the experiences of rural and urban family caregivers of the terminally ill. *Rural Remote Health.* 2013;13(1):2250.

117. Rural Assistance Center (RAC). *Rural Health Disparities.* 2013. www.raconline.org/topics/rural-health-disparities. Accessed May 7, 2014.

118. Duggleby WD, Penz K, Leipert BD, Wilson DM, Goodridge D, Williams A. 'I am part of the community but . . .' The changing context of rural living for persons with advanced cancer and their families. *Rural Remote Health.* 2011;11(1733):online.

119. Kelley ML, Williams A, DeMiglio I, Mettam H. Developing rural palliative care: validating a conceptual model. *Rural Remote Health.* 2011;11:1717.

120. Buehler JA, Malone M, Majerus-Wegerhoff JM. Patterns of responses to symptoms in rural residents: the symptom-action-timeline process. In: Winters CA, ed. *Rural Nursing: Concepts, Theory, and Practice.* 4th ed. New York, NY: Springer Publishing Company; 2013:131-139.

121. Ceronsky L, Shearer J, Weng K, Hopkins M, McKinley D. Minnesota rural palliative care initiative: building palliative care capacity in rural Minnesota. *J Palliat Med.* 2013;16(3):310-313. doi: 10.1089/jpm.2012.0324.

122. Mayer DM, Murphy R. Palliative care at the end of life: a rural family perspective. In: Winters CA, ed. *Rural Nursing: Concepts, Theory, and Practice.* 4th ed. New York, NY: Springer Publishing Company; 2013:119-129.

123. Fink RM, Oman KS, Youngwerth J, Bryant LL. A palliative care needs assessment of rural hospitals. *J Palliat Med.* 2013;16(6):638-644. doi: 10.1089/jpm.2012.0574.

124. Oliver DP Demiris G, Wittenberg-Lyles E, Washington K, Day T, Novak H. A systematic review of the evidence base for telehospice. *Telemed J E Health.* 2012;18(1):38-47.

125. Jablonski K, Duke G. Pain management in persons who are terminally ill in rural acute care: barriers and facilitators. *J Hosp Palliat Nurs.* 2012;14(8):533-540.

126. U.S. Department of Veterans Affairs (VA). *Disability Compensation: "Presumptive" Disability Benefits.* 2011. www.benefits.va.gov/BENEFITS/factsheets/serviceconnected/presumption.pdf. Accessed October 6, 2014.

CHAPTER IX

ADVANCE CARE PLANNING AND GOALS OF CARE

Beverly J. Douglas, MSN, GNP-BC, ACHPN®, ARNP
Catherine Parsons Emmett, PhD, ARNP, ACHPN®

I.   Introduction

   A.   Advance care planning (ACP) enables individuals who are no longer able to speak for themselves convey their preferences for medical treatment.[1] ACP has been identified as a process that can involve steps, including initiation of the topic, disclosure of information, identification of a surrogate decision-maker, discussion of treatment options, and elicitation of patient values in collaboration with healthcare professionals and significant others.[2] Nurses play a crucial role in ACP as an advocate to elicit the patients' autonomous preferences as well as assisting in clarifying treatment options that patients may not understand[3]

II. Goals of Advance Care Planning

   A.   Enhance patient and family knowledge about their illness, including prognosis and likely outcomes of alternative care plans

   B.   Define key priorities in end-of-life care and develop a plan that addresses these issues

   C.   Shape future clinical care to fit the patient's preferences and values[4]

III. Definitions

   A.   Advance directives
      1.   A way for adults (18 years and older with capacity to make decisions) to communicate their wishes regarding treatment decisions and/or to designate a decision-maker when they may lack capacity or ability to speak for themselves, thus maintaining their autonomy[5]
      2.   May be communicated orally and/or in writing

3.   Living wills are a form of an advance directive that may specify whether life-sustaining treatments should be maintained or implemented in certain situations (e.g., terminal illness, persistent vegetative state, end stage disease); does not require a provider signature

4.   Many states allow the designation of a substitute decision-maker, referred to as the surrogate or proxy, or through a power of attorney that designates healthcare decision-making[6]

5.   Physician/Provider/Medical Orders for Life-Sustaining Treatments (POLST/MOLST) Paradigm Program

   a)   The program seeks to improve quality of life at the end of life, through communication of patient's wishes, documentation of medical orders on a standardized form that is transferable and recognized by healthcare professionals across different healthcare settings

   b)   This form differs from an advance directive in that it is a provider order form that requires a provider signature; who can sign a POLST/MOLST form varies from state to state; sometimes printed on brightly colored paper, but this also varies from state to state

   c)   Designed for individuals who are chronically ill, frail, and elderly or whose death in the next year would not be a surprise

   d)   This medical order form addresses four categories of treatment: cardiopulmonary resuscitation (CPR); medical interventions; antibiotics; and medically administered nutrition and hydration

   e)   Form is currently recognized in 15 states and is in development/pilot in 29 states[7]

   f)   A recent study demonstrated that this tool has been useful in ensuring that individual treatment preferences are honored[8]

B.   **ACP—a process that includes**

1.   Discussing goals of care based on the patient's current health situation

2.   Conversations regarding knowledge and attitudes toward life-sustaining treatments such as mechanical ventilation

3.   Providing information and documenting preferences for care (e.g., location of care, symptom management)

4.   May or may not include the completion of an advance directive, but can also include review and updating of documents with final application in identified situations

C.   **The process of ACP should include information sharing and decision-making**

1.   Information sharing

2.   Gather information—what does the patient know about his/her medical condition?

3.   Any ACP conversations in the past?

4.   Has a decision-maker been appointed? If so, have they had a conversation with their decision-maker about goals and preferences?

5. What has been his/her end-of-life experiences, if any, with other family members or close others?

6. Clarify goals and priorities of care

7. Estimate of prognosis, including if possible, an estimation of time remaining

8. Description of disease progression, including symptoms, and available treatments (e.g., artificial nutrition and hydration, pacemaker and/or defibrillator)

9. Acceptable quality of life (e.g., desired balance of pain and symptom relief with sedation)

10. Preferred place of death, organ/tissue donation, funeral arrangements

11. Educate the patient and family about disease progression, benefits and burdens of treatment, and what is possible given diagnosis and prognosis

12. Decision-making

13. Find out what the patient understands about available treatment options (e.g., palliative and hospice care)

14. Find out what the patient knows about his/her condition and what he/she expects to happen

15. Explain the risks and benefits of possible treatments that may be offered, may be in place for that patient's medical situation

16. Answer questions[9]

17. Speak in easily understood terminology and language, ask patient to repeat their understanding of what is being said

18. Provide information specific to the patient's situation

19. Identify a healthcare decision-maker should the patient be unable to speak for themselves

20. Determine goals of care[4]

21. Life-prolonging treatment

22. Limited life-prolonging treatment with defined trial of therapy discussed

23. Comfort-oriented treatment

D. Explore other ACP issues as appropriate (assisted living facility [ALF], nursing home, hospice, organ donation) and collaborate with other healthcare providers as needed

E. Document all discussions in the medical record; assist in the completion of advance directives per state law

1. Many states recognize an out-of-hospital do-not-resuscitate (DNR) order

2. How it is communicated varies from state to state (i.e., bracelets, signed forms); in many states, POLST/MOLST forms are taking the place of out-of-hospital DNR orders

3. Signed by the patient's provider; varies from state to state

4. Is recognized by emergency medical providers

IV.   Barriers to Completion of Advance Directives

    A.   Only 23% to 54% of Americans have an advance directive.[10] Several factors contribute to the lack of completion of either a living will or a proxy document[11]

        1.   Fear of having care withheld and of being abandoned by the medical community. People also fear that care would be withheld too soon

        2.   People with less education, lower socioeconomic group, or historically disenfranchised are suspicious of what they perceive as efforts to deny care

        3.   Patients assume providers should initiate a discussion about advance directives, while providers often assume the patient should. Therefore this discussion is delayed

        4.   Many people procrastinate due to the emotional implications of the topic

V.   Case Law and Legislation

    A.   Karen Ann Quinlan case raised awareness of decision-making at the end of life and that patients are not required to continue with treatments that may not be of benefit[12]

    B.   Nancy Cruzan case established that patients can refuse life-sustaining treatment such as medically-administered nutrition and hydration, and can preserve this right even when lacking capacity through an advance directive. However, the state can require clear and convincing evidence of the patient's wishes[13]

    C.   Terri Schiavo case illustrated the right to refuse medical treatment even if incapacitated, "artificial nutrition and hydration are medical treatments and may be legally and ethically withdrawn under appropriate circumstances"[14, p. 297]

    D.   The Patient Self-Determination Act was passed as a result of the Cruzan case. This law requires that healthcare organizations accepting Medicare must

        1.   Inquire upon admission whether the patient has an advance directive

        2.   Offer the patient information on advance directives

        3.   Provide information to staff, patients, and the community about advance directives[15]

VI.   Institute of Medicine (IOM) Report—*Dying in America: Improving Quality and Honoring Individual Preferences Near the End of Life*[10]

    A.   The focus of the 2014 report from the IOM is on opportunities for the improvement of end-of-life care, specifically with advance care planning and medical/provider orders to ensure that these preferences are honored

    B.   Two of the committee's recommendations directly impact advance care planning

        1.   Clinician-Patient Communication and Advance Care Planning

        2.   Public Education and Engagement

VII. The Nurse's Role in Advance Care Planning

A. Nurses are in a unique position to advocate on behalf of their patients' wishes[16]

B. Nurses should facilitate the ACP process with their patients

1. Through the development of a therapeutic relationship with their patients, nurses can initiate discussions regarding future healthcare decisions

2. This process is dynamic and should begin prior to crisis situations

3. ACP conversations should be revisited with changes in condition

4. Discussions should include desires for treatment options as well as designation of healthcare decision-maker, should the patient no longer possess medical decision-making capacity[3]

C. Failure of healthcare providers to initiate conversations regarding ACP has been frequently cited as a barrier for patients[17]

D. Nurses need to be familiar with state and federal laws regarding advance directives and other forms of ACP such as DNRs

E. The nurse should initiate and complete their own ACP prior to initiating conversations with patients. The more experience the nurse has with ACP, the more comfortable he/she may be with facilitating these discussions[17]

VIII. The Benefits of Advance Care Planning

A. Allows patients to make informed decisions

B. Allows expression of wishes for medical treatment to healthcare providers and family/ surrogates

C. Allows for wishes to be honored in the event of being unable to participate or speak for themselves

D. Provides family members/surrogates peace of mind that the patient's wishes have been honored[18]

IX. Special Considerations

A. Advance care planning/goals of care discussions. In particular, conducting family meetings is often out of the scope of the generalist hospice and palliative nurse. The nurse is in a prime position, however, to advocate for the patient and family/surrogate and ensure accurate and timely information is provided

B. **Individuals with chronic and terminal illness should receive disease-specific information, including understanding their illness, treatment expectations, emerging symptoms, benefits and burdens of possible treatment, communication with health professionals, and ACP specific to their disease process. For example, preferences regarding**

1. Cardiomyopathy—deactivation of automatic implantable cardioverter defibrillator (AICD), DNR

2. Chronic obstructive pulmonary disease—do not intubate

3. End stage renal disease—discontinuation of dialysis

4. Cognitive impairment—preferences regarding medically administered nutrition and hydration[19,20]

C. **ACP is a dynamic process, and the patient's desires may change over time. ACP should be reviewed on a regular basis as well as with any changes in condition, family situation (i.e., new diagnosis, appointed healthcare decision-maker no longer available)**

D. **The nurse should maintain sensitivity to elements of diversity (i.e., race, culture, ethnicity, and religion) during ACP discussions[3]**

CITED REFERENCES

1. Hirschman KB, Abbott KM, Hanlon AL, Prvu Bettger J, Naylor MD. What factors are associated with having an advance directive among older adults who are new to long-term care services? *J Am Med Dir Assoc*. 2012;13(1):82.e7-e11. doi: 10.1016/j.jamda.2010.12.010. Epub February 26, 2011.

2. Sudore RL, Fried TR. Redefining the "planning" in advance care planning: preparing for end-of-life decision making. *Ann Intern Med*. 2010;153(4):256-261. doi: 10.7326/0003-4819-153-4-201008170-00008.

3. Hospice and Palliative Nurses Association (HPNA). *The Nurse's Role in Advance Care Planning* [Position Statement]. 2013. Pittsburgh, PA; Hospice and Palliative Nurses Association. hpna.advancingexpertcare.org/education/position-statements/. Accessed October 20, 2014.

4. Davison SN. Advance care planning in chronic illness. Fast Facts #162. *J Palliat Med*. 2008;11(2): 243-244. doi: 10.1089/jpm.2008.9972.

5. Escher M, Perneger TV, Rudaz S, Dayer P, Perrier A. Impact of advance directives and a health care proxy on doctors' decisions: a randomized trail. *J Pain Symptom Manage*. 2014;47(1):1-11. doi: 10.1016/j.jpainsymman.2013.03.010. Epub June 4, 2013.

6. Pollack KM, Morhaim D, Williams MA. The public's perspectives on advance directives: implications for state legislative and regulatory policy. *Health Policy*. 2010;96(1):57-63. doi: 10.1016/j.healthpol. 2010.01.004. Epub January 27, 2010.

7. Natinal Physician Orders for Life-Sustaining Treatment Paradigm (POLST). *Programs in Your State*. 2014. www.polst.org/programs-in-your-state/. Accessed October 7, 2014.

8. Hickman SE, Nelson CA, Moss AH, Tolle SW, Perrin NA, Hammes BJ. The consistency between treatments provided to nursing facility residents and orders on the physician orders for life-sustaining treatment form. *J Am Geriatr Soc*. 2011;59(11):2091-2099. doi: 10.1111/j.1532-5415.2011.03656.x. Epub October 22, 2011.

9. Jacobsen J, Robinson E, Jackson VA, Meigs JB, Billings JA. Development of a cognitive model for advance care planning discussions: results from a quality improvement initiative. *J Palliat Med*. 2011;14(3):331-336. doi: 10.1089/jpm.2010.0383. Epub January 19, 2011.

10. Institute of Medicine (IOM). *Dying in America: Improving Quality and Honoring Individual Preferences at the End of Life*. Washington DC: National Academic Press; 2014.

11. Perrin KO. Legal aspects of end-of-life decision making. In: Matzo M, Sherman DW, eds. *Palliative Care Nursing: Quality Care to the End of Life*. New York, NY: Springer Publishing Company; 2015:61-87.

12. *Quinlan*, 355 A.2d 647. 70 (NJ 10, 1976).

13. *Cruzan v. Director of Missouri Department of Health*. 497 U.S. 261. (US Supreme Court, 1990).

14. Kenny NP. Responding to requests for euthanasia and physician-assisted suicide. In: Emanuel LL, Librach SL, eds. *Palliative Care: Core Skills and Clinical Competencies*. 2nd ed. St. Louis, MO: Elsevier Sanders; 2007:284-299.

15. Patient Self-Determination Act (PSDA), 42 U.S.C. 1395. §§4206 et seq. United States Congress, 1990. Vol. 42.

16. American Nurses Association (ANA). *Nursing Care and Do Not Resuscitate (DNR) and Allow Natural Death (AND) Decisions* [Position Statement]. 2012. www.nursingworld.org/MainMenu Categories/EthicsStandards/Ethics-Position-Statements/Nursing-Care-and-Do-Not-Resuscitate-DNR-and-Allow-Natural-Death-Decisions.pdf. Accessed July 10, 2014.

17. Wenger B, Asakura Y, Fink RM, Oman K. Dissemination of the Five Wishes advance directive at work. *J Hosp Palliat Nurs.* 2012;14(8):551-558.

18. Fried TR, Drickamer M. Garnering support for advance care planning. *JAMA.* 2010;303(3):269-270. doi: 10.1001/jama.2009.1956.

19. Schellinger S, Sidebottom A, Briggs L. Disease specific advance care planning for heart failure patients: implementation in a large health system. *J Palliat Med.* 2011;14(11):1224-1230. doi: 10.1089/jpm.2011.0105. Epub August 26, 2011.

20. Hajizadeh N, Crothers K, Braithwaite RS. Informing shared decisions about advance directives for patients with severe chronic obstructive pulmonary disease: a modeling approach. *Value Health.* 2012;15(2):357-366. doi: 10.1016/j.jval.2011.10.015. Epub January 30, 2012.

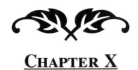

CHAPTER X

CARE OF THE PATIENT AND FAMILY IN THE FINAL DAYS

Karen A. Kehl, PhD, RN, ACHPN®, FPCN®
Patricia Berry, PhD, RN, ACHPN®, FPCN®, FAAN

I. Introduction

A. Care in the final days of life shifts and changes rhythm as the patient's condition changes

1. Nurses should facilitate open and honest communication between the patient (as able), the family, and the healthcare team[1] (e.g., role model slowed pace, longer pauses if patient is trying to respond, gentle touch)

2. The patient's goals, values, and preferences should be included in the plan of care for the final days to make the quality of their death optimal[1,2]

   a) This includes discussion about place of death,[1] who should be present, symptom management,[2] resuscitation, and other life-sustaining measures[3]

   b) Gentle anticipatory guidance to allow the family time to "feel" their emotions

B. Care should be focused on patient's goals of care and providing comfort

1. Ensure that the environment is as comfortable as possible for the patient and family

   a) Privacy and personalization of the environment

2. Avoid care that does not promote the patient's goals or comfort

   a) Discontinue routine assessments or tests that will not alter the course of care or provide information to improve the patient's comfort. Hygiene and oral care remain priorities to communicate to the patient and family that they are being cared for and about

II. Nurse's Role When a Patient Is in His/Her Final Days

A. Normalize the Experience for the Patient and the Family

1. Outline normal changes of dying

   a) What patient may experience

b)   What family may see

c)   Reasons for the changes

d)   How they relate to the timeline of dying. Use general terms as the family may be searching for "how much longer?" and no one really knows

2.   Facilitate expression of emotions

a)   Refer to social worker and/or chaplain as needed

B.   Interpret Symptoms and Guide Family in Symptom Management

1.   Thoroughly assess the patient for early indications of symptoms[1]

a)   Reassessment may need to be done more frequently if the patient's condition is changing rapidly

b)   Anticipate patient and family needs

2.   Provide information on common signs and symptoms

a)   Teach family to recognize symptoms and signs of distress

 i.   Most signs of dying are not distressing to the patient but can be to the family, especially respiratory changes (noisy breathing), changes in how the patient communicates, decreased intake, and incontinence

 ii.   Vocalization is not always a sign of distress

 iii.   Distress can usually be recognized by changes in behavior or expression

 iv.   Distressing symptoms often include

   (a)   Pain

   (b)   Dyspnea

   (c)   Restlessness

   (d)   Delirium

   (e)   Nausea

   (f)   Vomiting

   (g)   Bleeding/hemorrhaging

   (h)   Increased respiratory secretions

b)   Anticipate common symptoms and be prepared for their management

 i.   Prepare patients for what they may experience

 ii.   Prepare families for what they are likely to see and what they should do

 iii.   Assess for common symptoms with every visit

 iv.   Have appropriate medications for common symptoms available 24 hours a day (e.g., opioids, benzodiazepines, antiemetics)

C.   Commonly Occurring Distressing Symptoms When Death Is Nearing

1.   Pain

    a)   Patients who have not experienced pain prior to the final days are unlikely to experience pain at that point. If pain occurs suddenly or increases dramatically, a new problem should be suspected

    b)   May change in the days before death[4-6]

    c)   Patients may not be able to participate in a 0 to 10 pain rating scale. As the patient approaches death, they will be less able to communicate their pain

        i.   Behavior change is generally the best indicator of pain in a nonverbal patient (e.g., restlessness, grimacing, rubbing, shifting positions, screaming, moaning, guarding, muscular rigidity, diaphoresis, irritability, oppositional, combative, quiet passivity, tearfulness)

    d)   Administration of oral or transdermal medications may not be optimal

        i.   Patients may not be able to swallow oral medications[7] or they may not be consistently absorbed[4]

        ii.   Decreased circulation and increased diaphoresis in the final days means that transdermal medications may not be absorbed as they were earlier in the disease trajectory[8]

        iii.   Have a plan for sublingual, subcutaneous, rectal, or intravenous (IV) routes for pain medication in the final days

2.   Dyspnea

    a)   Dyspnea is prevalent in about 62% of dying individuals.[7] It is a subjective sensation of shortness of breath

    b)   Position the patient with the head of the bed elevated, with pillows behind the patient, or sit the patient up in a reclining chair.[9] Direct a fan toward the patient's face or open a window to move air through the room and trigger baroreceptors that initiate bronchial dilation and may reduce dyspnea[10]

    c)   Oxygen may be useful if the patient is hypoxic. If they do not have hypoxia, it is unlikely to decrease the sensation of dyspnea.[9] However, if it is already in the home, the nasal cannula may also trigger the baroreceptors

    d)   Short-acting opioids provide the best relief.[9] Be ready to reassure family about addiction and that treating symptoms does not hasten death

    e)   Benzodiazepines are a useful adjunct medication that increases relaxation and decreases anxiety[9]

3.   Restlessness

    a)   Assess for reversible causes[11]

        i.   Bladder distention

        ii.   Bowel distention

        iii.   Nicotine withdrawal

        iv.   Pain

        v.   Dehydration

        vi.   Anxiety

        vii. Drug withdrawal

        viii. Alcohol withdrawal

        ix.   Pruritus

        x.   Insomnia/sleep deprivation

b)   Provide calm, comforting environment

        i.   Avoid bright lights, loud sounds

        ii.   Continue modalities that the patient has been comfortable with (e.g., aroma and music therapies, Reiki)

        iii. Limit visitors

            (a)   Observe if certain visitors are calming or agitating to patient

c)   Administer medications as ordered[11,12]

        i.   Haloperidol

        ii.   Atypical neuroleptics

            (a)   Olanzapine

            (b)   Quetiapine

            (c)   Risperidone

        iii. Sedatives

            (a)   Chlorpromazine

            (b)   Propofol

        iv.   Benzodiazepines—not preferred due to paradoxical effects (i.e., can worsen restlessness)

d)   Delirium

        i.   Delirium may be hyperactive, hypoactive, or mixed

            (a)   All types of delirium include a change in level of arousal

            (b)   Additional features that may be present in either type include sleep–wake disturbances, perceptual changes, hallucinations, and/or delusions

            (c)   Hyperactive delirium may include restlessness, agitation, calling out, or trying to get out of bed

            (d)   Hypoactive delirium is difficult to distinguish in the final days. This may include lethargy, somnolence, and stupor

            (e)   Mixed delirium may include signs or symptoms from either of the other types

(f)   Treatment of delirium includes

   (i)   Environmental care such as dimming lights at night and lighting the room during the day

   (ii)   Administration of antipsychotics if indicated

      a.   Haloperidol is most common in the final days[12]

      b.   Benzodiazepines may be used with caution[12]

      c.   Benzodiazepines should be discontinued if a paradoxical reaction occurs

D.   Non-Distressing Symptoms When Death Is Nearing

1.   Cardiovascular signs and symptoms

   a)   Cold extremities

   b)   Mottling

      i.   Blue or purple color usually noted in dependent areas or lower extremities

      ii.   Circumoral cyanosis

   c)   Changes in pulse and blood pressure. Reinforce why it isn't necessary to measure pulse and blood pressure

2.   Respiratory signs and symptoms

   a)   Audible respiratory secretions

      i.   Noise is usually more distressing to family than to the patient

      ii.   May be managed with[13]

         (a)   Discontinuation of IV or other medically-administered fluids

         (b)   Positioning the patient on his/her side, keep the head flat or elevated as tolerated to reduce noisy breathing

         (c)   Drying agents

            (i)   Scopolamine

            (ii)   Hyoscyamine

            (iii)   Glycopyrrolate

            (iv)   Atropine sulfate

            (v)   Antihistamines (often diphenhydramine)

         (d)   Gentle (bulb) suctioning of the oropharynx is recommended if needed after the use of drying agents; only suction what can be seen[14]

   b)   Change in breathing patterns—these do not require action and are not uncomfortable for the patient

      i.   Apnea

         (a)   Periods with no breathing. May be short at first and often lengthens as death approaches

ii.   Shallow breathing

iii.   Cheyne-Stokes—periods of breathing (often shallow and/or fast) that alternate with periods of apnea

iv.   Panting—sometimes seen as a very late breathing pattern

v.   Mandibular breathing

   (a)   Occasional, often deep breaths where the jaw is noted to move

   (b)   Often periods of apnea noted between breaths

3.   Neurologic signs and symptoms

a)   Confusion

   i.   Confusion may be noted along with restlessness or delirium or as a separate condition

   ii.   "Seeing" people who have died is common as death nears and should not be considered confusion

b)   Sensory changes

   i.   Increased sensitivity to light

   ii.   Decreased visual acuity

   iii.   Increased or decreased sensation of touch

c)   Semi-comatose or comatose state

4.   Metabolic signs and symptoms

a)   Fatigue

b)   Surge of energy

c)   Increased temperature—administration of antipyretics may not be effective in the final days as the hypothalamus loses the ability to regulate temperature

d)   Diaphoresis—keep the skin as clean and dry as possible

5.   Gastrointestinal signs and symptoms

a)   Changes in intake

b)   Nausea

c)   Vomiting

d)   Diarrhea

e)   Constipation

f)   Bowel incontinence

6.   Urinary signs and symptoms

a)   Decreased urinary output—urine is often dark and concentrated

b)   Incontinence

7. Communication

    a) Social withdrawal, reassure family and friends

    b) Decreased talking

    c) Symbolic communication

    d) Patients often use metaphors or allegory when communicating. Common symbolism relates to travel (getting ready to go on a trip), going home, or standing in line

    e) Emotional changes

    f) Patients may express fear of

       i. The unknown

       ii. Being abandoned

E. Communication with Patient and Family

1. Emphasize the fact that each death is unique. Some of the common signs and experiences will likely occur, but there is no way to anticipate exactly what will happen

    a) Avoid giving absolute time lines. It is very difficult to prognosticate exactly when death will occur

       i. Discuss impending death in terms of days to weeks, hours to days, minutes to hours, etc.

       ii. Encourage family to have important conversations while the patient is able to participate

       iii. Encourage the patient and family to say goodbye in their own way and do not push

       iv. If it is culturally acceptable to the patient and family, you may support the family in giving the patient permission to die and reassuring the patient that, while they will be missed, the family will be fine

    b) Explain that while some patients will want to have family present at the time of death, others prefer to die alone. These deaths often occur in the few minutes when everyone has left the room. It is important if this occurs to reinforce that the patient knew how the family cared for them

F. Assessing Family Readiness and Understanding

1. Assess family readiness to learn before providing education about care in the final days

    a) Consider characteristics of the family member such as

       i. Caregiving experience in general and specifically at the end of life

       ii. Experience providing end-of-life care

       iii. Cultural background

       iv. Education

       v. Resources

vi. Family preferences for knowledge

(a) Ask them what they want more information about

(b) Remember that "they don't know what they don't know" so do not rely solely on family request for information to prepare them

2. Assess family desire and ability to provide care

a) Regardless of setting, if family desires to participate in caregiving they should be encouraged to do so

b) If family does not wish to provide care or is emotionally or physically fatigued, give them permission to take a break and discuss other options for care provision (e.g., read a chapter from a favorite book, listen to music, reminisce)

c) For the families that do provide the care, support and assurance that they are doing a good job can help them feel more confident and to do a better job of caregiving

3. Assess family understanding

a) Ask family to return demonstrate techniques, such as dissolving medications in a small amount of water, positioning patient to relieve dyspnea, administering medications by the rectal or sublingual route, use of draw sheet, changing adult briefs

b) Ask family to repeat what you have taught them or ask them to teach another family member while you are present

c) Ask if they have any questions or if any information was not clear

4. Echoing family language—use the family's terminology whenever possible when discussing patient symptoms and death

5. Confirm plans and actions by the family and/or caregivers for time of death

6. Confirm placement of relevant orders (physician/medical orders for life-sustaining treatment [POLST/MOLST], out of hospital do not resuscitate [DNR]) in the home or facility

III. Recognition of Death

A. Signs that Death has Occurred

1. Lack of the following signs, although rarely does the nurse need to measure blood pressure, test blinking, or corneal reflex

a) Pulse

b) Blood pressure

c) Respirations

d) Response to stimuli

e) Blinking/corneal reflex

2. These signs occur in some patients

a) Bowel or bladder incontinence

b) Eyelids slightly open

        c)   Jaw relaxed and mouth slightly open

        d)   Waxy appearance to skin

B.   Prepare Family for What they Should do When Death Occurs

1.   As death is not an emergency in the home setting, families are encouraged to take time to say goodbye or be with the person's body after death; encourage touch, reassure family it is permissible to do so

2.   Call hospice or notify the provider

      a)   The death of a patient with a DNR (do not resuscitate) or AND (allow natural death) order does not require emergency intervention

      b)   The hospice nurse will take care of notifying the physician and funeral home

           i.   In some states, home hospice nurses can pronounce death. In other settings, the nurse will relay the lack of vital signs to the physician and obtain an order to release the body

          ii.   Notify the coroner or verify that the coroner does not need notification before moving the patient, removing any tubes or equipment, or calling the funeral home

               (a)   Be mindful of cultural and/or religious practices regarding handling of the body and removing tubes; consult the family or a faith leader

      c)   Encourage family to call other family or friends who may want to say goodbye

C.   Registered Nurse's Role at the Time of Death

1.   Assist with facilitating any cultural or religious rituals that the family desires, if appropriate

2.   Encourage family to spend time with the body, saying goodbyes, prayers, or other rituals meaningful to them

3.   Ask if other family, friends, or clergy need to come to view or attend to the body before postmortem care is performed

4.   Offer chaplain or other staff support, being mindful of maintaining the family's need for support and privacy

5.   Generally, the body should not be moved until the family is ready and feel they have been given enough time to say goodbye. However, nurses should know if local laws, institutional regulations, or customs are in conflict with this

6.   Interpret and normalize postmortem changes (see Table 10-1)

D.   Postmortem Care of the Body after Death

1.   Handle the body with the same respect you would if the person were alive; model this behavior for family and close others present

2.   Bathe body and groom as appropriate; place either an adult brief or a waterproof pad under the patient to catch urinary and bowel leakage and to minimize odor; allowing body fluids to drain in a confined space reduces bacteria proliferation and odor

3.   Ask if the family would like to participate in postmortem care; some family members find it comforting to perform this last act of care; in some cultures and for some relationships (e.g., the death of a child), family participation in preparation of the body may be very important for the grieving process; if the family participates gently remind them that when a body is being turned, air escapes from the lungs, producing a "sighing" sound

4.   Prepare family members for the removal of the body from the room or home, as this is often a difficult process to observe. Give families the option of leaving the area prior to the body being removed

    a)   At times, families, especially in the home care setting, wish to keep the person's body at home

        i.   If the family wishes the body to be embalmed, this is generally best done within 12 hours[15]

        ii.   If embalming is not desired, the body can, in most cases, remain in the home for approximately 24 hours before further decomposition and odor production occur; state laws vary on the amount of time a body can remain in the home and not be refrigerated

        iii.   Advise the family, if possible, to reduce the ambient temperature in the room and remove heavy blankets or coverings

5.   For home (including some facilities) death

    a)   Arrange for the removal of durable medical equipment and medical supplies; be sure to schedule to accommodate the family's needs and schedule

    b)   Dispose of unused medications

        i.   Make sure unneeded drugs are disposed of properly and document in patient's medical record

        ii.   Destroy controlled substances so that they are "nonretrievable" (i.e., the substance be permanently rendered in an unusable state) using "methods that are secure, convenient, and responsible, consistent with preventing the diversion of such substances"[16] in all settings

            (a)   Be knowledgeable of federal, state, local, and agency guidelines[16]

            (b)   Dispose discontinued or no longer needed drugs in a manner that protects the environment[16]

            (c)   Document patient/family compliance or refusal in patient's medical record

    c)   Educate patient and family by providing written guidelines in their language, if available

        i.   Modify drugs for proper disposal

        ii.   According to the Drug Enforcement Agency (DEA) "sewering (disposal by flushing down a toilet or sink) and landfill disposal (mixing controlled substances with undesirable items such as kitty litter or coffee grounds and depositing in a garbage collection) are examples of current methods of disposal that do not meet the nonretrievable standard"[16]

        iii.   The DEA lists three voluntary options for disposal—take-back events, mail-back programs, and collection receptacles[16]

        iv.   Needles and syringes require puncture-proof containers

    d)   Giving postmortem care provides an important opportunity for nurses and other caregivers to say their goodbyes to the patient and is an important role for nursing[17]

6.   After the body has been transported to the morgue or funeral home

    a)   Assess family and caregivers needs

    b)   Allow the family and caregivers to voice their experience of caregiving and the death

    c)   Acknowledge the loss

    d)   Offer support through presence

    e)   Introduce information about bereavement services and follow-up services that will be provided if any. If a hospice patient, provide bereavement counseling as per the Medicare Hospice Benefit for up to 1 year following the death for family and/or residents and employees of where the patient had been living

    f)   Ascertain safety of caregivers and family members' ability to drive if the death did not occur in their home

    g)   Staff may find it useful to have a debriefing meeting on the death[18]

    h)   Staff may wish to participate in formal closure activities (e.g., attend visitation at the funeral home, attend funeral/memorial services, send a card)

Table 10-1. Normal Postmortem Physiological Changes and Their Implications for Nursing and Care of the Body after Death[adapted from 19]

Change	Underlying Mechanisms	Nursing Implications
Rigor mortis	• Approximately 2–6 hours after death, adenosine phosphate (ATP) ceases to be synthesized due to the depletion of glycogen stores • ATP is necessary for muscle fiber relaxation, so the lack of ATP results in an exaggerated contraction of the muscle fibers that eventually immobilizes the joints • Rigor begins in the involuntary muscles (i.e., heart, gastrointestinal tract, bladder, arteries) and progresses to the muscles of the eyelids, head and neck, trunk, and lower limbs • After approximately 96 hours, however, muscle chemical activity totally ceases, and rigor passes • Persons with large muscle mass (e.g., body builders) are prone to more pronounced rigor mortis. Conversely, frail elderly persons and persons who have been bed-bound for long periods are less subject to rigor mortis[15]	• The guiding principle is to understand rigor mortis is a natural and temporary postmortem change and immediate positioning of the deceased does not impact the appearance of the body long term • After death, position the person in a relaxed and peaceful manner as is possible. For example, close the eyes (using petroleum jelly on the eyelids can help to keep them closed), position the patient with the head on a pillow or on his/her side so the jaw does not hang open, and fold the hands • If rigor mortis does occur, it can often be "massaged out" by the funeral director[15] • Finally, by understanding this physiology, the nurse can also reassure the family about the myth that due to rigor mortis, muscles can suddenly contract and the body can appear to move
Algor mortis	• After the circulation ceases and the hypothalamus stops functioning, internal body temperature drops by approximately 1° C or 1.8° F per hour until it reaches room temperature. As the body cools, skin loses its natural elasticity • If a high fever was present at death, the changes in body temperature are more pronounced and the person may appear to "sweat" after death. Body cooling may also take several more hours[15]	• The nurse can prepare family members for the coolness of the skin to touch or the increased moisture by explaining the changes that happen after death • The nurse may also suggest kissing the person on their hair instead of their skin • The skin, due to loss of elasticity, becomes fragile and easily torn • If dressings are to be applied, it is best to apply them with either a circular bandage or paper tape • Handle the body gently as well, being sure to not place traction on the skin

Table 10-1. Normal Postmortem Physiological Changes and Their Implications for Nursing and Care of the Body after Death[adapted from 19] *(continued)*

Change	Underlying Mechanisms	Nursing Implications
Postmortem decomposition or "liver mortis"	• Discoloration and softening of the body are caused largely by the breakdown of red blood cells and the resultant release of hemoglobin that stains the vessel walls and surrounding tissue • This staining appears as a mottling, bruising, or both in the dependent parts of the body as well as parts of the body where the skin has been punctured (e.g., intravenous or chest tube sites)[15] • Often this discoloration becomes extensive in a very short time. The remainder of the body has a gray hue. In cardiac-related deaths, the face often appears purple in color regardless of the positioning at or after death[15]	• As the body is handled (e.g., while bathing and dressing), the nurse informs the family member about this normal change that occurs after death • Prop the body up with pillows under the head and shoulders or raise the head of the bed approximately 30° • Remove heavy blankets and clothing and cover the deceased with a light blanket or sheet

CITED REFERENCES

1. National Consensus Project for Quality Palliative Care (NCP). *Clinical Practice Guidelines for Quality Palliative Care*. Pittsburgh, PA: NCP; 2013. www.nationalconsensusproject.org/Guidelines_ Download2.aspx. Accessed September 24, 2014.

2. Kehl KA. Moving toward peace: an analysis of the concept of a good death. *Am J Hosp Palliat Care*. 2006;23(4):277-286. doi: 10.1177/1049909106290380.

3. Silveira MJ, Kim SY, Langa KM. Advance directives and outcomes of surrogate decision making before death. *N Engl J Med*. 2010;362(13):1211-1218. doi:10.1056/NEJMsa0907901.

4. Glare P, Dickman A, Goodman M. Symptom control in care of the dying. In: Ellershaw J, Wilkinson S, eds. *Care of the Dying: A Pathway to Excellence*. 2nd ed. New York, NY: Oxford University Press; 2011:33-62.

5. Kehl K, Roberts T. Documented symptom changes in the last week of life (739). *J Pain Symptom Manage*. 2012;43(2):443.

6. Seow H, Barbera L, Sutradhar R, et al. Trajectory of performance status and symptom scores for patients with cancer during the last six months of life. *J Clin Oncol*. 2011;29(9):1151-1158. doi: 10.1200/jco.2010.30.7173.

7. Kehl KA, Kowalkowski JA. A systematic review of the prevalence of signs of impending death and symptoms in the last 2 weeks of life. *Am J Hosp Palliat Care*. 2013;30(6):601-616. doi: 10.1177/ 1049909112468222.

8. Näf E. Evidence based use of fentanyl patches in adult cancer patients. *Schweizer Krebsbulleitn Bulletin Suisse du Cancer*. 2011(4):341-346.

9. Campbell ML. Dyspnea. *AACN Adv Crit Care*. 2011;22(3):257-264. doi: 10.1097/NCI.1090b1013e 318220bc318224d.

10. Galbraith S, Fagan P, Perkins P, Lynch A, Booth S. Does the use of a handheld fan improve chronic dyspnea? A randomized, controlled, crossover trial. *J Pain Symptom Manage*. 2010;39(5):831-838. doi: 10.1016/j.jpainsymman.2009.09.024.

11. Kehl KA. Treatment of terminal restlessness: a review of the evidence. *J Pain Palliat Care Pharmacother*. 2004;18(1):5-30.

12. Quijada E, Billings JA. Pharmacologic management of delirium; update on newer agents. 2nd ed. *Fast Facts and Concepts*. 2009; 60. www.eperc.mcw.edu/EPERC/FastFactsIndex/ff_060.htm. Accessed October 15, 2014.

13. Bickel K, Arnold R. Death rattle and oral secretions. 2nd ed. *Fast Facts and Concepts*. 2009; 109. www.eperc.mcw.edu/EPERC/FastFactsIndex/ff_109.htm. Accessed October 15, 2014.

14. Bennett M, Lucas V, Brennan M, Hughes A, O'Donnell V, Wee B. Using anti-muscarinic drugs in the management of death rattle: evidence-based guidelines for palliative care. *Palliat Med*. 2002;16(5): 369-374.

15. Tjaarda N. Licensed Funeral Director and Embalmer, Young's Funeral Home, Tigard, OR, personal communication, June, 2014.

16. Drug Enforcement Administration. *Disposal of Controlled Substances*. 2014. www.federalregister.gov/ articles/2014/09/09/2014-20926/disposal-of-controlled-substances. Accessed September 9, 2014.

17. Olausson J, Ferrell BR. Care of the body after death: nurses' perspectives of the meaning of post-death patient care. *Clin J Oncol Nurs*. 2013;17(6):647-651.

18. Zerwekh JV. *Nursing Care at the End of Life: Palliative Care for Patients and Families*. Philadelphia, PA: F. A. Davis Company; 2006.

19. Berry PH, Griffie J. Planning for the actual death. In: Ferrell BR, Coyle N, Paice J, eds. *Oxford Textbook of Palliative Nursing*. 4th ed. New York, NY: Oxford University Press; in press.

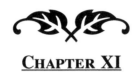

CHAPTER XI

ETHICAL ISSUES IN END-OF-LIFE CARE

Karen Wahle, RN, MSN, JD, CHPN®
Susan Lysaght Hurley, PhD, GNP-BC, ACHPN®

I.   **Introduction**

A.   **What Is Ethics?**[1]

1.   General term for methods used to understand and examine the moral life; also a branch of philosophy that focuses on the moral life

2.   Morality—social customs, norms, and rules that define "right" and "wrong" behavior; includes common morality and particular moralities, which individuals and groups may or may not accept

3.   Healthcare ethics (also called bioethics, medical ethics)—the study of moral obligations of healthcare providers and society in preventing and treating disease and injury and in caring for people with illness and injuries

4.   Nursing ethics—the reflection on and study of the moral norms for the professional practice of nursing

5.   Ethics and legality

a)   Ethics can guide the development and enforcement of laws

b)   Some legal actions are considered immoral by some people (e.g., capital punishment, apartheid)

c)   Some illegal actions can be viewed as moral by some people (e.g., active, voluntary euthanasia)

6.   Ethics is not static; it is influenced by societal norms and changes over time; although the principles and methods generally are fairly constant, sociocultural trends and scientific advances alter the way ethical principles are applied to a given situation

B.   **Ethical Principles**[1]

1.   Principles—concepts that form a framework and are used to evaluate and decide the morality of an action, commonly used to frame and deliberate about specific bioethical issues

2. Four major bioethical principles

   a) Autonomy

      i. From the Greek *autos* (self) and *nomos* (rule, law, governance); person's right to choose freely

      ii. In American society, which is based on individual rights, autonomy greatly influences how healthcare decisions are made

      iii. Autonomy depends on

         (a) Liberty—ability to make a choice that is not overly influenced or coerced by others

         (b) Agency—capacity to understand relevant information, consider the options, evaluate risks and benefits, make and communicate a decision

         (c) Having information necessary to make the decision (e.g., information about diagnosis, prognosis, treatment options)

         (d) Analysis of the moral requirements of respect for autonomy includes[1]

            (i) Intentionality—is the act intentional or unintentional?

            (ii) With understanding—sometimes varying levels of understanding are taken into account (e.g., children, persons with dementia)

            (iii) Without controlling influences that determine their action—must be a substantial degree of freedom from coercion, persuasion, and/or manipulation[1]

         (e) Informed consent depends on autonomy

         (f) Autonomy includes the right to choose or refuse therapies

   b) Beneficence

      i. Obligation to "do good," to act for another's benefit

      ii. In clinical practice, it is usually necessary to consider benefits, burdens, and costs of a particular action (treatment) to ensure beneficence

   c) Nonmaleficence

      i. Obligation not to inflict harm; the basis for the phrase "first, do no harm"

      ii. In palliative care, nonmaleficence is most commonly invoked when deliberating about life-prolonging therapies that can harm a patient by causing increased suffering without increasing the patient's quality of life; nonmaleficence can offer justification for withholding/withdrawing futile treatments

      iii. Futility

         (a) Refers to a situation in which irreversibly-dying patients have reached a point where further treatment provides no physiological benefit or is hopeless and becomes optional[1]

         (b) Used to justify withholding/withdrawing of therapies

         (c) Determining futility involves making a judgment based on both values and scientific evidence[2]

(d) Because the value judgment is based on clinicians' or societal perspectives, determining the patient's goals for treatment and values should *precede* any judgment about the futility of a particular therapy whenever possible[2]

d) Justice

    i. Fair, equitable, and appropriate treatment in light of what is due or owed to persons[1]

    ii. Distributive justice

        (a) Distribution of societal rights and responsibilities

        (b) Allocation of scarce healthcare resources

    iii. Vulnerability

        (a) Focuses on a person's susceptibility—whether as a result of internal (e.g., age) or external (e.g., socioeconomic status) factors—to inducement or coercion, on the one hand, or to harm, loss, or indignity, on the other[1]

        (b) Concept of vulnerability has evolved to a "condition of vulnerability" versus speaking of vulnerable groups because labels may overprotect or stereotype and not everyone in a labeled group is categorically vulnerable

e) Bioethical principles guide reflection and discussion about ethical issues but do not provide answers; sound ethical reasoning and action depends on clinicians who understand and evaluate their beliefs and values in light of societal norms, laws, professional obligations, and values and goals of patients and families

II. Ethics of Care[1]

A. The ethics of care is a form of virtue ethics and calls attention to what health professionals do, and to how and why they do it

1. Emphasizes the underlying commitment of healthcare professionals to care about the interpersonal relationships between themselves, patients, and families. Caring is the fundamental orienting virtue in healthcare[1]

    a) For example, the ethics of care would require paying particular attention to when and how a conversation about introducing hospice care is conducted with patients and families

B. Five Focal Virtues of an Ethics of Care

1. Compassion—the development among healthcare professionals of compassion balanced with detachment; allowing a professional distance, but deep concern beyond empathy for patients and families

    a) See Chapter II, *Interdisciplinary Collaborative Practice in the Hospice and Palliative Settings*, for more information on professional boundaries

2. Discernment—the ability to reach conclusions about ways to proceed in difficult situations "without being unduly influenced by extraneous considerations, fears, personal attachments"[1]

3.   Trustworthiness—to have confidence that someone will act in a moral way and maintain trust

4.   Integrity—being aware of and consistently standing up for moral values

5.   Conscientiousness—the manifestation of acting in the right, of acting in support of one's conscience

III.   Ethical Dilemmas and Conflicts

A.   Dilemmas arise when evidence suggests that a particular act is viewed by different individuals and groups as both morally right and morally wrong (e.g., assisted suicide/ death or when a person feels morally compelled to do 2 or more mutually exclusive actions, such as palliative sedation to control refractory symptoms even if the unintended consequence is that death is hastened)[1]

B.   Ethical Conflicts[3]

1.   Arise when there is disagreement

   a)   About goals of care (e.g., curative treatment, life-prolonging treatment at all costs versus care aimed at quality of life and comfort)

   b)   Whether or not specific medical treatments are futile

   c)   About what the incapacitated patient would want

   d)   When a team member expresses discomfort with the plan of care

2.   Involve disagreements between or among

   a)   Healthcare team members

   b)   Family members

   c)   Patient (or surrogate)

C.   Process to resolve ethical dilemmas and conflicts is similar to other problem-solving methods[4]

1.   Identify the issue—what is it about the clinical situation that is causing distress or conflict?

2.   Gather data—seek information on the following

   a)   Information about the clinical situation—patient's clinical status (e.g., diagnosis, prognosis), burdens, benefits of all treatment options

   b)   Patient and family's understanding of the situation and their values, goals of care, and wishes; if the patient is unable to voice preferences and values, seek information from patient's advance directives, if available, or from others who know the patient well

   c)   Who are the decision-makers in the situation and what are their opinions, beliefs, and values? Who else will be affected by the decision and what are *their* opinions, beliefs, and values?

   d)   What are the ethical principles and/or values that are in conflict?

3.   Identify options—what are all the possible courses of action? What are the possible outcomes of these actions?

4.   Evaluate options—evaluate the possible courses of action with input from

    a)   Statutory law

    b)   Case law

    c)   Ethics and healthcare literature

    d)   Position and consensus statements from professional organizations (e.g., Hospice and Palliative Nurses Association, American Nurses Association, American Medical Association)

    e)   Institutional or agency policies

    f)   Formal ethics consultation

5.   Decide on course of action—make a decision and implement the plan

6.   Evaluate the plan—were acceptable outcomes achieved? Does the plan need to be changed?

7.   Open and respectful communication that reflects cultural sensitivity, negotiation, and consensus building must occur throughout the process of resolving conflicts[5]

IV.   Common Ethical Issues at the End of Life

A.   Truth-Telling (Veracity)[4]

1.   Current ethical and legal obligations require that healthcare providers ensure that patients are fully informed about their conditions, including diagnosis, prognosis, and potential risks and benefits of all treatment options (e.g., curative/life-prolonging treatment if available)

2.   Providing complete, accurate information is necessary to ensure that patients and families are able to make informed decisions and provide informed consent or refusal

3.   There sometimes is tension between what healthcare providers need to tell patients and families and what they want to hear

    a)   Some patients do not wish to be burdened with all the information, or wish to have others (family or healthcare providers) make decisions for them

    b)   Some families do not want the patient to know the details of the illness for fear of having the patient become upset or hopeless

    c)   Some families, especially those from non-European-American cultures, consider it the responsibility of the adult children to receive information and make decisions for their elderly parents

    d)   In some cultures, giving ill people negative information about their condition is considered rude and/or emotionally destructive

    e)   In cases where tension exists about disclosure of health-related information

        i.   Clinicians must "offer" truth rather than "inflict" truth; patient should be offered information but if she/he freely chooses not to receive the information, the clinician should honor this. Deferring one's autonomy is an act of autonomy. Clinicians should continue to offer information, always giving the patient the option to defer or refuse it and/or request that the information be given to others whom the patient trusts

B. Confidentiality[5]

   1. Patients have the right to expect privacy of their personal health information through the Health Insurance Portability and Accountability Act (HIPAA) of 1996[6]

      a) Clinicians must maintain security of all patient records, including electronic medical records

      b) Clinicians must obtain patient's consent to share information with family members

C. Determination of Capacity[5]

   1. "The ability to understand relevant information, to appreciate the medical situation and its possible consequences, to communicate a choice, and to engage in rational deliberation about one's own values in relation to the [provider's] recommendations about treatment options"[5, p. 66]

   2. Patients may clearly lack capacity or it may be more difficult to assess capacity because of acute illness, delirium, or medications clouding their judgment

   3. Determination of decisional capacity is usually made by trained clinicians speaking with the patient, family members, or others involved in the patient's care. Sometimes the determination of decisional capacity may require patient evaluation by psychiatrists or other mental health counselors

   4. Decisional capacity may also vary with the gravity and significance of the decision to be made (e.g., refusing a bath versus refusing hemodialysis)

D. Surrogate Decision-Making[5]

   1. A patient without decisional capacity may need a surrogate decision-maker

   2. Advance care planning usually involves naming an individual who will become a surrogate decision-maker in these instances

   3. Standards of surrogate decision-making involve "substituted judgment" and "best interests"

      a) Substituted judgment occurs "when a surrogate relies on known preferences of the patient to reach a conclusion about medical treatment"[5, p. 88]

      b) Best interests can also be relevant because "if the patient's own preferences are unknown or are unclear, the surrogate must consider the best interests of the patient . . . defined as making those choices, namely, about relief of suffering, preservation, or restoration of function and the extent and sustained quality of life, that reasonable persons in similar circumstances would be likely to choose"[5, p. 90]

E. Withholding and Withdrawing Life-Sustaining Therapies

   1. Also referred to as letting or allowing a patient to die, as death would naturally occur without the therapy; terms distinguish these actions from actions that are generally seen as ethically *unjustified* (see section on Assisted Death)[7]

   2. Generally, a therapy may be withheld/withdrawn if the patient (or designated surrogate) refuses it and/or if the treatment is medically futile; ideally, the concept of futility is not invoked without consent of the patient/family.[2] This may vary based on individual state law; understanding the law of the state in which you practice is critical

3. Courts, professional healthcare organizations, and many religions recognize patients' ethical and legal right to refuse life-sustaining therapies[8-10]

4. The American Nurses Association has published the following guidance for nurses dealing with this issue—"The American Nurses Association (ANA) believes that adults with capacity or, in the event of incapacity, their surrogates are in the best position to weigh the harms and benefits of nutrition and hydration as evaluated and discussed with them by the healthcare team. The acceptance or refusal of food and fluids, whether delivered by normal or artificial means, must be respected"[11]

5. Two highly publicized court cases, those involving Karen Ann Quinlan[12] and Nancy Cruzan,[13] were instrumental in establishing the legal right to withhold/withdraw life-prolonging therapies; the case of Terri Schiavo[14] reinforced the legality of withdrawal of artificial nutrition and hydration

6. The Patient Self Determination Act of 1990[15] reaffirmed the right of patients to choose or refuse therapies, requiring healthcare agencies to inform patients of this right. It was a catalyst for discussions on this topic. All 50 states have enacted laws that allow adults with decisional capacity to document their wishes for treatment, should they be unable to communicate these wishes at the time due to incapacity

    a) Advance directives—state law governs the use of advance directives, a mechanism through which persons can communicate their wishes in the event they are unable to communicate them directly. It is also referred to as a plan for future medical care created for some yet uncertain future. This plan can be communicated orally (verbal expressions to loved ones, friends, or healthcare providers); in formal written documents that meet statutory requirements (living will, power of attorney for healthcare); or in informal documents (letter to physician, values history) that may not meet statutory requirements but provide evidence of preferences

    b) Advance care planning (ACP)—a process of assisting individuals to understand why advance directives are important; to reflect on personal beliefs, cultural or religious norms, and goals; to discuss these choices, values, and beliefs, with others; and to develop a plan for communicating preferences (i.e., an advance directive)[16]

    c) Refer to Chapter IX, *Advance Care Planning and Goals of Care*, for an in-depth discussion of this topic

7. Contrasting withholding versus withdrawing therapies[17]

    a) No moral or legal differences between withholding and withdrawing treatments

    b) Some clinicians and family caregivers report greater emotional distress when *withdrawing* therapy

    c) To alleviate distress around initiating and withdrawing life-prolonging therapies, experts recommend initiating a time-limited trial, which involves starting a treatment only with specific criteria and a timeline for achieving clinical goals; at established times, treatment efficacy, burdens, and benefits are evaluated vis-à-vis criteria; if goals are not met, therapy is discontinued[18,19]

    d) There is variation in state law regarding situations under which therapies may be withheld or withdrawn

    e) Some cultural/religious groups will have specific decision-makers for treatments, especially regarding basic nutrition and hydration and life-prolonging treatments

8. Life-prolonging treatments include

    a) Cardiopulmonary resuscitation (CPR)

    b) Mechanical ventilation

    c) Dialysis

    d) Medically-administered enteral and parenteral nutrition and hydration (note that hydration, in rare cases, may provide comfort and to flush medication metabolites)

    e) Antibiotics (note that antibiotics can be used, when appropriate, for the provision of comfort)

    f) Oxygen—high-flow, bilevel positive airway pressure (BiPAP) (note that oxygen can be used for the provision of comfort)

    g) Implantable cardioverter defibrillators (ICD)

    h) Left ventricular assist device (LVAD)

9. Deactivation of implanted cardioverter defibrillators (ICD) and pacemakers[20]

    a) A patient or surrogate decision-maker has the legal right to request the withdrawal of ICD/pacemaker therapy, regardless of the reason and regardless of whether it prolongs life

    b) Similar to other life-prolonging therapies, there is no legal or ethical difference between deactivating an ICD/pacemaker device, refusing insertion, or refusing a generator (i.e., battery) change

    c) Legally and ethically, fulfilling a patient's or surrogate's request to withdraw ICD/pacemaker therapy is neither euthanasia nor assisted suicide

    d) Ethical consultation is not required prior to device deactivation, but may be helpful where there is conflict

F. Administering opioids at the end of life—risk of hastening death

1. Healthcare workers are legally and ethically required to treat patients' pain and other symptoms adequately, including aggressive pain therapy at the end of life. This obligation has been voiced by professional nursing organizations[8,21,22]

2. Despite the fear that administering opioids to seriously ill patients can hasten death, there is limited empirical evidence to justify this concern[23]

3. If concerns remain despite the lack of evidence, administering aggressive opioid therapy is ethically and legally justified through the Rule of Double Effect (RDE).[1] The RDE is a bioethical concept that provides moral justification for an action that has 2 foreseen effects: one good and one bad. The key factor is the intent of the person performing the act. If the intent is good (e.g., relief of pain and suffering), then the act is morally justifiable even if it causes a foreseeable but unintended result (e.g., hastening of death)[21]

4. RDE—derived from the principle of nonmaleficence, RDE provides ethical justification for actions that have positive intended effects and negative unintended but foreseen effects[1]

5. RDE justification for administering opioids when there is a risk of hastening death involves four conditions[1]

    a) The action in question must be good or at least morally neutral—relieving pain by administering opioids is a morally and clinically accepted act

b)   The clinician must intend only the good effect—the nurse must administer the opioid with the intention of relieving pain (and not to end the patient's life)

c)   The bad effect must not be the means to the good effect—that is, it is not necessary to end the patient's life in order to relieve pain

d)   The good effect must outweigh the bad effect—that is, the good involved in relieving pain outweighs the minor (unproven) risk of hastening death

6.   The moral obligation to relieve pain and suffering should be the primary issue in administering palliative therapies at the end of life[24]

G.   Palliative Sedation[25]

1.   "The intentional administration of sedative drugs in dosages and combinations required to reduce the consciousness of a terminal patient as much as necessary to adequately relieve one or more refractory symptoms."[26, p. 329] Palliative sedation can be used intermittently or continuously until death, with varying depths of sedation

2.   Similar to administering opioids at the very end of life, palliative sedation is distinct from assisted death because the intent is not to end life,[27] and because the desired outcome is palliation rather than death. Nevertheless, reducing consciousness until death remains controversial

3.   There is little evidence to indicate whether the administration of artificial hydration during palliative sedation will either prolong life or hasten death[28]

a)   When a patient's life expectancy is already short, continuous deep sedation without hydration may have no effect on lifespan; the cause of death is the disease process, not the withholding of fluids. Moreover, the administration of fluids at end of life may be harmful and lead to discomfort

b)   Others argue that continuous deep sedation without hydration almost certainly hastens death by dehydration. Even though there is no or limited evidence to support this position, families often perceive the withholding of hydration as abandonment of the patient

c)   Some ethicists suggest a trial of fluids (e.g., subcutaneous fluids limited to 1 L per day) until it can be ascertained whether the fluids are causing harm or aiding comfort

d)   Families should be educated that decreasing oral intake is part of the dying process, and that reluctance by clinicians to give oral hydration is not abandonment

4.   Recent studies suggest that in the overwhelming majority of patients, palliative sedation does not hasten death.[29] Additional studies are needed to guide clinical practice

5.   The Hospice and Palliative Nurses Association (HPNA) "[a]ffirms the use of palliative sedation to manage refractory and unendurable symptoms in imminently dying patients as one method of aggressive and comprehensive symptom management. There is no legal barrier to its appropriate use." HPNA does, however, allow that nurses who object to participation in palliative sedation should be allowed to transfer care to another nurse[27]

6.   Decisions as to whether to institute palliative sedation should be made carefully and involve the patient if possible, the family/surrogate, and members of the interdisciplinary team

a)   Interdisciplinary assessment including medicine, nursing, psychiatry, ethicists, chaplains, social workers, and pharmacists as available and appropriate

b)   Conversations about artificial hydration and nutrition is a separate discussion

c)   Informed consent process

H. Assisted Death

1.   Term includes[30]

a)   Euthanasia—acting to end the life of a patient to relieve the patient's suffering; usually involves administration of a lethal injection

b)   Assisted suicide—providing a person with the means (usually a prescription for a lethal amount of a medication) knowing that the person intends to kill himself/herself by taking an overdose of the medication

2.   Unlike withholding/withdrawing life-prolonging therapies, euthanasia is generally not seen as ethically acceptable or justifiable

3.   Currently, euthanasia is illegal throughout the United States and Canada. Assisted suicide is legal only in the states of Oregon (1997),[31] Washington (2008),[32] and Vermont (2013).[33] Assisted suicide has also been approved by court ruling in Montana (2009)[34]

4.   Arguments in favor of assisted suicide are usually based in autonomy and state that a terminally ill individual who is in intense, intractable, and intolerable physical or psychological pain and wishes to end his/her suffering should be allowed to do so. Arguments against assisted suicide are usually based in nonmaleficence, and also include the argument that assisted suicide actually leads to loss of autonomy rather than support of it. Further, suicidal individuals should instead receive support services that will make them want to live[7,35]

5.   Many professional organizations have published position statements against the legalization of assisted suicide and euthanasia[30,36–38]

a)   The American Nurses Association published a revised position statement in 2013 that states: "The American Nurses Association (ANA) prohibits nurses' participation in assisted suicide and euthanasia because these acts are in direct violation of *Code of Ethics for Nurses with Interpretive Statements*, the ethical traditions and goals of the profession, and its covenant with society. Nurses have an obligation to provide humane, comprehensive, and compassionate care that respects the rights of patients but upholds the standards of the profession in the presence of chronic, debilitating illness and at end of life"[37]

b)   The Hospice and Palliative Nurses Association, in its 2011 position statement, opposes the legalization of assisted suicide but also notes that "nurses have important roles in supporting patients requesting assisted suicide, advocating for comprehensive palliative care for persons with life-limiting illnesses, providing accurate and complete information about assisted suicide to patients, families, colleagues, and the public, and understanding the legal and ethical implications of assisted suicide"[30]

6.   The Oregon Nurses Association position statement addresses nursing roles where assisted suicide is legal[39]

7.   The Vermont State Nurses Association published a position statement declaring that nurses must not deliver, administer, inject, or delegate administration of a medication prescribed by a physician for the purpose of ending a patient's life, which is prohibited by state law[40]

V.   **Cultural Issues in End-of-Life Ethical Decision-Making**

   A.   **Bioethics and healthcare systems generally reflect European-American values**

   B.   **In a diverse society, it is important to recognize variations in values and perspectives that can cause distress and conflict**

   C.   **Major differences between European-American values and those of the cultures that may influence decision-making**

      1.   Autonomy is highly valued in American society but less so in other cultures; for example, needs and wishes of the family or community may be more important than an individual's rights and wishes; family/community may expect to play a greater role in decision-making than is typical in American culture

      2.   Truth-telling is a moral and ethical imperative in American healthcare systems; however, some cultures view full disclosure as disrespectful and/or harmful

      3.   Personal control is desired by many patients, but some cultures and religions value trust in a deity, the healthcare team, or family over the need for personal control

      4.   For some cultural and racial groups, a history of discrimination and distrust of the healthcare system will affect end-of-life decision-making[41–43]

   D.   **Clinicians must never make assumptions about patient/family values and preference based on patient's/family's culture, religion, age or gender; individual assessment always is necessary[24]**

VI.   **End-of-Life Research[44,45]**

   A.   **Concerns about the ethics of conducting research on individuals at end-of-life presents a potential barrier to advancement of science in the area. As a result, many common interventions in palliative care have little or no support in the research**

      1.   Autonomy—individuals near end of life are often unable to consent to participation or may be overly susceptible to undue influence

      2.   Beneficence—evaluation of risks and benefits of participation in research are different for someone at end of life; for example, there may be no direct personal benefit

      3.   Nonmaleficence—there must be constant vigilance of patient's clinical status and ability to substitute research protocols when symptoms are not controlled

      4.   Justice—fair subject selection and equal opportunity to participate are not possible due to actions of gatekeepers who wish to protect the patient

   B.   **Recruitment of participants is often difficult due to a desire to avoid upsetting individuals and families at such a difficult time; clinicians are often reluctant to participate in end-of-life research for the same reason**

   C.   **Achieving a balance among these competing principles often requires methodological and ethical tradeoffs**

VII. Nursing Roles

A.   **Practice Self-Reflection**—awareness of one's values and beliefs and understanding how they influence one's behavior, particularly responses to patients, family members, and other healthcare team members

B.   **Maintain Clinical Competence**

C.   **Demonstrate Moral Integrity**—the consistent application of ethical norms; in other words, one's *basic* approach to ethical decision-making does not change depending on the situation or the specific patient or family[1]

D.   **Practice Conscientious Objection Responsibly**

   1.   Conscientious objection—the right of persons to refuse to participate in acts that they deem unethical. Examples of clinical situations in which nurses may practice conscientious objection include abortion, capital punishment, and assisted suicide

   2.   Clinicians may morally refuse to participate in care, but only on the grounds of a moral objection to a specific type of intervention; they may not refuse care on grounds of discomfort, lack of knowledge, or discrimination

   3.   Clinicians who refuse to provide specific care based on moral beliefs must assure that decisions of the patient/family are respected and that they are not abandoned if their goals differ from that of the healthcare team[39]

      a)   Keep current with ethical and legal issues related to end-of-life care

E.   **Provide information to assist in decision-making and resolving ethical conflicts**

F.   **Advocate for patients and families**

G.   **Participate in patient/family conferences that address ethical issues**

H.   **Ensure informed consent for clinical care and research participation**

I.   **Participate in institutional/agency committees and boards; for example**

   1.   Institutional Review Boards (IRB) for Human Subjects Protections

   2.   Ethics committees

J.   **Participate in networking opportunities (e.g., special interest groups [SIGs]) in person and online outside of one's agency**

Cited References

1. Beauchamp T, Childress JF. *Principles of Biomedical Ethics*. 7th ed. New York, NY: Oxford University Press; 2012.

2. Jox R, Schaider A, Marckmann G. Medical futility at the end of life: the perspectives of intensive care and palliative care physicians. *J Med Ethics*. 2012;38:540-545.

3. Kirsch NR. The multidisciplinary team: end-of-life ethical decisions. *Topics Geriatr Rehab*. 2009; 25(4):292-306.

4. Scanlon C, Fleming C. Ethics in palliative care. In: Panke J, Coyne P, eds. *Conversations in Palliative Care: Questions and Answers with the Experts*. 3rd ed. Pittsburgh, PA: Hospice and Palliative Nurses Association; 2011:139-146.

5. Jonsen AR, Siegler M, Winslade WJ. *Clinical Ethics: A Practical Approach to Ethical Decisions in Clinical Medicine*. New York, NY: The McGraw-Hill Companies, Inc.; 2010.

6. 104th Congress. *Health Insurance Portability and Accountability Act of 1996, Public Law 104-191*. 1996. aspe.hhs.gov/admnsimp/pl104191.htm. Accessed October 15, 2014.

7. Friend ML. Physician-assisted suicide: death with dignity? *J Nurs Law*. 2011;14(3):110-116.

8. American Nurses Association (ANA). *Registered Nurses' Roles and Responsibilities in Providing Expert Care and Counseling at the End of Life* [Position Statement]. 2010. www.nursingworld.org/MainMenuCategories/EthicsStandards/Ethics-Position-Statements/etpain14426.pdf. Accessed September 23, 2014.

9. Hospice and Palliative Nurses Association (HPNA). *Withholding and/or Withdrawing Life-Sustaining Therapies* [Position Statement]. 2011. hpna.advancingexpertcare.org/education/position-statements/. Accessed October 20, 2014.

10. Zamer JA, Volker DL. Religious leaders' perspectives on ethical concern at the end of life. *J Hosp Palliat Nurs*. 2013;15(7):396-402. doi: 10.1097/NJH.0b013e31829cffa4.

11. American Nurses Association (ANA). *Foregoing Nutrition and Hydration* [Position Statement]; 2011. www.nursingworld.org/MainMenuCategories/EthicsStandards/Ethics-Position-Statements/prtetnutr 14451.pdf. Accessed September 23, 2014.

12. *Quinlan*, 355 A.2d 647. 70 (NJ 10, 1976).

13. *Cruzan v. Director of Missouri Department of Health*. 497 U.S. 261. (US Supreme Court, 1990).

14. Quill TE. Terri Schiavo: a tragedy compounded. *N Eng J Med*. 2005;352(16):1630-1633.

15. Patient Self-Determination Act of 1990 (PSDA). *Sections 4206 and 4571 of the Omnibus Budget Reconciliation Act of 1990, PL 101-508*. 1991.

16. Hospice and Palliative Nurses Association (HPNA). *The Nurse's Role in Advance Care Planning* [Position Statement]. 2013. hpna.advancingexpertcare.org/education/position-statements/. Accessed October 20, 2014.

17. Winkler E, Hiddemann W, Marckmann G. Evaluating a patient's request for life-prolonging treatment: an ethical framework. *J Med Ethics*. 2012;38:647-651.

18. Warnock M, Macdonald E. *Easeful Death: Is There a Case for Assisted Dying?* New York, NY: Oxford University Press; 2008.

19. Scott H. Issues related to nutrition and hydration at the end of life. *End Life Care J*. 2010;4(3):6-12.

20. Wright GA, Klein GJ, Gula LJ. Ethical and legal perspective of implantable cardioverter defibrillator deactivation or implantable cardioverter defibrillator generator replacement in the elderly. *Curr Opin Cardiol*. 2013;28(1):43-49. doi: 10.1097/HCO.0b013e32835b0b3b.

21. Hospice and Palliative Nurses Association (HPNA). *The Ethics of Opiate Use at End of Life* [Position Statement]. 2013. hpna.advancingexpertcare.org/education/position-statements/. Accessed October 20, 2014.

22. American Society for Pain Management Nurses (ASPMN). *Pain Management at the End of Life* [Position Statement]. 2013. www.aspmn.org/documents/PainManagementattheEndofLife_August2013.pdf. Accessed September 24, 2014.

23. Hallenbeck J. Pathophysiologies of dyspnea explained: why might opioids relieve dyspnea and not hasten death. *J Palliat Med*. 2012;15(8):848-853. doi: 10.1089/jpm.2011.0167.

24. Dahlin CM, Sutermaster DJ, eds.; Hospice and Palliative Nurses Association, American Nurses Association. *Palliative Nursing: Scope and Standards of Practice—An Essential Resource for Palliative and Hospice Nurses*. Silver Spring, MD: nursesbooks.org; 2014.

25. Beland P. Ethical issues around continuous deep sedation without hydration. *Nurs Times*. 2012; 108(38):22-25.

26. Claessens P, Menten J, Schotsmans P, Broeckaert B. Palliative sedation: a review of the research literature. *J Pain Symptom Manage*. 2008;36(3):310-333. doi: 10.1016/j.jpainsymman.2007.10.004. Epub July 25, 2008.

27. Hospice and Palliative Nurses Association (HPNA). *Palliative Sedation* [Position Statement]. 2011. hpna.advancingexpertcare.org/education/position-statements/. Accessed October 20, 2014.

28. Maltoni M, Pittureri C, Scarpi E, et al. Palliative sedation therapy does not hasten death: results from a prospective multicenter study. *Ann Oncol*. 2009;20(7):1163-1169. doi: 10.1093/annonc/mdp0.

29. Olsen ML, Swetz K, Mueller P. Ethical decision-making with end-of-life care: palliative sedation and withholding or withdrawing life-sustaining treatments. *Mayo Clin Proc*. 2010;85(10):949-954. doi: 10.4065/mcp.2010.0201. Epub August 30, 2010.

30. Hospice and Palliative Nurses Association (HPNA). *Legalization of Assisted Suicide* [Position Statement]. 2011. hpna.advancingexpertcare.org/education/position-statements/. Accessed October 20, 2014.

31. Oregon Public Health Division. *Oregon's Death with Dignity Act—2013*. public.health.oregon.gov/ProviderPartnerResources/EvaluationResearch/DeathwithDignityAct/Documents/year16.pdf. Accessed October 7, 2014.

32. Washington State Department of Health. *Death with Dignity Act*. 2012. www.doh.wa.gov/dwda/. Accessed September 24, 2014.

33. Vermont Department of Health. No. 39. An act relating to patient choice and control at end of life (S.77). *Patient Choice and Control at End of Life*. 2013. www.leg.state.vt.us/docs/2014/Acts/ACT039.pdf. Accessed September 24, 2014.

34. Johnson K. Montana ruling bolsters doctor-assisted suicide. *New York Times*. December 31, 2009. www.nytimes.com/2010/01/01/us/01suicide.html. Accessed September 24, 2014.

35. Sjöstrand S, Helgesson G, Eriksson J, Juth N. Autonomy-based arguments against physician-assisted suicide and euthanasia: a critique. *Med Health Care Philos*. 2013;16(2):225-230. doi: 10.1007/s11019-011-9365-5.

36. American Academy of Hospice and Palliative Medicine (AAHPM). *Physician-Assisted Death* [Position Statement]. 2007. aahpm.org/positions/pad. Accessed September 24, 2014.

37. American Nurses Association (ANA). *Euthanasia, Assisted Suicide, and Aid in Dying* [Position Statement]. 2013. www.nursingworld.org/euthanasiaanddying. Accessed September 24, 2014.

38. National Hospice and Palliative Care Organization (NHPCO). *Commentary and Resolution on Physician Assisted Suicide* [Position Statement]. 2005. www.nhpco.org/sites/default/files/public/PAS_Resolution_Commentary.pdf. Accessed September 24, 2014.

39. Oregon Nurses Association. Assisted suicide: the debate continues. *The Oregon Nurse.* 1997;62(3): 1-7.

40. Vermont State Nurses Association. Patient choice at end of life: guidelines for nurses. *Vermont Nurse Connections.* 2013;16(4):6.

41. Allen RS, Allen JY, Hilgeman MM, DeCoster J. End-of-life decision-making, decisional conflict, and enhanced information: race effects. *J Am Geriatr Soc.* 2008;56(10):1904-1909. doi: 10.1111/j.1532-5415.2008.01929.x. Epub September 4, 2008.

42. Heyman JC, Gutheil IA. Older Latinos' attitudes toward and comfort with end-of-life planning. *Health Soc Work.* 2010;35(1):17-26.

43. del Rio N. The influence of Latino ethnocultural factors on decision making at the end of life: withholding and withdrawing artificial nutrition and hydration. *J Soc Work in End-of-Life Palliat Care.* 2010;6(3-4):125-149. doi: 10.1080/15524256.2010.529009.

44. Hickman SE, Cartwright JC, Nelson CA, Knafl K. Compassion and vigilance: investigators' strategies to manage ethical concerns in palliative and end-of-life research. *J Palliat Med.* 2012;15(8):880-889.

45. LeBlanc TW, Wheeler JL, Abernethy AP. Research in end of life settings: an ethical inquiry. *J Pain & Palliat Care Pharmacother.* 2010;24(3):244-250. doi: 10.3109/15360288.2010.493579.

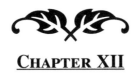

CHAPTER XII

POLICY AND ECONOMIC ISSUES IN PALLIATIVE CARE

Joy Buck, PhD, RN

Healthcare policy and economics are important to understand.

I. **Why Does Healthcare Policy Matter?**

   A. **Policy and associated regulations shape almost every aspect of the healthcare system and the provision of healthcare**

       1. Determines eligibility criteria for who has access to which programs under which circumstances

           a) The delivery of hospice care in the United States is defined largely by the Medicare Hospice Benefit and associated regulations[1]

               i. Eligibility criteria for hospice, including 6-month prognosis

               ii. Capitated payments for mandated services

       2. Regulates access to medications often used in palliative care, such as opioids and other controlled substances

           a) H.R. 4709, the Ensuring Patient Access and Effective Law Enforcement Act of 2014, seeks to strike the balance between access to controlled substances for those with legitimate need and efforts to curb illicit drug use, diversion, and other illegal activities[2]

       3. Determines scope of practice of healthcare professionals; sets parameters around what types of professionals will be reimbursed to perform certain functions; determines reimbursement rates for programs, healthcare facilities, and service provision

           a) Discrepancies exist in what nurses are licensed to do, best practices supported by evidence, and what insurers will reimburse nurses to do

           b) Financial penalties are associated with nonadherence to regulatory parameters (i.e., payments for services can be withheld [or withdrawn after payment has been made] and/or agencies can be fined for not following guidelines)

           c) Outcomes are or may be linked to reimbursement

4. Stipulates quality metrics and Conditions of Participation (CoPs), such as with Medicare-certified hospices and home health agencies

5. Stimulates and provides incentives for innovation and quality improvement (e.g., Center for Medicare and Medicaid Innovation, Medicare Care Choices Model, Advanced Chronic Illness Care Model) and research funding priorities

II. Why Do Healthcare Economics Matter?

A. The American healthcare system accounts for a large and growing share of all economic activity in the United States

1. Healthcare spending nearly doubled as a percent of the gross domestic product (GDP) between 1980 and 2012[3]

B. Medicare is the largest single purchaser of healthcare in the United States

1. The Centers for Medicare & Medicaid Services (CMS) estimates that American healthcare spending will reach almost $5 trillion by 2021[4]

2. Of the $2.4 trillion spent on personal healthcare in 2012, Medicare spending accounted for 23%, or $538 billion[3]

III. Healthcare Policy Is Determined at National, State, and Local Levels

A. Federal policy provides funding and regulations that guide

1. Federal programs, including Medicare and Medicaid, and the agencies that develop rules and administer such programs

2. Minimum requirements that must be met by states participating in programs (i.e., Medicaid programs [costs shared by state and federal governments] have requirements that all participating states must meet). Each state decides if they will add services and eligibility income levels above the federal mandate

3. Health professional training programs (Titles VII and VIII of the Public Health Service Act)

4. Basic, clinical (patient-focused), and health services research; research training priorities and funding

5. Demonstration projects for new programs (i.e., concurrent models of curative and palliative care among children and adults)

6. Medicare Payment Advisory Commission (MedPAC), which conducts analyses and provides guidance to Congress on Medicare payment issues[5]

B. State governments enact legislation and regulations for

1. Health professional licensure and scope of practice

2. Private health insurance industry, eligibility criteria for Medicaid (above federal minimums) and other state health programs

3.   Rules for healthcare facilities, Certificate of Need (some states are "CON" states), establish "state exchanges" and determine participation in expanded Medicaid programs under the Affordable Care Act

C.   **States often serve as breeding grounds for national policy. The Medicare Hospice Benefit enacted in 1982 was heavily influenced by the definition of hospice under Connecticut state statute enacted in 1978[6]**

D.   **Local and institutional policies interpret and apply regulations for day-to-day care delivery, reporting requirements, which professionals perform which functions, etc.**

IV.   **Healthcare Policy, Economics, and Healthcare Reform**

A.   **Traditional 3-Legged Stool of Healthcare Policy**

1.   Access to healthcare

2.   Cost of healthcare

3.   Quality of healthcare

B.   **Policy and regulations aim to get the "right person, in the right bed, being cared for by the right person, at the right time, at the right cost"**

1.   Impacts what will be reimbursed in different settings (i.e., skilled nursing for oral medication administration is not covered in the home but intravenous [IV] administration is because the expectation is that patients and/or caregivers should administer oral medications but might need additional training to administer medications by IV or injection)

C.   **Contemporary 3-Legged Stool of Healthcare Reform[7]**

1.   Access and expanded healthcare insurance coverage

2.   Improve quality and cost of healthcare. This is often referred to as the "value" of healthcare, a ratio of quality to cost (i.e., highest quality at the lowest cost)

a)   Research to document the comparative effectiveness of treatments, programs, and health professionals provides evidence for policy decision-making

b)   Reporting quality metrics provides evidence of the "value" of specific programs, such as hospice and palliative care

c)   Adherence to regulations and reporting is critical to organizational viability

3.   Assure consumer protections are in place

D.   **Healthcare reform and associated regulatory changes are ongoing and subject to change**

E.   **Resources are available to nurses to remain current with legislative and regulatory changes**

V. Economic Factors Influencing Healthcare for Persons with Serious or Life-Threatening Illness

A. **In 2010, the "costliest" 5% of beneficiaries accounted for 39% of annual Medicare fee-for-service (FFS) spending, and the costliest 25% accounted for 82% of FFS spending[3]**

   1. "Costly" beneficiaries tend to include those who have multiple chronic conditions, are using inpatient hospital services, are dually eligible for Medicare and Medicaid, and are in the last year of life

B. **Factors that increase healthcare spending include[8]**

   1. Fragmentation of healthcare delivery

   2. FFS reimbursement and high cost of medical services

      a) FFS means reimbursement at cost for individual services

   3. Scope of practice restrictions that favor payment for higher cost professionals (i.e., payment for physicians when advanced practice registered nurses [APRNs] are credentialed [the process of privileging to practice at a setting] and are prepared to provide comparable services)

   4. Administrative burden associated with third party payer requirements

   5. Population demographics including growth in numbers of older Americans and rising rates of chronic illness and comorbidity

   6. Advances in and demand for medical technology[8]

C. **Medicare spending varies significantly across regions of the United States, healthcare institutions, and settings of care[3]**

VI. Access to Palliative and Hospice Care

A. **Access to hospice has increased both in numbers of persons receiving hospice and the average and median length of stay (LOS) in hospice[9]**

   1. The number of Medicare beneficiaries receiving hospice services more than doubled between 2000 and 2011 and continued to grow in 2012[9]

   2. Average hospice length of stay increased to 88 days in 2012, up from 86 days in 2011 and 54 days in 2000[9]

   3. There are disparities in access to hospice based on race and ethnicity. Non-Caucasians accounted for less than one-fifth of hospice patients in 2012[9,10]

B. **Access to palliative care in acute care settings (hospitals) grew substantially between 2000 and 2013 but gaps in other care settings remain**

   1. Sixty-three percent of hospitals report having a palliative care team; 85% of hospitals with 300 beds or more have palliative care teams[11]

   2. Little is known about disparities in access to and use of specialty palliative care among historically underserved populations with serious or life-threatening illness

C. **Provisions of the Affordable Care Act (ACA) and federal/state exchange insurance programs hold promise for palliative care for persons with serious or life-threatening illness**

    1. The implementation of the ACA and its impact is still unfolding

    2. Palliative care nurses at both the generalist and advanced practice levels are important to the provision of quality palliative care in diverse settings

D. **Policy initiatives to establish the value of, and reimbursement for, specialty palliative care services and nursing in hospice and nonhospice settings are supported by national organizations such as**

    1. Hospice and Palliative Nurses Association (HPNA) and American Academy of Hospice and Palliative Medicine (AAHPM)

    2. National Coalition for Hospice and Palliative Care (NCHPC)

    3. Center to Advance Palliative Care (CAPC) and Palliative Care Research Center (PCRC)

    4. National Hospice and Palliative Care Organization (NHPCO)

VII. The Role of Nurses and Research in Healthcare Reform

A. **Nurses have played and continue to have a central role in the development of hospice and palliative care in the United States[6]**

B. **Healthcare reforms evolve over time and are influenced by national, state, and professional politics[1,6]**

    1. The Institute of Medicine's (IOM) *Report on the Future of Nursing* recommendations include the following[12]

        a) Nurses should practice to the full extent of their education and training

        b) Nurses should achieve higher levels of education and training through an improved education system that promotes seamless academic progression

        c) Nurses should be full partners, with physicians and other health professionals, in designing and redesigning healthcare in the United States

        d) Effective workforce planning and policy-making require better data collection and an improved information infrastructure

        e) In March 2014, the Federal Trade Commission issued a white paper that called for caution when evaluating proposals to limit the scope of practice of APRNs at the state level. Such limitations of the range of services APRNs *may* provide, and the extent to which they can practice independently, may reduce competition that benefits consumers and violate federal trade laws[13]

    2. In 1997, the IOM released its first report on end-of-life care, *Approaching Death: Improving Care at the End of Life*. The IOM Committee on Care at the End of Life included one nurse[14]

3.   In 2014, the IOM revisited the topic of end of life and palliative care, noting that "a substantial body of evidence shows that broad improvements to end-of-life care are within reach" and released the report *Approaching Death: Addressing Key End-of-Life Issues.* The Committee included 2 nurses and noted the continued need for preparation and certification of nurses and other healthcare specialties in palliative care. Key findings included a focus on[15]

a)   Delivery of person-centered, family-oriented care

b)   Clinician–patient communication and advance care planning

c)   Professional education and development

d)   Policies and payment systems

e)   Public education and engagement

C.   **Research provides an evidence base for clinical practice and continuous quality improvement**

1.   Comparative effectiveness research (CER) can document the "value" of the nurse to hospice and palliative care teams and subsequent health outcomes, alternative approaches to pain and symptom management, and effective communication

2.   Certification research can provide an evidence base for the links between licensing and higher value in healthcare. It may also serve as evidence to support higher wages for certified individuals

D.   **Membership and active engagement in nursing specialty organizations such as HPNA helps to advance expert care in serious or life-threatening illness at local, state, and national levels[16,17]**

E.   **The American Nurses Association sets standards and advocates on behalf of nurses[17]**

VIII. Standards of Palliative Nursing Practice[16]

A.   **The standards set forth in *Palliative Nursing: Scope and Standards of Practice—An Essential Resource for Hospice and Palliative Nurses* provides authoritative statements about the responsibilities that hospice and palliative nurses are held accountable**

B.   **Standards of practice are based on the nursing process, which includes**

1.   Assessment; diagnosis; outcomes identification; planning; and implementation of nursing interventions (based on level of practice, licensure, and regulatory standards) and evaluation

2.   Nursing interventions may include but are not limited to skilled care, care coordination, teaching, advocacy, consultation, health promotion, and harm reduction

C.   **Standards of Professional Performance[16]**

1.   Standards of Professional Performance and accompanying measurement criteria describe "competent" professional roles related to: ethics, education, evidence-based practice and research, quality of practice, communication, leadership, collaboration, professional practice evaluation, resource utilization, and environmental health

IX. Affordable Care Act has Provisions that Impact Palliative Care[3,7]

    A. Hospice-specific provisions, including payment adjustments, "concurrent" care demonstrations for adults and children, and quality reporting mandates

    B. Value-based purchasing and pay-for-performance (P4P) in acute care and other skilled nursing facilities (SNF) and home health

        1. Quality performance including quality measurement, patient-centered care research, and comparative effectiveness research

        2. Incentives such as P4P provide financial rewards for achieving quality metrics. Penalties are leveled when such metrics are not achieved

    C. Care coordination and delivery systems, including accountable care organizations (focused on coordinated and quality of care), independence at home demonstrations, community-based care, and care transitions demonstration projects, etc.

    D. Workforce, including creation of National Healthcare Workforce Commission, student loans and repayment programs, and similar programs

X. Economic Outcomes for Hospice and Palliative Care

    A. Why Measure Economic Outcomes?

        1. To demonstrate the value of palliative care in diverse care settings

        2. To inform health policy, regulations, and reimbursement rates

        3. To control costs associated with care for persons with serious or life-threatening illness

        4. To benchmark for creative management

        5. To demonstrate the comparative effectiveness and relative value of health professionals, use of medical technologies and alternative modes of pain and symptom management, certification, and models of care delivery

XI. Economic Evaluation of Therapies for Palliation of Symptoms

    A. Palliative care, including hospice, is often a sound economic choice[10,18]

        1. Reduced symptom burden and associated hospitalizations or hospital readmissions and higher quality of life

        2. Reduced caregiver burden and distress accompanied by increased productivity among those caregivers who work outside the home

        3. Potential reduction of out-of-pocket costs and healthcare utilization

    B. The following may influence cost outcomes and quality

        1. Reimbursement for "skilled" care in the least expensive setting

a) Institutional care is typically more expensive than noninstitutional care

b) Home opioid infusions are less expensive than hospital infusions; outpatient chemotherapy is less expensive than inpatient chemotherapy

c) Tensions between best practices and reimbursement for "skilled" care in the least expensive setting exist

   i. Oral medication administration is considered skilled need in an institution but not in homes, even when patient or caregiver are unable to self-manage medications

   ii. Transitioning persons with mental illness from institutions to the community may require both medication management and cognitive behavioral therapy (CBT) before the move can occur. However, CBT is not a reimbursable service in long-term care settings

2. Care coordination/care or case management[19]

a) Reduces hospitalizations and associated costs

b) Increases patient and family satisfaction

c) Improves communication among patient care provider (PCP) and specialists

d) Enhances treatment adherence and medication reconciliation

e) Can improve patient and caregiver knowledge, skill, and self-efficacy to manage illness and associated treatments

3. Pain and symptom management programs may lead to[19]

a) Reductions in admissions and readmissions

b) Market cost savings

c) Improved quality of life

4. Advance directives, including Physician/Provider/Medical Orders for Life-Sustaining Treatment (POLST/MOLST) forms, or equivalent (refer to Chapter IX for a complete discussion of advance care planning and determining goals of care)

5. Ethics and teaching consultations

a) Can lead to reductions in futile care

b) Assures the benefits and burdens of treatment options are discussed

c) Possible settings include intensive care, neonatal intensive care, prenatal when fetal life-limiting conditions are identified, long-term care, including assisted living settings, dedicated dementia units, and prisons, to name a few

XII. Access to Healthcare for Serious or Life-Threatening Illness

A. Factors influencing access may vary from state to state and setting to setting

1. Scope of benefits is restricted for serious or life-threatening illness care in nonhospice settings

a) Medicare hospice benefit eligibility criteria limits access, except for persons with 6-month prognosis or less

b) Eligibility for nonhospice home care restricted by "homebound," "skilled nursing," and "face-to-face" requirements (only PCP may certify)

2. Incentives for practitioners to provide more cost-effective care, which can translate into "less" care

3. Insurance and Medicaid preauthorization requirements; medication formularies that may or may not be responsive to individual response variation

4. Access disparities among poor, marginalized, and historically underserved populations, including persons living in rural and frontier areas

5. Delayed referral to hospice and/or palliative care

6. Cultural issues relating to end-of-life care and decision-making

B. **Factors Originating Within the Healthcare System**

1. Patients discharged "quicker and sicker"

2. Increased use of medical technology in the home

3. Functionally disabled and cognitively impaired are increasingly admitted to long-term care facilities

4. Stress on ambulatory and home care services to meet needs of population demographics and health trends

5. Financial rewards and penalties associated with hospital readmissions

C. **Financial Burden of Serious or Life-Threatening Illness**

1. Real and potential cuts in benefits (Medicare, Medicaid, Social Security, disability)

2. Impact on families and informal caregivers

a) Healthcare reforms shift the cost and burdens of caregiving to the family and local communities

i. Lost work hours

ii. Out-of-pocket expenses, including time off from work, travel time to medical appointments, and for associated lab work, etc.

iii. Care hours by family members/close others not compensated or reimbursed

iv. Caregiver stress, fatigue, and resultant poor health outcomes lead to increased use of healthcare system

3. Reported healthcare savings and costs for the system (Medicare spending, etc.) do not fully reflect the "actual cost" (direct and indirect out-of-pocket costs) of care for the full length of the illness

XIII. Palliative Care Settings

A. **Palliative Care is Provided in Three Settings**

    1.   Hospice—hospice at home or institution-based

    2.   Hospital-based palliative care—most common type of palliative care in nonhospice setting

    3.   Community-based palliative care[18]

        a)   Range of care delivery models, including advanced illness management (AIM) programs, supportive care programs, and "post-acute" transitional care programs

        b)   Large insurance companies such as Aetna, Excellus, BlueCross BlueShield, and Highmark have done extensive work evaluating the effectiveness (value) of palliative care programs in diverse settings

B. **No federal formal reimbursement system exists for palliative care in nonhospice settings, though some states are reimbursing for palliative care through managed care programs**

    1.   Palliative care diagnosis-related group (DRG)

        a)   DRG codes are used by CMS to define how Medicare funds are reimbursed

        b)   In 1996, an ICD-9-CM "v66.7" code for palliative care was developed; does not actually bring reimbursement, but allows data to be collected about the provision of palliative care services to determine if a new code is needed to pay hospitals, and to determine if it is feasible to reimburse for palliative care

XIV. Reimbursement Sources for Serious or Life-Threatening Illness and End-of-Life Care[3,19]

A. **Common Payer Sources for Serious or Life-Threatening Illness Care in the United States**

    1.   Medicare and Medicaid, including expanded Medicaid in certain states

    2.   Federal and state healthcare exchanges (state healthcare exchanges are only available in participating states)

    3.   Veterans Administration and federal health programs

    4.   Private insurance, either employer-based or purchased by individuals

    5.   Federal and state correctional systems

    6.   Private pay for those without any form of health insurance

B. **Medicare is the most common source of payment for hospice care[3,19]**

    1.   The proportion of Medicare beneficiaries using hospice services at the end of life continues to grow, and average length of stay increased in 2012

        a)   In 2012, 46.7% of Medicare beneficiaries who died that year used hospice, up from 45.2% in 2011 and 22.9% in 2000[3]

        b)   The median length of stay for hospice decedents was 18 days in 2012 and has remained stable at approximately 17 or 18 days since 2000

    c) Total Medicare payments to hospices increased from just under $3 billion in 2000 to just over $15 billion in 2012 due to increased hospice enrollment and longer lengths of stay[9]

XV. Medicare Hospice Reimbursement via the Medicare Hospice Benefit

A. In June, 2008, CMS and the Department of Health and Human Services issued the newly revised *Medicare and Medicaid Programs: Hospice Conditions of Participation; Final Rule* (42 CFR Part 418)[20]

    1. Overall, the changes reflect focus on patient- and family-centered care and are organized under 4 core conditions that are vital to the delivery of high-quality care

        a) Patient rights

        b) Patient and family assessment

        c) Interdisciplinary care planning and coordination of services

        d) Quality assessment and performance improvement (QAPI)

    2. There are also changes addressing drugs and durable medical equipment, inpatient care, hospice care provided to residents of facilities, and the requirement for a master's-prepared social worker to either provide care directly or supervise social workers prepared at the bachelor's level

    3. The basics of the Medicare Hospice Benefit, however, largely remain the same

B. Hospice care is an elected benefit covered under Medicare Part A for a patient who meets all of the following requirements[21]

    1. The individual is eligible for Part A

    2. The individual is certified as having a terminal illness with a medical prognosis of 6 months or less if the illness runs its normal course

    3. The individual receives care from a Medicare-approved hospice program

    4. The individual signs a statement (informed consent) indicating that he/she elects the Medicare Hospice Benefit and waives all other rights to Medicare payment for services that are related to the treatment of the terminal illness and related conditions

        a) Essential elements of an informed consent for hospice admission (either patient or surrogate, if appropriate)

            i. Comfort-oriented nature of services and definition of the services covered

            ii. Service settings

            iii. Specific services covered/not covered and financial responsibility, including co-pay

            iv. Withdrawal or discharge criteria and processes

        b) If the patient has capacity to make healthcare decisions, he/she must sign the consent form

            i. If the patient lacks decision-making capacity, a surrogate decision-maker must provide the informed consent

C.   **Important note: the Medicare hospice regulations** *apply to the care of all patients* **in a Medicare-certified hospice, regardless of payer, or lack of a payer source**

D.   **Benefit Periods**

1.   There are two 90-day benefit periods and unlimited 60-day periods, as long as the patient remains appropriate for hospice care

2.   Patients may sign-off of or revoke the Medicare hospice benefit and resume traditional Medicare coverage for the terminal illness. Any remaining days in that benefit period are forfeited

E.   **For Recertifications after January 1, 2011[22]**

1.   A hospice physician or hospice nurse practitioner (NP) must have a face-to-face encounter with each hospice patient prior to the beginning of the patient's third benefit period, and prior to each subsequent benefit period

2.   Failure to meet the face-to-face encounter requirements results in a failure by the hospice to meet the patient's recertification of terminal illness eligibility requirement, and the patient would cease to be eligible for the benefit

F.   **Hospices are required to continue to provide services regardless of ability to pay or bill a third party payer**

G.   **Hospice "core services" is a term used by Medicare to designate "core" team member services that must be provided by the agency**

1.   With the exception of physician services, all core services must be provided by the hospice and not contracted out. This in no way negates the requirement for a more comprehensive team

H.   **Core services include**

1.   Physician services

2.   Nursing services (routinely available on a 24-hour basis, 7 days a week) provided by or under the supervision of a registered nurse (RN) functioning within a plan of care developed by the hospice interdisciplinary group (IDG) in consultation with the patient's attending physician, if the patient has one

3.   Medical social services by a qualified social worker

4.   Counseling (spiritual, bereavement, dietary)

a)   The hospice must make bereavement services available to the family and other individuals identified in the bereavement plan of care up to 1 year following the death of the patient

5.   Hospice *may* contract for the services of a registered nurse if the services are highly specialized and provided nonroutinely

a)   Highly specialized services are determined by the nature of the service and the nursing skill level required to be proficient in the service. For example, a pediatric nurse may be needed if a hospice cares for pediatric patients infrequently, and if employing a pediatric nurse would be impracticable or cost-prohibitive

b)   NOTE: continuous care is not a highly specialized service, because while time intensive and costly, it is not necessarily highly-specialized care

6.   Hospices must also provide "noncore" therapy services (e.g., physical therapy [PT], occupational therapy [OT], speech-language pathology), hospice aide, and homemaker services

I.   Levels of Care in Medicare Hospice Program

1.   Routine home care day—a day in which a hospice patient receives care at home and is not receiving continuous care

2.   Continuous home care day—a day in which a hospice patient receives care at home for brief periods of crisis necessary to maintain the patient at home

a)   Continuous care is furnished during brief periods of crisis and only as necessary to maintain the terminally ill patient at home

b)   Care is provided for at least 8 hours a day in order to qualify for the continuous home care reimbursement rate (Medicare defines the "day" as one that starts and ends at midnight)

c)   Care must consist of predominantly (more than 50%) skilled nursing care (i.e., RN or licensed practical/vocational nurse [LP/VN])

3.   Inpatient respite care—a day in which a hospice patient receives care in an approved facility on a short-term basis for respite of family or other caregivers

a)   The hospice will not be reimbursed for respite care more than 5 days consecutively

b)   Payment to the hospice program for the sixth and any subsequent day of respite care is made at the routine home care rate

4.   General inpatient care—a day in which a hospice patient receives care in an approved facility for pain control or symptom management when care is not feasible in other settings (home or continuous care)

a)   Inpatient caps

i.   Medicare has established a limit to the number of total patient care days that will be reimbursed at either the general inpatient or inpatient respite care rates

ii.   The total inpatient days for Medicare patients may not exceed 20% of the total days for all the patients cared for by the hospice program who elect the Medicare hospice benefit in any Medicare fiscal year (this is sometimes described as the 80/20 rule)

5.   Change in level of care within the Medicare Hospice Benefit

a)   Transfer to another level of care is based on the medical needs of the patient (e.g., uncontrolled pain)

b)   Change in level of care requires a discussion with the patient and family and the IDG, changes in the plan of care, the primary physician's order, documentation in the patient's record

J.   Guidance was provided by CMS in 2014 on medication coverage as it related to Medicare Part D as follows[23]

1.   Federal regulations require that Medicare hospice providers conduct and document a readily-producible, patient-specific, comprehensive assessment in writing that identifies the patient's need for hospice care and services as well as any need for physical, psychosocial, emotional, and spiritual care

2.   The assessment must include

a)   All areas of hospice care related to the palliation and management of the terminal illness and related conditions

b)   A drug profile with all of the patient's prescription and over-the-counter (OTC) drugs, herbal remedies, and other alternative treatments that could affect drug therapy

3.   The hospice plan of care is based on the needs identified in the initial and updated plan of care assessments, including medication documentation

K.   Medicare Part D Guidelines (July 2014)[23]

1.   Medication information obtained through the assessments, including *whether the medications are related or unrelated* to the terminal illness and related conditions, should be provided to the Part D sponsor *before* a hospice beneficiary presents a prescription for fill—or, failing proactive provision of the information by the hospice, should be provided to the Part D sponsor, after the Part D sponsor contacts the hospice provider during the prior authorization (PA) process

2.   Hospices are strongly encouraged to provide a "compassionate first fill" for any medication needed by a beneficiary who is experiencing difficulty in accessing the drug at point of service (POS)

a)   If the drug provided is unrelated to the terminal illness and related conditions, the *hospice provider* should contact the Part D sponsor to negotiate recovery of the hospice's payment to the pharmacy

L.   Patient Coinsurance Payments

1.   Under specific circumstances, hospices may bill coinsurance for

a)   Prescription drugs or biologicals—coinsurance may be billed the amount for each palliative drug or biological prescription when he/she is not an inpatient (i.e., when the patient is receiving routine or continuous home care)

i.   When a patient is receiving general inpatient care or respite care, there is no coinsurance for covered prescriptions

b)   Respite care—coinsurance may be billed the amount for each respite care day equal to 5% of the payment made by Medicare for a respite care day

M.   Caps on Hospice Payments

1.   Two caps affect Medicare payments under the Hospice Benefit

a)   The number of days of inpatient care furnished is limited to not more than 20% of total patient care days (the inpatient cap)

b)   An aggregate payment amount that hospices may receive in Medicare payments for services provided in the cap year is limited to the cap amount times the number of Medicare patients served by the hospice program (the aggregate cap)

2.   The hospice aggregate cap amount is adjusted annually by the medical expenditure category of the Consumer Price Index for all Urban Consumers (CPI-U) published by the Bureau of Labor Statistics

N.   Volunteer Services

1.   Volunteer service hours must account for 5% of all direct patient care hours for all paid hospice employees and contract staff in a Medicare-certified hospice program

2.   The volunteer hours may be accumulated as direct patient care hours or indirect, administrative support hours

O.   Discontinuation of Hospice Services

1.   Patient and family initiated actions

a)   Transfers occur when a patient moves out of the service area of one hospice and into another hospice's service area, or chooses a different provider in the area. Patient remains in the current benefit period and loses no days in that period, but a transfer is allowed only once per benefit period

b)   Role of the transferring hospice is to

i.   Assure care continuity measures are in place and coordinate any referrals for provision of ongoing care (medical, nursing, social services, etc.)

ii.   Notify the patient's primary physician of the change in service area and/or service provider

2.   Withdrawal—any patient and family can choose to discontinue all services of the hospice for any reason

a)   Role of the hospice in facilitating patient and family withdrawal from service is to

i.   Notify primary physician of change and initiate any paperwork necessary for the change

ii.   Assure continuity measures and coordinate any referrals for provision of ongoing care

3.   The choice to withdraw from hospice care requires the patient or their legal representative to *revoke* the hospice benefit

a)   Revocation may be chosen in order to receive treatment not covered under the hospice plan of care, to receive care from a different service provider (e.g., SNF, noncontracted hospital) or because of dissatisfaction with the service being provided

b)   Revocation may occur any time during a benefit period; a patient or legal representative must *choose* to revoke his/her Medicare hospice (i.e., the hospice program may not instruct patient/family to revoke)

P. **Hospice Program Initiated Actions (Live Discharges)**

1. Discharge—a patient who no longer meets the Medicare criteria may be discharged; otherwise this action is only used in extraordinary circumstances such as when a threat to the safety of staff is posed

2. A patient MAY NOT be discharged

   a) Because of inability to pay for services

   b) If the management of the illness and palliative treatment is too expensive for the hospice

   c) If the primary physician orders expensive, "high tech" palliative care or if they are "difficult" to care for

3. Nonrecertification—also referred to as "decertification"

   a) At the end of a benefit period, the hospice interdisciplinary team, with the patient's primary physician, determines the patient no longer has a prognosis of 6 months or less (if the disease runs its normal course); a change in the status of the patient's terminal condition is the *ONLY consideration justifying nonrecertification*

Q. **Role of the hospice program in discontinuation of care; the hospice program is responsible to**

1. Notify the patient and family of the reasons for discontinuation of services

2. Inform the patient and family that the hospice benefit is still available to them if the need arises later

3. Provide for continuity of care to the degree possible

XVI. Medicaid Reimbursement under the Medicaid Hospice Benefit

A. **Hospice is an optional benefit under the Medicaid program and not all states choose to provide it**

B. **The Medicaid hospice benefit is modeled after the Medicare Hospice Benefit; Medicaid regulations differ by state and some state regulations are not current**

XVII. Reimbursement for Palliative Care under Medicare

A. **There currently is no direct reimbursement for nonhospice specialty palliative care under the Medicare program**

1. Demonstration projects evaluating value of palliative care

   a) Medicare Care Choices Model (MCCM) provides a new option for persons with advanced cancers, chronic obstructive pulmonary disease, congestive heart failure, and human immunodeficiency syndrome (HIV)/acquired immune deficiency syndrome (AIDS) who meet eligibility requirements under the Medicare Hospice Benefit to receive palliative care services from certain hospice providers while concurrently receiving curative care

2. Demonstration project eligibility

    a) Medicare certified hospices that are able to demonstrate experience providing coordination services and/or case management for beneficiaries *prior* to electing hospice

    b) MCCM hospices will provide services for routine home care and inpatient respite levels of care under the hospice benefit that cannot be separately billed under Medicare Parts A, B, and D

    c) CMS will pay a $400/beneficiary/month fee for these services. Participating curative service providers will be able to continue to bill Medicare for the "reasonable and necessary" services

XVIII. Reimbursement for Hospice and Palliative Care under Private Insurance[20]

A. Hospice Reimbursement under Private Insurance Benefit Plans

1. About 80% of private insurance plans have a hospice benefit; most others will negotiate a rate for hospice; some use a home health benefit

2. If a program is Medicare-certified, *all patients must receive all the services available to a Medicare beneficiary* whether or not the insurance company pays

B. Types of Plans

1. Per diem—similar to Medicare Hospice Benefit in that it is on a daily basis and includes all services

2. Per visit—insurance company authorizes the number of visits and the disciplines visiting

3. Dollar caps—the benefit is limited to a specific amount

4. Negotiated rates—rate of reimbursement is individualized according to the plan of care and agreement reached between the hospice and the insurance provider

XIX. Palliative Care Reimbursement under Private Insurance Benefit Plans[19]

A. Palliative care services (nonhospice benefits) generally are reimbursable under various parts of the patient's medical insurance (e.g., hospital medical services, skilled nursing at home, physician medical services)

B. Palliative nurses in nonhospice settings also may be providing symptom management and other key components of palliative care that are reimbursed but not call it "palliative care"

XX. Relevant Economic Issues in Serious or Life-Threatening Illness Care

A. In the Hospital Setting

1. Diagnosis-related group (DRG) prospective payment system

    a) Hospital stays are paid on a prospectively-determined, diagnosis-related basis (i.e., hospitals get paid a specific amount of money for specific diagnoses, based on average length of stay for those diagnoses) b)　Hospitals are reimbursed the same amount whether or not patients with a specific DRG have longer or shorter stays

c)　"Outlier" or "high cost patients"—hospital costs for these patients must reach designated levels before the hospital is reimbursed

2.　The Affordable Care Act requires hospitals to report hospital readmissions for specific conditions[7]

a)　Many patients are readmitted to hospitals repeatedly due to unmet palliative care and care coordination needs

b)　Hospitals are charged up to 1% of their annual Medicare reimbursement if their readmission rates rise above a national benchmark

B.　**Actual or potential effects of the prospective payment system on serious or life-threatening illness care in the hospital setting**

1.　Shorter hospital stays have not been offset by increased admissions

2.　Shorter stays have put increased burden on the family

3.　Premature discharge from hospital may leave families without adequate support systems to manage care

a)　Home care system not in place or inadequate

b)　Increased medical technology in home without adequate supports or education

c)　Symptom management expertise may vary

d)　Hospice coverage for inpatient care is limited

C.　**Issues for Palliative Care in the Hospital Setting**

1.　Intended to improve outcomes for persons with serious or life-threatening illness

a)　Clarification of, or determining the goals of care

b)　Enhanced symptom management

c)　Earlier hospice referral

2.　How to identify homogeneous care resources (not tied to diagnosis) that can be reimbursed and outcomes that can be quantified

a)　"Measuring What Matters" initiative supported by HPNA and AAHPM

b)　Quality Forum measures for palliative care

c)　How to balance reducing futile care while respecting patient and family wishes if they prefer to continue aggressive care or life-sustaining treatments

XXI. Issues for Physicians and Advanced Practice Nurses Who Care for Persons Who Are Imminently Dying

A.　**Different visit codes exist for brief, limited, extended, and other classes**

1.　Importance of coding visits for "evaluation and management" versus procedures and tests

2. Codes do not differentiate between classes of patients

3. May discourage care of those with special needs

    a) Hearing/vision/cognitively impaired

    b) Those with linguistic needs (non-English speaking)

    c) Those requiring special symptom management

    d) Those with needs for emotional support

4. Nursing home visits not reimbursed at same level as hospital visits

XXII. Palliative Care and Nursing Homes

A. **Barriers to palliative care in nursing homes include factors such as**

1. Regulations that favor rehabilitation over palliative care

2. Inadequate staff knowledge and skill in palliative care

3. Financial disincentives (e.g., higher reimbursement for skilled nursing care and invasive therapies)

4. Misconceptions about palliative care

5. Lack of reimbursement for specialized palliative care

B. **Issues in the Nursing Home Facility Where Most Funding Comes from Medicaid**

1. Seven of 10 residents receive some funding from Medicaid

2. State cuts to Medicaid impacting the quality of care nursing homes can provide

3. Nursing home populations are more ill and impaired and more demanding of resources due to

    a) Reduced hospital lengths of stay

    b) Demand for increased access to technologically-sophisticated care in the nursing home

    c) Increasing resident age and disability

C. **Data on Medicare hospice care in nursing home facilities demonstrated**

1. Hospice care is associated with less hospitalization for Medicare hospice patients

2. Diffusion of palliative care philosophy and practices with care of nonhospice residents resulted in lower rates of end-of-life hospitalizations as well

XXIII. Issues for Home Healthcare in Providing Palliative Care Services

A. **Eligibility Requirements**

1. Patient must be homebound. "Homebound" means that an individual is considered to be "confined to his/her home" if

a)   The individual has a condition due to an illness or injury that restricts the ability to leave his/her home except with the assistance of another individual or the aide of a supportive device (e.g., crutches, a cane, a wheelchair, or a walker)

b)   The individual has a condition due to an illness or injury such that leaving his/her home is medically contraindicated

c)   The condition should be such that there exists a normal inability to leave home—that leaving the home requires a considerable and taxing effort

2.   Patient must need part-time or intermittent skilled nursing care, or physical or speech therapy, or continued occupational therapy

3.   A physician must order Medicare home health services and must certify a patient's eligibility for the benefit at start of care. This face-to-face requirement ensures that the orders and certification for home health services are based on a physician's current knowledge of the patient's clinical condition

B.   Growth in Home Care Expenditures

1.   Changes in Medicare home care policies

2.   Earlier discharge from hospitals

3.   Increased feasibility of providing advanced technology in the home

C.   Palliative Care in Home Care Settings

1.   Barriers include

a)   Eligibility criteria

b)   Lack of reimbursement

c)   Emphasis on "rehabilitation potential"

d)   Cultural barriers of health professionals, patients, and family

2.   Opportunities include

a)   Improve symptom management

b)   Ease transition into hospice, if appropriate

c)   Provide more intensive services, education, and family support

d)   Care coordination, medication reconciliation, and other supportive services

XXIV. Economic Value of the Advanced Practice Nurse (APN) in Hospice and Palliative Care

A.   Two Levels of Advanced Practice Palliative Nursing[16]

1.   Graduate-level prepared specialty nurse—educated at the master's or doctoral level and are essential to advance palliative care in roles other than direct care (e.g., education, research, administration)

2. Advanced practice registered nurse—clinically educated at the master's level or above, providing patient care in one of four roles: clinical nurse specialist (CNS), nurse practitioner (NP), certified nurse midwife (CNM), or certified registered nurse anesthetist (CRNA). Most hospice and palliative APRNs are CNSs and/or NPs. Though all APRNs have the knowledge, skills, abilities, and competency to perform all aspects of basic palliative nursing, additional graduate education and preparation enable the APRN to practice at an advanced specialty level

B. Practice Models

1. Should provide clarity and direction to the field

2. Purposes served are determined by the concepts delineated in the framework (i.e., practice competencies)

3. Competency is core concept in several APN practice models

C. Factors Indicating a Need for Advanced Practice Nurses Who Specialize in Serious or Life-Threatening Illness and Palliative Care

1. Studies increasingly are demonstrating the APN role can improve quality of life in a cost-effective way[24–26]

2. Palliative care services research reflects growing gap in supply and demand for palliative care professionals

3. Increasing evidence to support specialty certification in hospice and palliative care at the generalist and advanced practice levels[27,28]

CITED REFERENCES

1. Buck J. Policy and the reformation of hospice: lessons from the past for the future of palliative care. *J Hosp Palliat Nurs.* 2011;13(6):S35-S43.

2. 113th Congress, 2nd Session. *H.R. 4709, Ensuring Patient Access and Effective Drug Enforcement Act of 2014.* www.gpo.gov/fdsys/pkg/BILLS-113hr4709rfs/pdf/BILLS-113hr4709rfs.pdf. Accessed August 20, 2014.

3. Medicare Payment Advisory Commission (MedPAC). *Report to the Congress: Medicare Payment Policy.* 2014. www.medpac.gov/documents/mar14_entirereport.pdf. Accessed June 30, 2014.

4. Centers for Medicare & Medicaid Services (CMS). *National Health Expenditure Projections 2011–2021.* 2011. www.cms.gov/Research-Statistics-Data-and-Systems/Statistics-Trends-and-Reports/NationalHealthExpendData/Downloads/Proj2011PDF.pdf. Accessed August 20, 2014.

5. Medicare Payment Advisory Commission (MedPAC). *About MEDPAC.* 2014. www.medpac.gov/about.cfm. Accessed August 20, 2014.

6. Buck J. Home hospice versus home health: cooperation, competition, and co-optation. *Nurs Hist Rev.* 2004;12:25-46.

7. Schultz HK. *Implementation of the Affordable Care Act: Opportunities for Collaboration and Partnership.* Presented at 33rd Congressional Council Town Hall. 2011. bass.house.gov/sites/karenbass.house.gov/files/documents/Affordable%20Care%20Act%20101%20-%20Herb%20Schultz.pdf. Accessed June 10, 2014.

8. Adler L, Hoagland GW; Bi-Partisan Policy.Org. *What is Driving U.S. Health Care Spending? American's Unsustainable Health Care Cost Growth.* 2012. bipartisanpolicy.org/library/what-driving-us-health-care-spending-americas-unsustainable-health-care-cost-growth/. Accessed December 12, 2014.

9. Medicare Payment Advisory Commission (MedPAC). *A Data Book: Health Care Spending and the Medicare Program.* 2014. www.medpac.gov/documents/publications/jun14databookentirereport.pdf?sfvrsn=1. Accessed August 20, 2014.

10. Meier DE. Increased access to palliative care and hospice: opportunities to improve value in health care. *Millbank Q.* 2011;89(3):343-380. doi: 10.1111/j.1468-0009.2011.00632.x.

11. Center to Advance Palliative Care (CAPC). *A State-by-State Report Card on Access to Palliative Care in Our Nation's Hospitals.* 2011. www.capc.org/reportcard/summary. Accessed May 29, 2014.

12. Institute of Medicine (IOM). *The Future of Nursing: Leading Change, Advancing Health.* 2010. www.iom.edu/Reports/2010/the-future-of-nursing-leading-change-advancin-health.aspx. Accessed February 23, 2014.

13. Federal Trade Commission (FTC). *Policy Perspectives: Competition and the Regulation of Advanced Practice Nurses.* 2014. www.ftc.gov/system/files/documents/reports/policy-perspectives-competition-regulation-advanced-practice-nurses/140307aprnpolicypaper.pdf. Accessed May 21, 2014.

14. Institute of Medicine (IOM). *Approaching Death: Improving Care at the End of Life.* Washington, DC: The National Academies Press; 1997.

15. Institute of Medicine (IOM). *Dying in America: Improving Quality and Honoring Individual Preferences Near the End of Life.* Washington, DC: The National Academies Press; 2014.

16. Dahlin CM, Sutermaster DJ, eds.; Hospice and Palliative Nurses Association, American Nurses Association. *Palliative Nursing: Scope and Standards of Practice—An Essential Resource for Palliative and Hospice Nurses.* Silver Spring, MD: nursesbooks.org; 2014.

17. American Nurses Association (ANA). *Health Care Reform*. 2014. www.nursingworld.org/
    MainMenuCategories/Policy-Advocacy/HealthSystemReform/AffordableCareAct.pdf. Accessed
    August 20, 2014.

18. Coyne P, Lyckholm L, Smith TJ. Clinical interventions, economic impact, and palliative care. In:
    Ferrell BR, Coyle N, eds. *Oxford Textbook of Palliative Nursing*. 3rd ed. New York, NY: Oxford
    University Press; 2010:487-499.

19. Center to Advance Palliative Care (CAPC). *Payer-Provider Partnerships: A Palliative Care Toolkit
    and Resource Guide*. www.capc.org/payertoolkit/. Accessed June 2, 2014.

20. Centers for Medicare & Medicaid Services (CMS). Medicare and Medicaid programs: hospice
    conditions of participation. Final rule. *Fed Regist*. 2008;73(109):32088-32220.

21. Center for Medicare & Medicaid Services (CMS). *Payment System Fact Series*. 2013. www.cms.gov/
    Outreach-and-Education/Medicare-Learning-Network-MLN/MLNProducts/downloads/hospice_pay_
    sys_fs.pdf. Accessed May 29, 2014.

22. Center for Medicare & Medicaid Services (CMS). *Medicare Learning Network Matters: Hospice
    Policy Manual Update (MM7337)*. 2012. www.cms.gov/Outreach-and-Education/Medicare-Learning-
    Network-MLN/MLNMattersArticles/Downloads/MM7337.pdf. Accessed, May 29, 2014.

23. Center for Medicare & Medicaid Services (CMS). *Guidance Memo: Part D Payment for Drugs for
    Beneficiaries Enrolled in Medicare Hospice*. July 18, 2014. www.cms.gov/Medicare/Medicare-Fee-
    for-Service-Payment/Hospice/Downloads/2014-PartD-Hospice-Guidance-Revised-Memo.pdf.
    Accessed August 21, 2014.

24. Hospice and Palliative Nurses Association (HPNA). *Value of the Advanced Practice Registered Nurse
    in Palliative Care* [Position Statement]. 2013. hpna.advancingexpertcare.org/education/position-
    statements/. Accessed October 20, 2014.

25. American Academy of Nurse Practitioners (AANP). *Quality of Nurse Practitioner Practice*. 2013.
    www.aanp.org/images/documents/publications/qualityofpractice.pdf. Accessed August 21, 2014.

26. American Academy of Nurse Practitioners (AANP). *Nurse Practitioner Cost-Effectiveness*. 2013.
    www.aanp.org/images/documents/publications/costeffectiveness.pdf. Accessed August 21, 2014.

27. Hospice and Palliative Nurses Association (HPNA). *Value of Hospice and Palliative Nursing
    Certification* [Position Statement]. 2012. hpna.advancingexpertcare.org/education/position-statements/.
    Accessed October 20, 2014.

28. American Board of Nursing Specialties (ABNS). *Nursing Certification Bibliography*. 2014.
    www.nursingcertification.org/pdf/ABNS%20Cert%20bib%202014.pdf. Accessed August 22, 2014.

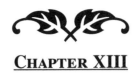

CHAPTER XIII

NATIONAL GUIDELINES AND RN PRACTICE

Constance Dahlin, ANP-BC, ACHPN®, FPCN®, FAAN
Judith C. Lentz, RN, MSN, FPCN®

Preface

There are two national documents that delineate expectations, guidelines, and preferred practices for palliative care. These are the National Consensus Project (NCP) for Quality Palliative Care's *Clinical Practice Guidelines for Quality Palliative Care*,[1] and the National Quality Forum's *A National Framework and Preferred Practices for Palliative and Hospice Care Quality: A Consensus Statement*.[2] Both provide a comprehensive framework to evaluate quality palliative care. They serve as the basis for the performance measures used in Palliative Care Certification by The Joint Commission.

The National Consensus Project *Clinical Practice Guidelines* were first developed in 2004, but were revised in 2009 and 2013. The National Quality Forum's *A Framework* was produced in 2006, using the 2004 edition of the National Consensus Project *Clinical Practice Guidelines* as a foundation. However, the Preferred Practices have not been updated to reflect the revisions of the *Clinical Practice Guidelines*. This chapter offers the registered nurse (RN) recommendations on applying the *Clinical Practice Guidelines* and the 38 Preferred Practices (PP) to promote the highest provision of quality palliative nursing. Therefore, the language of the 2013 National Consensus Project frames the role of the RN. Most of Preferred Practices are applicable to the palliative care RN, although not necessarily in the order of *A Framework*.

Throughout this chapter, there has been an effort to provide consistency and congruency between the National Consensus Project for Quality, *Care Clinical Practice Guidelines*; the National Quality Forum, *A National Framework and Preferred Practices for Palliative and Hospice Care Quality: A Consensus Statement*; the American Nurses Association and Hospice and Palliative Nurses Association's, *Palliative Nursing: Scope and Standards—An Essential Resource for the Hospice and Palliative Nurse*; and Hospice and Palliative Nurse Association, *Competencies for the Generalist Hospice and Palliative Nurse*.

The *Clinical Practice Guidelines* describe how the plan of care is individualized to the patient and family, occurring in the context of initiation of services within the disease trajectory.[1] For the purposes of this document, plan of care is used throughout the chapter to reflect its use. The American Nurses Association and Hospice and Palliative Nurses Association document *Palliative Nursing: Scope and Standards* defines palliative nursing as the specialty under which hospice and palliative nurses practice.[3] Thus, throughout this chapter, palliative nursing is used to indicate all hospice and palliative care programs, units, and agencies. For simplicity, the term palliative RN includes both hospice and palliative nurses.

DOMAIN 1: Structure and Processes of Care

GUIDELINE 1.1—A comprehensive and timely interdisciplinary assessment of the patient and family forms the basis of the plan of care.

Criteria

1. Assessment by the palliative RN is consistent with education and within the limits of licensure. Assessment is reviewed on a regular basis and systematically documented, reflecting coordinated interdisciplinary perspectives.

2. The palliative RN, within state statutes of scope of practice, completes an initial assessment and subsequent reevaluation through patient assessment.

3. The palliative RN assessment process includes documentation of disease status, including diagnoses; comorbid medical and psychiatric disorders; physical and psychological symptoms; functional status; social, cultural, and spiritual strengths; values, practices, concerns, and goals; advance care planning concerns, preferences, and documents; and appropriateness of hospice referral including Domain 2, *Physical Aspects of Care*; Domain 3, *Psychological and Psychiatric Aspects of Care*; Domain 4, *Social Aspects of Care*; Domain 5, *Spiritual, Religious, and Existential Aspects of Care*; and Domain 8, *Ethical and Legal Aspects of Care*.

4. The palliative RN performs appropriate assessment of children with consideration of age and stage of neurocognitive development and within scope of practice.

5. The palliative RN documents assessment of the patient and family perception and understanding of the serious or life-limiting illness including patient and family expectations of treatment, goals for care, quality of life, as well as preferences for the type and site of care.

6. The palliative RN performs an assessment of the elements of quality of life defined by the 4 domains of physical, psychological, social, and spiritual aspects of care.[4]

7. This palliative RN performs assessment on a regular basis and in subsequent intervals or in response to significant changes in the patient's or family's status or goals.

Preferred Practice Examples for the Palliative RN under DOMAIN 1/GUIDELINE 1.1

PP 1—The palliative RN provides palliative and hospice care as part of the interdisciplinary team who collaborates with primary healthcare professional(s).

PP 2—The palliative RN assures availability of qualified nursing professionals 24/7 to meet the needs of the patient–family.

PP 3—The palliative RN educates patient, family, and co-team members about hospice and palliative care.

PP 10—The palliative RN empowers patients and caregivers to make informed decisions about their care by offering information about their disease and benefits and burdens of care.

GUIDELINE 1.2—The plan of care is based on the identified and expressed preferences, values, goals, and needs of the patient and family and is developed with professional guidance and support for patient-family decision making. *Family* is defined by the patient.

Criteria

1. The palliative RN formulates a nursing plan based on an ongoing assessment and reflects goals set by the patient and family or surrogate in collaboration with the interdisciplinary team (IDT).

2. In collaboration with the patient, family, and other involved healthcare providers, the palliative RN develops the nursing plan with the additional input, when indicated, of other providers in the community, such as school professionals, community service providers, and spiritual leaders.

3. The palliative RN changes the plan based on the evolving needs and preferences of the patient and family and recognizes the complex, competing, and shifting priorities in goals of care. The evolving care plan is documented over time.

4. The palliative RN provides support for patient–family decision making and implements and coordinates the plan in collaboration with the patient and family. The RN promotes patient and family education of the plan and assures communication of the plan to all involved health professionals. Particular attention is necessary when a patient transfers to a different care setting to communicate with the receiving provider.

5. The palliative RN documents responses to treatment and care setting alternatives and communicates with the patient and family in a manner that promotes informed decision making.

6. The palliative RN assures that treatment decisions are based on goals of care established by the patient, family, and IDT; assessment of risk and benefit; and best evidence. Reevaluation of patient–family goals and choices is documented.

Preferred Practice Examples for the Palliative RN under DOMAIN 1/GUIDELINE 1.2

PP 6—The palliative RN regularly reviews a plan based on values, preferences, goals, and needs of patient–family and communicates with the entire IDT.

PP 11—The palliative RN provides education and support to families and caregivers to promote a safe and appropriate individualized care plan.

GUIDELINE 1.3—An interdisciplinary team provides services to the patient and family consistent with the plan of care. In addition to chaplains, nurses, physicians, and social workers, other therapeutic disciplines who provide palliative care services to patients and families may include: child-life specialists; nursing assistants; nutritionists; occupational therapists; recreational therapists; respiratory therapists; pharmacists; physical therapists; massage; art and music therapists; psychologists; and speech and language pathologists.

Criteria

1. A palliative RN provides specialist-level palliative care as a member of an IDT.

2. The palliative RN is part of a team that includes palliative care professionals with the appropriate patient population-specific education, credentialing, experience, and the skills to meet the physical, psychological, social, and spiritual needs of both patient and family. The palliative RN has undergraduate or associate nursing education and is certified by the Hospice and Palliative Credentialing Center (HPCC) in hospice and palliative nursing. Palliative RNs should be expected to have current certification as a CHPN® or seek certification within 2 years of employment.

3. The interdisciplinary palliative care team involved in the care of children, whether the child is a patient or a family member of either an adult or pediatric patient, has expertise in the delivery of services for such children.

4.   The palliative RN is part of the team that provides palliative care expertise. The palliative RN is knowledgeable about access to respite services available for the families and caregivers of children or adults with serious illnesses.

5.   The patient and family have access (either by phone or in person) to palliative care expertise and staff 24 hours a day, 7 days a week. Respite services are available for the families caring for either children or adults with serious or life-threatening illnesses.

6.   The palliative RN participates in regular IDT communication (at least weekly or more often as required by the clinical situation) to plan, review, evaluate, and update the plan, with input from both the patient and family. The palliative RN is an essential part of quality care, providing input on policy development, and assisting in the development of clinical practices.

Preferred Practice Examples for the Palliative RN under DOMAIN 1/GUIDELINE 1.3

PP 4—The palliative RN receives adequate training to be confident in his/her care.

PP 5—The palliative RN is a certified hospice and palliative nurse (CHPN®), a certified hospice and palliative pediatric nurse (CHPPN®), certified in perinatal loss (CPLC®) or other Hospice and Palliative Credentialing Center certifications and demonstrates leadership according to standards of professional performance.

GUIDELINE 1.4—The palliative care program is encouraged to use appropriately trained and supervised volunteers to the extent feasible.

Criteria

1.   For programs utilizing volunteers, the palliative RN participates in the development of policies and procedures to assure safe and quality volunteer programs, such as recruitment; screening (including background checks); training; job descriptions; role clarification; work practices; support; supervision; and performance evaluation, in addition to clarity of the responsibilities of the program to its volunteers.

2.   A program that uses volunteers has policies and procedures outlining the program's responsibilities to its volunteers. The palliative RN assures appropriate use of volunteers.

3.   The palliative RN may participate in screening, educating, coordinating, and collaborating with volunteers.

Preferred Practice Example for the Palliative RN under DOMAIN 1/GUIDELINE 1.4

The palliative RN participates in the creation of policies and procedures, in the development of volunteer programs, supervises appropriately-screened volunteers, and participates in education for volunteers as appropriate.

GUIDELINE 1.5—Support for education, training, and professional development is available to the interdisciplinary team.

Criteria

1.   The minimum orientation for the palliative RN as delineated in the NCP Guidelines as the attitudes, knowledge, and skills in the domains of palliative care (i.e., pain and symptom assessment and

management; communication skills; medical ethics; grief and bereavement; family and community resources; and hospice care including philosophy, eligibility, and core features of the Medicare Hospice Benefit). It may include advance care planning and coordination of care with primary care teams as well.

2. Palliative RN education and training occurs in various venues such as baccalaureate education, practicums, or palliative RN shadowing in compliance with federal and state licensure and credentialing regulations.

3. The palliative care program supports the palliative RN's professional development through mentoring, preceptorship, and supervision.

4. Palliative RNs participate in essential continuing palliative care education, and their participation is documented accordingly. Educational resources, focused on the domains listed in this document, are available and provided to palliative RNs in a number of venues.

5. Palliative care programs assure appropriate education for palliative RNs, specifically undergraduate degrees in clinical nursing, and appropriate professional experience.

6. Palliative care programs encourage palliative RN discipline-specific certification, or other recognition of competence, as part of the educational support for the IDT. Educational resources, education, and support are provided specifically to enhance IDT communication and collaboration.

7. Education regarding effective team management, human resource management, budgets, and strategic planning is available to support palliative RN leadership.

Preferred Practice Example for the Palliative RN under DOMAIN 1/GUIDELINE 1.5

The palliative RN is expected to participate in educational programming based on his/her level of care responsibilities and with the financial support by the organization of these efforts.

GUIDELINE 1.6—In its commitment to quality assessment and performance improvement, the palliative care program develops, implements, and maintains an ongoing data-driven process that reflects the complexity of the organization and focuses on palliative outcomes.

Criteria

1. The palliative care program commits to the pursuit of excellence and the highest quality of care and support for all patients and their families. The program determines quality by providing regular and systematic measurement, analysis, review, evaluation, goal setting, and revision of the processes and outcomes of care. The palliative RN participates in the quality process.

2. Quality care follows the national quality strategy set out by the U.S. Department of Health and Human Services in carrying out the provisions of the Patient Protection and Affordable Care Act. The strategy states

   • "Making care safer by reducing harm caused in the delivery of care.

   • Ensuring that each person and family is engaged as partners in their care.

   • Promoting effective communication and coordination of care.

   • Promoting the most effective prevention and treatment practices for the leading causes of mortality, starting with cardiovascular disease.

   • Working with communities to promote wide use of best practices to enable healthy living.

- Making quality care more affordable for individuals, families, employers, and governments by developing and spreading new healthcare delivery models."[5]

3. The palliative RN coordinates care continually focused on the illness trajectory, which offers the right care at the right time in the course of an individual's disease or condition.

4. The palliative RN participates in the quality assessment and performance improvement (QAPI) review done across all the domains including organizational structure, education, team utilization, assessment and effectiveness of physical, psychological, psychiatric, social, spiritual, cultural, and ethical assessment and interventions.

5. The palliative RN participates in QAPI process in which the palliative care program establishes quality improvement policies and procedures.

6. A process for quality improvement is documented and leads to change in clinical practice. The palliative RN participates in or develops quality improvement projects that might include the development and testing of screening, history, and assessment tools, and appropriate protocols for diagnoses, interventions, and outcomes. Some examples may include

   - Structure and Processes—development of outcomes for program development, education and training, development of quality measures, cost analysis.

   - Physical Aspects of Care—education and training, development and testing of evidence-based therapies.

   - Psychological and Psychiatric Aspects of Care—education and training, development and testing of bereavement and grief screening, assessment tools of types of grief, and development and testing of evidence-based therapies.

   - Social Aspects of Care—education and training, development and testing of social screening, assessment, and intervention tools; identification and enhancement of the evidence base within the social domain.

   - Spiritual, Religious, and Existential Aspects of Care—education and training, development and testing of spiritual screening, history, and assessment tools; and appropriate protocols for spiritual diagnoses, interventions, and outcomes.

   - Cultural Aspects of Care—education and training, development and testing of cultural assessment tools and culturally-appropriate interventions; evaluation of outcomes within and across cultural and linguistic communities.

   - Care of the Patient at the End of Life—education and training, appropriate protocols for the imminently dying patient.

   - Ethical and Legal Aspects of Care—education and training, appropriate protocols for ethical and legal occurrences, best practices for advance care planning.

7. Quality improvement activities are routine, regular, reported, and are shown to influence clinical practice. Designated staff, with experience in QAPI planning, including a palliative RN, operates the QAPI process in collaboration with leaders of the palliative care program.

8. The clinical practices of the palliative RN reflect the integration and dissemination of research and evidence of quality process.

9. Quality improvement activities for clinical services are collaborative, interdisciplinary, and focused on meeting the identified needs and goals of patients and their families.

10. Patients, families, health professionals, and the community participate in evaluation of the palliative care program.

> ## Preferred Practice Example for the Palliative RN under DOMAIN 1/GUIDELINE 1.6

The palliative RN participates in quality improvement policies and procedures for the palliative care program and evaluates the outcomes. The palliative RN assures that fellow nursing staff members comply as per policies.

GUIDELINE 1.7—The palliative care program recognizes the emotional impact of the provision of palliative care on the team providing care to patients with serious or life-threatening illnesses and their families.

Criteria

1   The program provides emotional support to palliative RNs to facilitate coping with the stress of caring for individuals and families affected by serious or life-threatening illness.

2   Support structure of palliative RNs includes regular meetings where review, impact, and processes of the provision of palliative care are discussed.

3   The program and IDT implements interventions to promote resiliency and sustainability of palliative RN team members.

> ## Preferred Practice Example for the Palliative RN under DOMAIN 1/GUIDELINE 1.7

The palliative RN serves as an emotional support to staff and volunteers. In addition, the palliative RN identifies and accesses further resources for emotional support per organizational policies.

GUIDELINE 1.8—Community resources ensure continuity of the highest quality palliative care across the care continuum.

Criteria

1.   Palliative care programs support and promote continuity of care throughout the trajectory of illness across all settings. The palliative RN plays a role in continuity and consistency across settings.

2.   Non-hospice palliative care programs have a relationship with one or more hospices and other community resources to ensure continuity of the highest-quality palliative care across the care continuum.

3.   Non-hospice palliative care programs and palliative RNs routinely inform patients and families about hospice and other community-based healthcare resources when such resources are consistent with the patient's and family's values, beliefs, preferences, and goals of care. Palliative RNs suggest referral only with patient and family consent.

4.   Referring clinicians, as described by Centers for Medicare & Medicaid Services (CMS), including other RNs, are routinely informed about the availability and benefits of hospice, as well as other appropriate community resources for their patients and families. The palliative RN understands these services, offers early discussion of these services, and promotes early referral to such services as hospices and community resources.

5.   The palliative RN participates and facilitates the work of hospice programs, non-hospice palliative care programs, and other major community service providers involved in the patient's care to establish policies for formal written and verbal communication about all domains in the plan of care.

6.   The palliative RN is aware of policies to enable timely and effective sharing of information among teams while safeguarding privacy.

7.   When possible, hospice and palliative program staff, including palliative RNs, participate in each other's team meetings to promote regular professional communication, collaboration, and an integrated plan of care on behalf of patients and families.

8.   Hospice and palliative programs, as well as other major community providers, routinely seek opportunities to collaborate and work in partnership to promote increased access to quality palliative care across the continuum.

Preferred Practice Examples for the Palliative RN under DOMAIN 1/GUIDELINE 1.8

PP 7—The palliative RN promotes a seamless patient transfer through various care settings with communication of patient values, preferences, and beliefs and suggests a hospice referral when appropriate.

PP 8—The palliative RN presents hospice as an option when appropriate.

PP 9—The palliative RN should promote skills and abilities in other healthcare providers to discuss hospice as an option.

GUIDELINE 1.9—The physical environment in which care is provided meets the preferences, needs, and circumstances of the patient and family, to the extent possible.

Criteria

1.   When feasible, care occurs in the setting preferred by the patient and his/her family and this preference is elicited by the palliative RN.

2.   When care is provided outside the patient's or family's home, the palliative RN collaborates with residential service providers to maximize the patient's safety. Flexible visiting hours, as appropriate, promote social interaction for the patient. A space is arranged for families to visit, rest, and prepare or eat meals, as well as to meet with palliative care providers and other professionals, along with other needs identified by the family.

3.   Providers in all settings address the unique care needs of children as patients, family members, or visitors.

Preferred Practice Example for the Palliative RN under DOMAIN 1/GUIDELINE 1.9

When feasible and safe, the palliative RN provides care as per the patient's preferences, meeting the needs of safety, visitation, family, comfort, privacy, and other needs as identified by the patient and/or family. The palliative RN elicits and advocates for preferences for care, participates in planning to honor these preferences, and provides care in accordance with the plan.

DOMAIN 2: Physical Aspects of Care

GUIDELINE 2.1—The interdisciplinary team assesses and manages pain and/or other physical symptoms and subsequent effects based upon the best available evidence.

Criteria

1. The goal of pain and symptom management is the safe and timely reduction of a physical symptom to an acceptable level to the patient, or surrogate if the patient is unable to report distress.

2. The palliative RN promotes symptom assessment and treatment as part of the IDT.

3. Palliative RNs demonstrate specialist-level skill in symptom control for all types of serious or life-threatening illnesses. Symptoms include but are not limited to pain, shortness of breath, nausea, fatigue, anorexia, insomnia, and constipation.

4. It is essential that healthcare organizations develop and utilize symptom assessment, treatment policies, standards, and guidelines appropriate to the care of patients with serious or life-threatening illnesses that conform to best palliative care practices.

5. The palliative RN promotes the use of such assessments, policies, standards, and guidelines.

6. The palliative RN documents regular, ongoing assessment of pain, other physical symptoms, and functional capacity. Validated symptom assessment instruments are utilized when available. Symptom assessment of adults with cognitive impairment and of children is performed by appropriately-trained professionals using validated instruments when available.

7. The palliative RN participates in the care of distressing symptoms and side effects, which includes the entire spectrum of effective pharmacological, interventional, behavioral, and complementary interventions and therapies that are supported by research, and refers to appropriate specialists.

8. Symptom assessment, treatment, and treatment outcome information, including side effects, is recorded in the medical record by the palliative RN and transmitted across healthcare settings during transitions.

9. The palliative RN identifies barriers related to the use of opiates and addresses misconceptions of the risks of side effects, addiction, respiratory depression, and hastening death.

Preferred Practice Example for the Palliative RN under DOMAIN 2/GUIDELINE 2.1

PP 12—The palliative RN documents all symptoms using available standardized scales.

GUIDELINE 2.2—The assessment and management of symptoms and side effects are contextualized to the disease status.

Criteria

1. The palliative RN implements treatment plans for physical symptoms in the context of the disease, prognosis, and patient functional limitations. The palliative RN assesses the patient, family, or surrogate's understanding of the illness in relation to patient-centered goals of care.

2. The palliative RN assesses the patient's or surrogate's understanding of the disease and its consequences, symptoms, side effects of treatments, functional impairment, and potentially beneficial treatments with consideration of culture, cognitive function, and developmental stage.

3. The palliative RN educates family and other healthcare providers to support safe and appropriate care of the patient. The palliative RN provides family with resources for response to urgent needs.

Preferred Practice Example for the Palliative RN under DOMAIN 2/GUIDELINE 2.2

PP 13—The palliative RN assesses and manages implementation of interventions to treat symptoms and side effects in a timely, safe, and effective manner with a goal of providing relief that is acceptable to the patient and family.

DOMAIN 3: Psychological and Psychiatric Aspects of Care

GUIDELINE 3.1—The interdisciplinary team assesses and addresses psychological and psychiatric aspects of care based upon the best available evidence to maximize patient and family coping and quality of life.

Criteria

1. The palliative RN has training and skills to identify the potential psychological and psychiatric impact of serious or life-threatening illness, on both the patient and family, including depression, anxiety, delirium, and cognitive impairment.

2. Based on patient and family goals of care, the palliative RN implements interventions that address psychological needs and psychiatric diagnoses, promote adjustment to the physical condition, and support opportunities for emotional growth, psychological healing, completion of unfinished business, and effective grieving.

3. The palliative RN performs and documents regular, ongoing assessment of psychological reactions related to the illness (including but not limited to stress, anticipatory grieving, and coping strategies) and psychiatric conditions. Whenever possible and appropriate, validated and context-specific assessment tools are used.

4. The palliative RN assesses psychological distress including patient and family understanding of the disease or condition, symptoms, side effects, and their treatments, as well as assessment of caregiving needs, decision-making capacity, and coping strategies.

5. The palliative RN effectively implements interventions to manage psychiatric diagnoses, with appropriate psychiatric collaboration.

6. The palliative RN provides family education that includes the provision of safe and appropriate psychological support measures to the patient.

7. The palliative RN skillfully communicates treatment alternatives, promoting informed decision making by the patient and family and documents these discussions.

8. The palliative RN bases implementation of treatment decisions on assessment of risk and benefit, evidence-informed practice, and patient–family preferences.

9. The palliative RN utilizes nonpharmacological, complementary, and interventional therapies for the treatment of psychological distress or psychiatric syndromes, as appropriate.

10. The palliative RN responds to psychological distress promptly, effectively reflecting patient–family choice. The palliative RN documents regular reassessment of treatment efficacy, response to treatment, and patient–family preferences.

11. The palliative RN promotes the use of appropriate healthcare professionals with specialized skills in age-appropriate psychological and psychiatric treatment (e.g., psychiatrists, psychologists, social workers).

12. The palliative RN provides developmentally-appropriate assessment and support to pediatric patients and children who are family members of pediatric or adult patients.

13. The palliative RN communicates with individuals using verbal, nonverbal, and/or symbolic means appropriate to the patient, with particular attention to patients with cognitive impairment and the developmental stage and cognitive capacity of children.

14. The palliative RN provides staff education regarding the recognition and treatment of anticipatory grief and common psychological and psychiatric syndromes (e.g., anxiety, depression, delirium, hopelessness), and professional coping strategies in managing difficult symptoms.

Preferred Practice Examples for the Palliative RN under DOMAIN 3/GUIDELINE 3.1

PP 14—The palliative RN measures and documents the presence of anxiety, depression, delirium, behavioral disturbances, and other psychological symptoms using available standardized scales.

PP 15—The palliative RN implements strategies to manage anxiety, depression, delirium, and behavioral disturbances in a timely, safe, and effective manner to achieve outcomes acceptable to the patient and family, and assess responses accordingly.

GUIDELINE 3.2—A core component of the palliative care program is a grief and bereavement program available to patients and families, based on assessment of need.

Criteria

1. The palliative RN demonstrates appropriate education and skill in the care of patients, families, and staff experiencing loss, grief, and bereavement.

2. The palliative RN identifies and recognizes loss and grief in patients and families living with serious or life-threatening illness at diagnosis. The palliative RN performs ongoing assessment and reassessment throughout the illness trajectory.

3. Staff and volunteers, including those who provide bereavement services, receive ongoing education, supervision, and support in coping with their own grief, and responding effectively to patients' and families' grief.

4. At the time of admission to hospice or palliative care, the palliative RN completes an initial, developmentally-appropriate, professional assessment to identify patients and families at risk for complicated grief, bereavement, and comorbid complications, particularly among older adults.

5. The palliative RN ensures that identified patients and families receive intensive support, and prompt referral to appropriate professionals as needed.

6. Bereavement services and follow-up are available to the family for a minimum of 12 months after the death of the patient.

7. The palliative RN ensures that culturally- and linguistically-appropriate information on loss, grief, and the availability of bereavement support services is routinely communicated to the family before and after the death of the patient. This includes community services such as support groups, counselors, and collaborative partnerships with hospice.

8. The palliative RN provides support and grief interventions in accordance with developmental, cultural, and spiritual needs; and the expectations and preferences of the family, with attention to children family members of any patient.

Preferred Practice Examples for the Palliative RN under DOMAIN 3/GUIDELINE 3.2

PP 16—The palliative RN assesses and manages the psychological reactions of patients and families to address emotional response to disease, functional impairment, and loss.

PP 17—The palliative RN may assist in the development of a grief and bereavement care plan for patients and families prior to, and for at least 12 months after, the death of the patient.

DOMAIN 4: Social Aspects of Care

GUIDELINE 4.1—The interdisciplinary team assesses and addresses the social aspects of care to meet patient–family needs, promote patient–family goals, and maximize patient–family strengths and well-being.

Criteria

1   The palliative RN facilitates and enhances patient–family understanding of, and coping with, illness and grief; supports patient–family decision making; discusses the patient's and family's goals for care; provides emotional and social support; and enhances communication within the family and between patient–family and the IDT.

2   The palliative RN collaborates with the IDT social worker with patient population-specific skills in the assessment of, and interventions to address, social needs during a serious or life-threatening illness.

3   Health professionals, including palliative RNs, skilled in assessment and intervention of the developmental needs and capacities of children, are available. This includes both pediatric patients and children who are family members of pediatric or adult patients.

Preferred Practice Example for the Palliative RN under DOMAIN 4/GUIDELINE 4.1

PP 18—The palliative RN initiates and participates in regularly scheduled patient and family conferences with the IDT to provide information, discuss goals of care, disease prognosis, advance care planning, and offer support.

GUIDELINE 4.2—A comprehensive, person-centered interdisciplinary assessment (as described in Domain 1, Guideline 1.1) identifies the social strengths, needs, and goals of each patient and family.

Criteria

1.   The palliative RN elicits a social assessment, including the following elements

- Family structure and function—roles, communication, and decision-making patterns.

- Strengths and vulnerabilities—resiliency; social and cultural support networks; effect of illness or injury on intimacy and sexual expression; prior experiences with illness, disability, and loss; risk of abuse, neglect, or exploitation.

- Changes in family members' schooling, vocational roles, recreational activities, and economic security.

- Geographic location, living arrangements, and perceived suitability of living environment.

- Patient's and family's perceptions about caregiving need, availability, and capacity.

- Needs for adaptive equipment, home modifications, and transportation.

- Access to medications (prescription and over-the-counter) and nutritional products.

- Need for and access to community resources, financial support, and respite.

- Advance care planning and legal concerns (See Domain 8: *Ethical and Legal Aspects of Care*, Guideline 8.1).

2. The palliative RN's social care plan reflects the patient's and family's culture, values, strengths, goals, and preferences, which may change over time.

3. The palliative RN implements interventions to maximize the social well-being and coping skills of both the patient and family, including education and family meetings.

4. The palliative RN refers the patient and family to appropriate resources and services, that address the patient's and family's identified social needs and goals, and support patient–family strengths.

Preferred Practice Example for the Palliative RN under DOMAIN 4/GUIDELINE 4.2

PP 19—The palliative RN implements a comprehensive social care plan, which addresses the social, practical, and legal needs of the patient and caregivers, including but not limited to relationships, communication, existing social and cultural networks, decision making, and work.

DOMAIN 5: Spiritual, Religious, and Existential Aspects of Care

GUIDELINE 5.1—The interdisciplinary team assesses and addresses spiritual, religious, and existential dimensions of care.

Criteria

1. Spirituality is recognized as a fundamental aspect of compassionate, patient- and family-centered care, honoring the dignity of all persons.

2. Spirituality is defined as, "the aspect of humanity that refers to the way individuals seek and express meaning and purpose and the way they experience their connectedness to the moment, to self, to others, to nature, and/or to the significant or sacred."[6, p. 887] The palliative RN is responsible for recognizing spiritual distress and for attending to the patient's and the family's spiritual needs[7] within their scope of practice.

3. The interdisciplinary palliative care team, in all settings, includes spiritual care professionals; specifically a board-certified professional chaplain, with skill and expertise in assessing and addressing spiritual and existential issues frequently confronted by pediatric and adult patients with serious or life-threatening illnesses and their families.

4. The palliative RN's communication with the patient and family is respectful of their religious and spiritual beliefs rituals, and practices. The RN does not impose his/her own spiritual, religious, or existential beliefs and practices on their patients, patients' families, and colleagues.

Preferred Practice Example for the Palliative RN under DOMAIN 5/GUIDELINE 5.1

PP 20—The palliative RN documents a plan based on assessment of religious, spiritual, and existential concerns using a structured instrument and integrates the information obtained from the assessment into the palliative care plan.

GUIDELINE 5.2—A spiritual assessment process, including a spiritual screening, history questions, and a full spiritual assessment as indicated, is performed. This assessment identifies the religious or spiritual/existential background, preferences, and related beliefs, rituals, and practices of the patient and family; as well as symptoms, such as spiritual distress and/or pain, guilt, resentment, despair, and hopelessness.

Criteria

1. Regular, ongoing exploration of spiritual and existential concerns occurs; including but not limited to, life review; assessment of hopes, values, and fears; meaning, purpose, and beliefs about afterlife; spiritual or religious practices; cultural norms; beliefs that impact understanding of illness; coping; guilt; forgiveness; and life-completion tasks. These spiritual themes are documented and communicated to the team. Whenever possible, a standardized instrument is used.

2. The palliative RN documents periodic reevaluation of the impact of spiritual/existential interventions and patient and family preferences.

3. As a member of the IDT, the palliative RN addresses spiritual/existential care needs, goals, and concerns identified by patients and family members according to established protocols, and documented in the interdisciplinary plan during transitions of care and/or in discharge plans. The palliative RN offers support for issues of life closure, as well as other spiritual issues, in a manner consistent with the patient's and family's cultural, spiritual, and religious values.

4. The palliative RN refers to appropriate community-based professionals with specialized knowledge or skills in spiritual and existential issues when appropriate (e.g., to a pastoral counselor or spiritual director). Spiritual care professionals are recognized as specialists who provide spiritual counseling.

5. The palliative RN supports and indicates the patient's spiritual sources of strength.

Preferred Practice Example for the Palliative RN under DOMAIN 5/GUIDELINE 5.2

PP 21—The palliative RN provides information about the availability of spiritual care services and offers resources for spiritual care.

GUIDELINE 5.3—The palliative care service facilitates religious, spiritual, cultural rituals or practices as desired by patient and family, especially at and after the time of death.

Criteria

1. Professional and institutional use of religious/spiritual symbols and language are sensitive to cultural and religious diversity.

2. The palliative RN supports the patient and family in their desires to display and use their own religious/spiritual and/or cultural symbols.

3. Healthcare chaplaincy and RNs facilitate contacts with spiritual/religious communities, groups, or individuals, as desired by the patient and/or family. Palliative care programs create procedures to facilitate patients' access to clergy, religious, spiritual, and culturally-based leaders, and/or healers in their own religious, spiritual, or cultural traditions.

4. Palliative RNs acknowledge their own spirituality as part of their professional role. The palliative RN participates in opportunities to engage staff in self-care and self-reflection on their beliefs and values as they work with seriously ill and dying patients. It is expected that RNs respect of spirituality and beliefs of all colleagues and the creation of a healing environment in the workplace.

5.   Non-chaplain palliative care providers obtain training in basic skills of spiritual screening and spiritual care.

6.   The palliative RN ensures follow up after the patient's death (e.g., phone calls, attendance at wake or funeral, scheduled visit) to offer support and identify any additional needs that require community referral, and help the family during bereavement.

Preferred Practice Examples for the Palliative RN under DOMAIN 5/GUIDELINE 5.3

PP 22—The RN assures that specialized palliative care teams include spiritual care professionals, who are appropriately educated and certified in palliative care. The RN builds relationships with community clergy, and provides education and counseling related to end-of-life care.

PP 23—The palliative RN participates in community partnerships to provide spiritual care.

DOMAIN 6: Cultural Aspects of Care

GUIDELINE 6.1—The palliative care program serves each patient, family, and community in a culturally- and linguistically-appropriate manner.

Criteria

1.   Culture is multidimensional.

2.   Culture is far reaching and may include many aspects such as "race, ethnicity, and national origin; migration background, degree of acculturation, and documentation status; socioeconomic class; age; gender, gender identity, and gender expression; sexual orientation; family status; spiritual, religious, and political belief or affiliation; physical, psychiatric, and cognitive ability; and literacy, including health and financial literacy."[8, pp. 15-16]

3.   During the assessment process, the palliative RN elicits and documents the cultural identifications, strengths, concerns, and needs of the patient and family, recognizing that cultural identity and expression vary within families and communities.

4.   The palliative RN implements a plan of care that addresses the patient's and family's cultural concerns and needs and maximizes their cultural strengths. Palliative RNs consistently convey respect for the patient's and family's cultural perceptions, preferences, and practices regarding illness, disability, treatment, help-seeking, disclosure, decision making, grief, death, dying, and family composition.

5.   The palliative RN communicates in a language and manner that the patient and family understand.

   •   Palliative RNs tailor their communication to the patient's and family's level of literacy, health literacy, financial literacy, and numeracy.

   •   For patients and families who do not speak or understand English, or who feel more comfortable communicating in a language other than English, the palliative care program makes all reasonable efforts to use professional interpreter services, accessed either in person and/or by phone. When professional interpreters services are unavailable, other healthcare providers, preferably those trained in palliative care, may interpret for patients and families. In general, family members are not placed in the role of interpreter. However, in the absence of all other alternatives, the palliative RN may use family members to interpret in an emergency situation only if the patient and family agree to this arrangement.

- In addition to interpreter services, the palliative care program endeavors to provide written materials in each patient's and family's preferred language. When translated written materials are not available, the program utilizes professional interpreter services as described above, to facilitate patient and family understanding of information provided by the program.

6. The palliative RN respects and accommodates dietary and ritual practices of patients and their families.

7. The palliative RN identifies community resources that serve various cultural groups, and refers patients and families to such services as appropriate.

Preferred Practice Examples for the Palliative RN under DOMAIN 6/GUIDELINE 6.1

PP 24—The palliative RN incorporates cultural assessment as a component of a palliative and hospice care assessment, including, but not limited to locus of decision making; preferences regarding disclosure of information, truth telling, and decision making; dietary preferences; language; family communication; desire for support measures such as palliative therapies and complementary and interventional therapies; perspectives on death, suffering, and grieving; and funeral/burial rites.

PP 25—The palliative RN provides professional interpreter services and education materials that are culturally sensitive and in the patient and family's preferred language.

GUIDELINE 6.2—The palliative care program continually strives to enhance its cultural and linguistic competence.

Criteria

1. *Cultural competence* refers to the process by which palliative RNs "respond respectfully and effectively to people of all cultures [and] languages . . . in a manner that recognizes, affirms, and values the worth of individuals, families, and communities."[9, pp. 12–13]

2. The palliative care program values diversity as demonstrated by creating and sustaining a work environment that affirms multiculturalism. The recruitment, hiring, retention, and promotion practices of the palliative care program reflect the cultural and linguistic diversity of the community it serves.

3. The palliative RN cultivates cultural self-awareness and recognizes how their own personal cultural values, beliefs, biases, and practices inform their perceptions of patients, families, and colleagues. RNs strive to prevent value conflicts from undermining their interactions with patients, families, and colleagues.

4. To reduce health disparities within and among the communities it serves, the palliative care program provides education to help palliative RNs increase their cross-cultural knowledge and skills.

5. The palliative care program regularly evaluates and, if needed, modifies its services, policies, and procedures to maximize its cultural and linguistic accessibility and responsiveness to a multicultural population. Input from patients, families, and community stakeholders is elicited and integrated into this process.

Preferred Practice Example for the Palliative RN under DOMAIN 6/GUIDELINE 6.2

The palliative RN promotes cultural competence and evaluates cultural competence within the organization.

DOMAIN 7: Care of the Patient at the End of Life

GUIDELINE 7.1—The interdisciplinary team identifies, communicates, and manages the signs and symptoms of patients at the end of life to meet the physical, psychosocial, spiritual, social, and cultural needs of patients and families.

Criteria

1. The palliative RN recognizes the need for higher intensity and acuity of care during the active dying phase.

2. Prior to and at onset of the dying process, the palliative RN routinely elicits and honestly addresses concerns, hopes, fears, and expectations about the dying process in a developmentally-appropriate manner, with respect for the social and cultural context of the family.

3. In collaboration with the patient and family and the IDT, the palliative RN provides care with respect for patient and family values, preferences, beliefs, culture, and religion.

4. The palliative RN acknowledges the patient's imminent death, and communicates signs and symptoms of approaching death to the patient and family, in culturally- and developmentally-appropriate language, with attention to population-specific issues and age appropriateness.

Preferred Practice Examples for the Palliative RN under DOMAIN 7/GUIDELINE 7.1

PP 26—The palliative RN recognizes and documents the transition to the active dying phase and communicates to the patient, family, and staff the expectation of imminent death.

PP 27—The palliative RN educates the family on a timely basis regarding signs and symptoms of imminent death in a developmentally-, age-, and culturally-appropriate manner.

GUIDELINE 7.2—The interdisciplinary team assesses and, in collaboration with the patient and family, develops, documents, and implements a plan of care to address preventative and immediate treatment of actual or potential symptoms, patient and family preferences for site of care, attendance of family and/or community members at the bedside, and desire for other treatments and procedures.

Criteria

1. The palliative RN assesses the patient for symptoms and proactively considers and implements symptom management according to the treatment plan.

2. With the patient and family, the palliative RN develops a plan to meet the unique needs of the patient and family during the actively dying phase and the needs of family immediately following the patient's death. The palliative RN reassesses and revises the plan in a timely basis.

3. The palliative RN documents in the medical record and communicates in a timely manner any inability to meet the patient's and family's expressed wishes for care immediately leading up to and following the death.

4. The palliative RN introduces or reintroduces a hospice referral, if such an option is congruent with the patient's and family's goals and preferences for patients who have not accessed hospice services.

5. Before the patient's death, the palliative RN educates the patient and family about autopsy, organ and tissue donation, and anatomical gifts, with respect to institutional and regional policies as appropriate.

Preferred Practice Examples for the Palliative RN under DOMAIN 7/GUIDELINE 7.2

PP 28—As part of the ongoing plan of care process, the palliative RN routinely ascertains and documents patient and family wishes about the site of death, and fulfills patient and family preferences when possible.

PP 29—The palliative RN administers adequate dosage of analgesics and sedatives as ordered to achieve patient comfort during the active dying phase and addresses concerns and fears about use of opioids and analgesics and hastening death.

GUIDELINE 7.3—Respectful postdeath care is delivered in a respectful manner that honors the patient and family culture and religious practices.

Criteria

1. The palliative RN assesses and documents cultural and religious practices particular to the postdeath period, and delivers care honoring those practices, and in accordance with both institutional practice and local laws and regulations.

Preferred Practice Example for the Palliative RN under DOMAIN 7/GUIDELINE 7.3

PP 30—The palliative RN promotes postdeath treatment of the body that is respectful and in accordance with the cultural and religious practices of the family and local law.

GUIDELINE 7.4—An immediate bereavement plan is activated postdeath.

Criteria

1. The palliative RN formulates and activates a postdeath bereavement plan of care based on a social, cultural, and spiritual grief assessment.

2. The palliative RN assures that a healthcare team member is assigned to the family in the postdeath period to support the family and assist with religious practices, funeral arrangements, and burial planning.

Preferred Practice Example for the Palliative RN under DOMAIN 7/GUIDELINE 7.4

PP 31—The palliative RN facilitates effective grieving by implementing in a timely manner a bereavement care plan after the patient's death when the family remains the focus of care.

DOMAIN 8: Ethical and Legal Aspects of Care

GUIDELINE 8.1—The patient or surrogate's goals, preferences, and choices are respected within the limits of applicable state and federal law, current accepted standards of medical care, and professional standards of practice. Person-centered goals, preferences, and choices form the basis for the plan of care.

Criteria

1. The palliative RN routinely seeks professionals with knowledge and skill in ethical, legal, and regulatory aspects of medical decision making in care planning.

2. The palliative RN educates the patient and family about advance care planning documents, including, but not limited to, designation of a surrogate healthcare decision maker for (except for minors) out of hospital do not resuscitate orders and advance directives.

3. The palliative RN sensitively elicits the patient or surrogate's expressed values, care preferences, religious beliefs, and cultural considerations, in collaboration with the family to assist in understanding patient and family decision making. The palliative RN confirms and routinely reviews these values, preferences, and considerations, with particular attention to changes in healthcare status or transitions of care, and assures they are documented.

4. The palliative RN routinely documents all expressed wishes, preferences, and values including the completion of clinician orders such as inpatient resuscitation status; out of hospital do not resuscitate orders; and healthcare surrogate declaration documents for adult patients. The palliative RN assists in completion of documents to promote communication and understanding of the patient's preferences for care across the healthcare continuum, and/or the preferences of the patient's designated surrogate.

5. The palliative RN documents and addresses the failure to honor the patient's or surrogate's preferences to assure it is accessible to other healthcare providers.

6. To determine decision-making capacity, the palliative RN assists with determining the ability of the patient and family to secure and accept needed care and to cope with the illness and its consequences. The adult patient with decisional capacity determines the level of involvement of the family in decision making and communication about the care plan. Patients with disabilities are assumed to have capacity unless determined otherwise.

7. In situations with pediatric patients, the palliative RN documents the child's views and preferences for medical care, including assent for treatment (when developmentally appropriate), and assures it is given appropriate weight in decision making. When the child's wishes differ from those of the adult decision maker, the palliative RN assures appropriate professional staff members are available to assist the family.

8. The palliative RN advocates for the observance of previously expressed wishes of the patient or surrogate in these situations. For patients unable to communicate or who have not previously expressed their values, preferences, or beliefs, the palliative RN seeks to identify advance directives, evidence of previously expressed wishes, values and preferences, and the designated surrogate decision maker(s).

9. The palliative RN provides assistance and guidance to surrogate decision makers about the legal and ethical basis for surrogate decision making, including honoring the patient's known preferences, substituted judgment, and best-interest criteria.

10. The palliative RN routinely encourages patients and families to seek professional advice on creating or updating legal and financial documents such as property wills, guardianship agreements, and custody documents.

Preferred Practice Examples for the Palliative RN under DOMAIN 8/GUIDELINE 8.1

PP 32—The palliative RN documents the designated surrogate decision maker in accordance with state law for every patient in primary, acute, and long-term care and in palliative and hospice care.

PP 33—The palliative RN documents the patient/surrogate preferences for goals of care, treatment options, and setting of care at first assessment and at frequent intervals as conditions change.

PP 34—The palliative RN promotes the conversion of the patient treatment goals into medical orders and ensures that the information is transferable and applicable across care settings, including long-term care, emergency medical services, and hospitals, such as the Physician/Provider/Medical Orders for Life-Sustaining Treatment (POLST/MOLST) programs.

PP 35—The palliative RN promotes advance directives and surrogacy designation availability and access across care settings, while protecting patient privacy and adherence to Health Insurance Portability and Accountability Act (HIPAA) regulations (e.g., by Internet-based registries or electronic personal health records).

PP 36—The palliative RN develops healthcare and community collaboration to promote advance care planning and completion of advance directives for all individuals (e.g., Respecting Choices, Community Conversations on Compassionate Care).

GUIDELINE 8.2—The palliative care program identifies, acknowledges, and addresses the complex ethical issues arising in the care of people with serious or life-threatening illness.

Criteria

1. The palliative RN, as part of the hospice and palliative care team, aims to prevent, identify, and resolve ethical dilemmas common to the provision of hospice and palliative care such as withholding or withdrawing treatments, instituting do not resuscitate (DNR) orders, and the use of sedation in hospice and palliative care.

2. The palliative RN has education in ethical principles guiding the provision of hospice and palliative care.

3. Ethical concerns commonly encountered in hospice and palliative care are identified, recognized, and addressed to prevent or resolve these concerns, using the ethical principles of beneficence, respect for individuals and self-determination, justice, and nonmaleficence with attention to avoidance of conflicts of interest.

4. The palliative RN documents ethical clinical issues and appropriately refers to ethics consultants or a committee for case consultation and assistance in conflict resolution.

5. Ethics committees are consulted in the appropriate manner to guide policy development, assist in clinical care, and provide staff education in common hospice and palliative care situations including, but not limited to, a patient's right to decline care, use of high dose medications, withdrawal of life-prolonging technology and treatments (e.g., ventilators, dialysis, antibiotics), palliative sedation, futile care, and cessation of artificial and oral nutrition and hydration.

Preferred Practice Example for the Palliative RN under DOMAIN 8/GUIDELINE 8.2

PP 37—The palliative RN assures establishment of/or access to ethics committees or ethics consultation across care settings to address ethical conflicts at the end of life.

GUIDELINE 8.3—The provision of palliative care occurs in accordance with professional, state and federal laws, regulations and current accepted standards of care.

Criteria

1. The palliative RN is knowledgeable about legal and regulatory aspects of hospice and palliative care and has access to legal and regulatory experts to guide the provision of his/her care in accordance with legal and regulatory aspects of hospice and palliative care.

2. The palliative RN models his/her hospice and palliative care practice on existing professional codes of ethics, scopes of practice, and standards of care for consistency.

3. The palliative RN is knowledgeable about federal and state statutes, regulations, and laws regarding disclosure of medical records and health information; medical decision making; advance care planning and directives; the roles and responsibilities of surrogate decision makers; appropriate prescribing of controlled substances; death pronouncement and certification processes; autopsy requests; organ and anatomical donation; and healthcare documentation.

4. The adherence to legal and regulatory requirements is expected for disclosure, decision-making capacity assessment, confidentiality, informed consent, as well as assent and permission for people not of legal age to consent.

5. The hospice and palliative care program establishes and implements policies outlining staff responsibility in regard to state and federal legal and regulatory requirements regarding patient and family care issues such as abuse, neglect, suicidal ideation, and potential for harm to others.

6. The palliative RN recognizes the role of cultural variation in the application of professional obligations, including information around diagnosis, disclosure, decisional authority, care, acceptance of and decisions to forgo therapy.

7. The palliative RN supports children and adolescents in decision making.

8. Legal counsel is accessible to the palliative RN particularly in common hospice and palliative care situations including but not limited to decision-making capacity, use of high dose medications, withdrawal of technology (e.g., ventilators, dialysis), palliative sedation, futile care, and cessation of artificial and oral nutrition and hydration.

Preferred Practice Examples for the Palliative RN under DOMAIN 8/GUIDELINE 8.3

The palliative RN participates in the development of policies on medical decision making, role of surrogate decision makers, legal requirements for use of controlled substances, death pronouncement, requests for autopsy, and organ transplantation consistent with federal and state statutes and regulations.

PP 38—For minors with decision-making capacity, the palliative RN documents the child's views and preferences for medical care, including assent for treatment, and assures that these are given appropriate weight in decision making. The palliative RN makes appropriate professional staff members available to both the child and the adult decision maker for consultation and intervention when the child's wishes differ from those of the adult decision maker.

CITED REFERENCES

1. National Consensus Project for Quality Palliative Care. *Clinical Practice Guidelines for Quality Palliative Care*. 3rd ed. Pittsburgh, PA: National Consensus Project for Quality Care; 2013. www.nationalconsensusproject.org/Guidelines_Download2.aspx. Accessed July 11, 2014.

2. National Quality Forum. *A National Framework and Preferred Practices for Palliative and Hospice Care Quality*. Washington, DC: National Quality Forum; 2006. www.qualityforum.org/Publications/2006/12/A_National_Framework_and_Preferred_Practices_for_Palliative_and_Hospice_Care_Quality.aspx. Accessed July 11, 2014.

3. Dahlin CM, Sutermaster DJ, eds.; Hospice and Palliative Nurses Association, American Nurses Association. *Palliative Nursing: Scope and Standards of Practice—An Essential Resource for Palliative and Hospice Nurses*. Silver Spring, MD: nursesbooks.org; 2014.

4. Ferrell BR, Coyle N. *The Nature of Suffering and Goals of Nursing*. New York, NY: Oxford University Press; 2008.

5. U.S. Department of Health and Human Services. *2013 Annual Progress Report to Congress: National Strategy for Quality Improvement in Health Care*. 2013. www.ahrq.gov/workingforquality/nqs/nqs2013annlrpt.htm. Accessed July 11, 2014.

6. Puchalski C, Ferrell B, Virani R, et al. Improving the quality of spiritual care as a dimension of palliative care: the Report of the Consensus Conference. *J Palliat Med*. 2009;12(10):885-904. doi: 10.1089/jpm.2009.142.

7. National Comprehensive Cancer Network. *NCCN Clinical Practice Guidelines in Oncology (NCCN Guideline®) Palliative Care*. Version 2. Fort Washington, PA: National Comprehensive Cancer Network; 2012. www.nccn.org/professionals/phsician-gls/pdf/palliative.pdf. Accessed February 15, 2013.

8. National Association of Social Workers. *NASW Standards for Social Work Case Management*. Washington, DC: National Association of Social Workers; 2013. www.socialworkers.org/practice/naswstandards/CaseManagementStandards2013.pdf. Accessed July 14, 2014.

9. National Association of Social Workers. *Indicators for the Achievement of the NASW Standards for Cultural Competence in Social Work Practice*. Washington, DC: National Association of Social Workers; 2007. www.socialworkers.org/practice/standards/NASWCulturalStandardsIndicators2006.pdf. Accessed July 14, 2014.

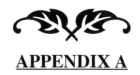

APPENDIX A

MEDICATIONS LISTED IN THE CORE CURRICULUM[1]

DRUG CLASS

Generic Drug Name.............   **Trade Drug Name**

ALCOHOL DETERENT
disulfiram.....................   Antabuse

ANALGESICS
acetaminophen.................   Tylenol
acetaminophen/codeine ....   Tylenol with codeine
buprenorphine ....   Butrans
capsaicin.....................   Capsaicin, Icy Hot PM, Zostrix
fentanyl citrate.................   Actiq
fentanyl transdermal system ....   Duragesic
hydrocodone/acetaminophen.......   Vicodin/Lorcet
hydromorphone ....   Dilaudid/Palladone
levorphanol ....   Levo-Dromoran
lidocaine.....................   Lidoderm HCl Topical
methadone ....   Dolophine
morphine ....   Avinza/Kadian/MS Contin/Oramorph SR/Roxanol
nalbuphine ....   Nubain
oxycodone ....   OxyContin/OxyFAST
oxycodone/acetaminophen.........   Percocet/Roxicet
pentazocine (G) ....   Talwin
tramadol (G)...................   Ultram

ANTACIDS/ANTIFLATULENTS/DIGESTANTS
simethicone ....   Mylicon

ANTI-ALZHEIMER'S DRUGS
donepezil ....   Aricept
galantamine ....   Cognex
memantine ....   Exelon
rivastigmine ....   Namenda

ANTIANGINAL
nifedipine (G)..................   Procardia

381

ANTIBIOTICS
demeclocycline . . . . Declomycin
Imipenem-cilastatin . . . . Primaxin

ANTICOAGULANTS
enoxaparin . . . . Lovenox
rivaroxaban . . . . Xarelto
warfarin . . . . Coumadin

ANTIDEPRESSANTS
amitriptyline (A, G) . . . . Elavil/Endep
bupropion (G) . . . . Wellbutrin
citalopram . . . . Celexa
desipramine (A) . . . . Norpramin
doxepin (A, G) . . . . Adapin, Sinequan
duloxetine . . . . Cymbalta
escitalopram . . . . Lexapro
fluoxetine . . . . Prozac
fluvoxamine . . . . Luvox
mirtazapine (G) . . . . Remeron
nefazodone . . . . Serzone
nortriptyline (A) . . . . Pamelor
paroxetine (A) . . . . Paxil
sertraline . . . . Zoloft
trazodone . . . . Desyrel
venlafaxine . . . . Effexor

ANTIDIARRHEAL
diphenoxylate/atropine (A) . . . . Lomotil
loperamide (A) . . . . Imodium
octreotide . . . . Sandostatin

ANTIEPILEPTIC
carbamazepine (G) . . . . Tegretol
clonazepam (B) . . . . Klonopin
gabapentin . . . . Neurontin
lamotrigine . . . . Lamictal
oxcarbazepine . . . . Oxtellar XR, Trileptal
phenytoin . . . . Dilantin
pregabalin . . . . Lyrica
tiagabine . . . . Gabitril Filmtabs
valproate . . . . Depacon
valproic acid . . . . Depakote

ANTIFUNGALS
clotrimazole . . . . Mycelex/Lotrimin
fluconazole . . . . Diflucan
metronidazole . . . . Flagyl
nystatin . . . . Mycostatin

ANTIGOUT
allopurinol . . . . Zyloprim/Lopurin

ANTIHISTAMINES
diphenhydramine (A, G) .... Benadryl
hydroxyzine (A, G) .... Atarax

ANTILIPIDEMIC
cholestyramine................. Prevalite

ANTIMANIC
lithium .... Lithobid

ANTINAUSEA/ANTIEMETIC/PROMOTILITY
metoclopramide (G)............. Reglan
ondansetron .... Zofran
perphenazine (G) .... Trilafon
prochlorperazine (G) .... Compazine
promethazine (G)............... Phenergan

ANTIOSTEOPOROTIC
alendronate................... Fosamax
calcitonin .... Fortical, Miacalcin
pamidronate .... Aredia
zoledronic acid................ Reclast, Zometa

ANTIPARKINSON AGENTS
benztropine (A, G).............. Cogentin
carbidopa/levodopa .... Sinemet
trihexyphenidyl (A, G)........... Artane

ANTIPSYCHOTICS
aripiprazole (G) .... Abilify
chlorpromazine (A, G)........... Thorazine
clozapine (A, G)............... Clozaril
fluphenazine (A, G) .... Prolixin
haloperidol (G)................ Haldol
olanzapine (A, G)............... Zyprexa
paliperidone (G)............... Invega
perphenazine (A, G)............ Trilafon
quetiapine (G) .... Seroquel®
risperidone (G)................ Risperdal
ziprasidone (G) .... Geodon

ANTISECRETORY/ANTICHOLINERGICS
atropine (A) .... AtroPen, Sal-Tropine
glycopyrrolate .... Robinul
hyoscyamine (A, G)............. Levsin
scopolamine (A, G) .... Transderm-Scop

ANTITUSSIVES
dextromethorphan .... Robitussin

ANXIOLYTICS

alprazolam (B, G)	Xanax
buspirone	BuSpar
chlordiazepoxide (B, G)	Librium
clorazepate (B)	Tranxene
diazepam (B, G)	Valium
lorazepam (B, G)	Ativan
midazolam (B)	Versed
oxazepam (B, G)	Serax
perphenazine/amitriptyline (A, G)	Etrafon/Triavil
zolpidem (G)	Ambien

APPETITE STIMULANTS

megestrol (G)	Megace

CARDIAC GLYCOSIDES

digoxin (G)	Lanoxin

CORTICOSTEROIDS

dexamethasone	Decadron
prednisone	Deltasone

H$_2$ RECEPTOR ANTAGONIST

cimetidine	Tagamet

HYPNOTICS

propofol	Diprivan

LAXATIVES

bisacodyl	Dulcolax
docusate sodium	Colace/Surfak/Regutol
lactulose	Chronulac
magnesium citrate	Citro-Mag
magnesium hydroxide	Magnesia
methylcellulose	Citrucel
polyethylene glycol	MiraLAX
psyllium	Metamucil
senna	Senokot

MUSCLE RELAXANTS

baclofen	Lioresal
tizanidine (A)	Zanaflex

NONSTEROIDAL ANTI-INFLAMMATORY DRUGS (NSAIDS)

celecoxib (G)	Celebrex
ibuprofen (G)	Motrin
naproxen (G)	Naprosyn

PROTON PUMP INHIBITORS

dexlansoprazole	Dexilant
esomeprazole	Nexium
lansoprazole	Prevacid
omeprazole	Prilosec
pantoprazole	Protonix

PSYCHOSTIMULANTS

methylphenidate (G)	Ritalin
modafinil	Provigil

KEY: A = anticholinergic properties, B = benzodiazepine, G = geriatric precautions as per the Beers list[2]

CITED REFERENCES

1.   Hallowell L, Comerford KC, eds. *Nursing 2015 Drug Handbook*. Philadelphia, PA: Wolters Kluwer: 2015.

2.   American Geriatric Society. *2012 Beers Criteria for Potentially Inappropriate Medication Use in Older Adults*. 2012. www.americangeriatrics.org/files/documents/beers/2012AGSBeersCriteria Citations.pdf. Accessed October 17, 2014.

INDEX

A

Abuse, 196–200, 249, 279. *See also* Substance abuse

Access to services (medications, supplies, durable medical equipment [DME]), 283, 335, 337–339, 342–343, 345, 348

Acetaminophen, 83–84, 90

Acquired immunodeficiency syndrome (AIDS), 6, 67

Activity intolerance (deconditioning), 59, 82, 157

Acute kidney injury, 61

Acute pain, 83, 247

Addiction, 77–79, 81, 204, 208, 218, 230–231, 283, 305, 367

Adjuvant
analgesics/medications, 80, 83, 88–89, 95–96, 104
treatment, 77–78

Advance care planning (e.g., advance directives, life-sustaining, DNR status), 10, 22, 24, 56, 61, 66, 68, 214–216, 218, 222, 224, 228–229, 238, 253, 255–256, 262, 276, 295–299, 303, 310, 322, 324–325, 340, 342, 360, 363–364, 370, 377–379

Agency for Healthcare Research and Quality (AHRQ), 10

Aggression, 183, 198–199

Agitation, 56, 107, 135, 160, 164–165, 167–168, 182–183, 205–206, 219, 274, 306

Alzheimer's disease, 54–55, 103, 188, 256–257, 262

American Academy of Hospice and Palliative Medicine (AAHPM), 10, 14, 339

Amyotrophic lateral sclerosis (ALS), 51, 55, 82, 101, 275, 286

Anemia, 38, 41–42, 61, 126, 157–159, 162–163, 166

Anger, 113, 189, 203, 206–207, 218, 232, 235, 274

Angina, 50, 82, 110–111, 160

Anorexia, 38, 40–42, 44–46, 48, 64–66, 84, 109, 120, 131, 136, 146, 152–153, 156, 367

Antidepressants, 88, 95, 187, 194, 196, 201, 206
Serotonin-norepinephrine reuptake inhibitors, 89, 192
Serotonin selective reuptake inhibitors, 88, 192
Tricyclic antidepressants, 88, 103, 106, 120, 141, 192

Antiepileptic, 88, 95, 105–107, 132, 134

Anxiety, 192–195, 204–208, 233, 235, 251, 274, 305–306, 368–369

Aphasia, 51–52. *See also* Nonverbal

Ascites, 40–41, 43, 48, 66–67, 109, 127–130, 138, 155, 236

Assistive personnel. *See* Nursing assistant, hospice aide, home health aide, certified nursing assistant

Automatic implantable cardioverter defibrillator (AICD), 51, 300

B

Benefit and burden, 47, 320

Bereavement services, 4, 313, 346, 369

Bipolar disorders, 184–186

Bladder spasms, 139

Bleeding, 40–42, 44, 46, 141, 147–149, 161–164, 304

Boundaries, 20, 202, 216, 281, 321

Bowel incontinence, 43, 55, 308

Bowel obstruction, 37, 40–41, 83, 123–124, 134, 137–139

Brain tumors, 44, 105

Breakthrough doses, 89, 90, 91, 95

Breast cancer, 33, 37, 39–40, 43, 188

Burden, 18, 36, 37, 47, 62, 99, 115, 117, 141, 215, 219, 220, 227, 228, 270, 338
Caregiver, 84, 227, 260, 341, 343, 352, 360
Financial, 343
Symptom, 56, 66, 68, 341
Treatment, 297, 300, 320, 322, 325, 342

C

Cachexia, 41–42, 62, 64, 66, 68, 146, 152–153

Cancer, 33–47
End-of-life considerations, 47
Epidemiology, 33–34
Genetics, 35–36
Process of disease progression, 34
Prognostication, 39–40
Psychosocial issues, 46–47
Treatment, 36–39, 157–158

Cardiac tamponade, 45

Caregiver, 11, 47, 56, 84, 94, 130, 168, 197, 213–237, 341–343
Burden, 84, 227, 341
Confidence and ability to provide care, 180, 322
Fatigue, 218, 232

Centers for Medicare & Medicaid Services (CMS), 3, 20, 248, 257, 336, 365

Cerebrovascular accidents (CVA). *See* stroke

Certification, 246–248, 257–258, 340–341, 354–355, 359, 361, 363, 379

Certified nursing assistant, 22, 247

Chronic obstructive pulmonary disease (COPD), 58, 111, 116, 152, 256, 350

Chronic pain, 80–81, 85

Chronic renal failure, 61

Coagulation, 40, 42, 46, 62, 129, 140, 161

Collaboration, 3, 19–21, 220, 228, 232, 244, 340, 361, 363–364, 366, 368, 375, 377–378

Communication, 243–244, 249, 296, 342, 361–363, 365–366, 370–371, 374, 377

Community resources, 227, 229, 279, 363, 365, 374

Compassion fatigue, 29, 226

Complementary therapies
Acupressure, 37, 92
Hypnosis, 39, 92
Music therapy, 135, 263
Reiki, 39, 92, 306

CPSIA information can be obtained
at www.ICGtesting.com
Printed in the USA
LVHW021511260321
682558LV00001B/1